# Mosby's
# Handbook of Patient Teaching

# Mosby's
# Handbook of Patient Teaching

**MARY M. CANOBBIO**, MN, RN

Cardiovascular Clinical Specialist
Assistant Clinical Professor
School of Nursing
University of California, Los Angeles
Los Angeles, California

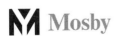 Mosby

St. Louis  Baltimore  Boston
Carlsbad  Chicago  Naples  New York  Philadelphia  Portland
London  Madrid  Mexico City  Singapore  Sydney  Tokyo  Toronto  Wiesbaden

Vice-President and Publisher: Nancy L. Coon
Senior Editor: Sally Schrefer
Developmental Editor: Gail Brower
Project Manager: Patricia Tannian
Design Manager: Gail Morey Hudson
Manufacturing Manager: Dave Graybill
Cover Designer: Teresa Breckwoldt

Printed in the United States of America
Composition by Clarinda Company
Printing/binding by R.R. Donnelley & Sons Company

Mosby–Year Book, Inc.
11830 Westline Industrial Drive
St. Louis, Missouri 63146

**Library of Congress Cataloging in Publication Data**

Canobbio, Mary M.
    Mosby's handbook of patient teaching / Mary M. Canobbio.
        p.    cm.
    Includes bibliographical references and index.
    ISBN 0-8151-1537-7
    1. Patient education.    2. Nurse and patient.    3. Nursing—Study
and teaching.      I. Title.
    [DNLM:    1. Patient Education—methods—handbooks.
    2. Patient Education—nurses' instruction.      W 49 C227m 1996]
RT90.C36 1996
615.5′07—dc20
DNLM/DLC
for Library of Congress                                                96-15637
                                                                                        CIP

96  97  98  99  00  /  9  8  7  6  5  4  3  2  1

# Contributors

**ANNE E. BELCHER, PhD, RN, FAAN**

Associate Professor
Chairperson, Department of Acute and Long-Term Care Nursing
University of Maryland School of Nursing
Baltimore, Maryland

**LEONOR C. CANCINO, MN, BS, RNC, OCN**

Clinical Instructor, Medical/Surgical Nursing
School of Nursing
University of California, Los Angeles
Staff Nurse, Coronary Observation Unit
UCLA Medical Center
Center for Health Sciences;
Private Consultant
Administration and Management/Health Care Services
Los Angeles, California

**PATRICIA CARTER, MN, RN**

Doctoral Student
Research Assistant
UCLA School of Nursing
Los Angeles, California

**BETTY Y.F. LEE, MN, RN, CCRN**

UCLA Medical Center
Los Angeles, California

**MARISE C. MAGSARILI, MN, RN, CCRN**

Clinical Nurse Specialist/Clinical Coordinator
University of Southern California School of Medicine
Division of Cardiothoracic Surgery
Los Angeles, California

**MARGARET MARINOW, BSN, RN**
Commander (retired)
United States Navy Nurse Corps
Long Beach, California

**CANDACE WEIGAND, MN, RN, CNS, FNP**
St. Joseph's Medical Center
Burbank, California

**ESTHER WINTHROP, RN, BS, MSE**
Education Nurse Clinician
Saint Mary's Medical Center
Duluth, Minnesota

# Reviewers

**SUSAN CHASE BALTRUS, MS, RNC**

Senior Level Coordinator
School of Nursing
Central Main Medical Center
Lewiston, Maine

**ELLEN CARSON, PhD, RNCS**

Associate Professor
Department of Nursing
Pittsburg State University
Pittsburg, Kansas

**MARY ANNE DUMAS, PhD, RN, C, FNP**

Associate Professor
Department of Nursing
SUNY Stony Brook
Stony Brook, New York

**JOYCE MULHOLLAND, MA, MS, RNC**

Nursing Education Consultant
Phoenix, Arizona

**JOAN MURPHY, RN, MS**

Associate Professor
Department of Nursing
Utica College of Syracuse University
Utica, New York

**GERVAISE E. NICKLAS, RN, MS, BSN**

Assistant Professor
School of Nursing
Northern Illinois University
DeKalb, Illinois

**ELIZABETH OUTLAW, RN, MA**
Staff Registered Nurse
Medical Oncology
Stamford Hospital
Stamford, Connecticut

**SANDRA SOLBERG, RN**
Instructor/Counselor
Student Services
Madison, Wisconsin

**ANITA LEE WYNNE, PhD**
Associate Professor
School of Nursing
University of Portland
Portland, Oregon

# Preface

As the climate of health care continues to change, the shift of care moves toward earlier discharges, placing more responsibility onto patients, their families, and home-based caretakers. Consequently, ensuring that patient education takes place becomes a greater responsibility for health care providers.

Assessing and meeting informational needs of patients and their families are integral parts of health care practice. In the past, the focus of patient education has been largely on the pathophysiology and treatment of disease. Today, however, patients are being asked to assume greater responsibility for all aspects of their care, including caring for their incisions and catheters and practicing disease prevention and health promotion. Therefore the intent of this book is to help health care providers ensure that their patients are well informed about every aspect of home care management.

As hospital lengths of stay decrease and same-day surgeries increase, it becomes essential to maintain safe and consistent standards of practice that lead to positive patient outcomes within any health care delivery system. The Joint Commission on Accreditation of Healthcare Organizations (JCAHO) has long recognized the importance of organizational delivery systems for patient and family education. A number of JCAHO standards statements* for patient education have been incorporated into this text and are summarized here.

1. Provide the patient and family with information that will enhance their knowledge and skills necessary to promote recovery and improve function.
2. Encourage patient participation in decision making and include the family in the teaching process.
3. Use an educational program that begins with an assessment

---

*Joint Commission on Accreditation of Healthcare Organizations: *The Joint Commission's 1996 accreditation manual for hospitals: the new care of the patient standards,* Washington, DC, 1996, American Hospital Association.

and addresses the identified learning needs, abilities, and preferences.

4. Educate patients about the safe and effective use of their medications.

5. Educate patients about the safe and effective use of equipment and supplies and means of obtaining them.

6. Counsel patients as to foods and diets appropriate to illness, as well as possible food-drug interactions.

7. Provide patients leaving a facility with information on obtaining follow-up care and accessing community resources.

Based on the preceding standards, this text provides guidelines for information the caregiver should cover with the patient and his or her family or primary caregiver. The guidelines are written as broad statements that will remind the health care provider of what to include in the individualized educational discharge plan. For example, because occupation varies from patient to patient, a reminder statement is made to "urge the patient to ask questions about occupational as well as recreational activities." In this way, patients are assured of receiving important information about allowances or limitations related to their clinical problems.

It is not the intent of this book to teach readers about diseases, disorders, or procedures. This knowledge is assumed. The purpose is simply to remind health care providers of what is essential to discuss with the patient. Each disease or procedure discussion begins with a brief **Definition. Signs/Symptoms** of the disease or disorder are those a patient would be taught to expect or observe for. Similarly, the **Complications** are those directly associated with the disease, that is, complications for which the patient should be alert. **Diagnostic Tests** are listed with a brief explanation of their purpose. A reminder to provide detailed information about each of the ordered tests is given at the beginning of each list. A general listing of **Medical Management** specific to the disease, disorder, or procedure follows.

The **Home Care** section includes key points to teach, review, and discuss with the patient in home care management. Using principles of adult education, the text's consistent, structured format serves to remind the health care provider to include the patient's family or caregiver in the teaching and to provide supportive materials such as written information and telephone numbers for follow-up questions. When demonstrating care is important in preparing the patient, the text reminds the reader to do so.

To assist health care workers in preparing the patient for discharge, the home care section addresses the elements to include in every discharge plan: description of the disorder or procedure, causes or risk factors, symptoms to report, diet counseling, medications, activities, and any specific instructions related to the disease or procedure. Finally, readers are reminded to provide home care referral, including community resources. A list of organizational resources for patient information is provided in Appendix H.

I gratefully acknowledge and thank Ginni McCanne, RN, BSN, Utilization Management Coordinator at Foothill Presbyterian Hospital, Glendora, California, for consulting and sharing her expertise. Thanks also to Pauline Nguyen, student volunteer at the University of California, for helping with manuscript preparation.

**Mary M. Canobbio**

# Contents

# Teaching Guidelines

Although patient education has long been a cornerstone of health care practice, the shortening of stays has increased the need for a discharge teaching plan that includes home care. Today's patients are assuming responsibility for aspects of care previously handled in the hospital. Therefore health care providers must broaden their assessment of patients' educational needs to include not only the disease or disorder, but also the environment to which patients will be returning and the available resources.

In developing an individual teaching plan, the care provider must incorporate basic principles of adult learning into the assessment of the patient.[2,3] Some of the issues to be considered in developing an educational discharge plan for home care follow.

## EDUCATIONAL ASSESSMENT

Patient education begins with an assessment of what the patient *needs to know* to achieve recovery and return to function. Because of anxiety and discomfort, patients retain little of the instruction in the hospital. Therefore nurses should limit the information to specific content, skills, and behaviors necessary to learn before discharge. What the patient *wants* to know and what can be learned in the limited time available should be factored into the assessment of necessary information to cover.

An assessment plan considers all factors that will influence the teaching and learning process. Age, gender, education, cultural and religious practices, occupation, and previous life experiences influence the patient's ability and readiness to learn. The nurse must attempt to assess the patient's life-style, preferences, and attitudes toward health and illness. Barriers to learning, such as physical limitations, finances, and type of health care coverage, must also be evaluated, particularly when prescribing home care equipment and supplies and making referrals.

## ENVIRONMENTAL ASSESSMENT

In preparing the patient for home care, the nurse must assess the physical and community environment to which the patient will be discharged. If the patient is discharged to home, the nurse must make certain that the home environment is safe and suitable for the patient to carry out the instructions given. For example, can the patient maneuver safely, or does he live in a second-story apartment with no elevator to reach the ground floor? If instructed to weigh daily, does the patient own a scale? The external environment includes both hospital-based and community resources available and affordable to the patient. The health care provider must become familiar with community resources, such as self-help programs, home health agencies, and professional organizations to which the patient can be referred. Appendix H provides a partial list of resources available to patients.

## LEVEL OF INFORMATION

The information given to the patient should be appropriate for the patient's age, literacy level, education, and language skills. Patient materials should be geared between sixth- and eighth-grade reading levels. Use of medical terminology or jargon should be avoided. For example, the terms "myocardial infarction" and "MI" should not be used in place of "heart attack" unless they have already been defined for the patient.

## USE OF PATIENT EDUCATION MATERIALS

With shorter lengths of stay and limited time for teaching, print and audiovisual materials are important adjuncts for any discharge teaching plan. They are, however, just adjuncts and should not replace individualized instruction.

Printed material can vary from comprehensive booklets to single-topic tearsheets. Printed materials are useful for reinforcing information provided to patients while in the hospital and also serve as a ready resource. Because of the low retention and recall levels of hospitalized patients, printed material is an important reminder of key points after patients return home.

## FAMILY PARTICIPATION

As hospital stays shorten, discharged patients may not feel prepared for or physically capable of performing self-care activities. Consequently, family members are the vital links in the transition from hospital to home care. Families must be included in all discussions and demonstrations.

For purposes of this book the term "family" is used in the broadest sense to include any person who plays an important role in the patient's life. The "family member" may not be an individual who is legally related to the patient but simply the one who will assume primary responsibility for the care of the patient at home. Therefore it is important to apply the previously discussed principles of learning to this family member, who now also becomes a client.

## TEACHING OF SKILLS

To maximize patient self-care skills, the health care provider must permit sufficient time and opportunity for the patient to practice the skills. Practice should be integrated into all encounters with the patient, not saved up until the patient is ready for discharge. Every effort must be made to ensure that learning takes place in incremental steps and that patients are not overwhelmed with too much information at one time.

## REFERENCES

Johnson EA, Jackson JE: Teaching the home care client, *Nurse Clin North Am* 24:687-693, 1989.

Joint Commission on Accreditation of Healthcare Organizations: *The Joint Commission's 1996 accreditation manual for hospitals: the new care of the patient,* Washington, DC, 1996, American Hospital Association.

Knowles MS: The modern practice of adult education. In *Pedagogy to andragogy,* ed 2, Chicago, 1980, Follett.

Redman B: *The process of patient education,* ed 7, St Louis, 1993, Mosby.

Ruzicki DA: Realistically meeting the educational needs of hospitalized acute and short-stay patients, *Nurs Clin North Am* 24:629-637, 1989.

Winthrop E: *Mosby's patient teaching tips,* St Louis, 1994, Mosby.

# Mosby's
# Handbook of Patient Teaching

# Abdominal Aneurysm

—**Abdominal aneurysm: an outpouching sac that forms at a weak point in the aortic wall. Most abdominal aneurysms are found below the bifurcation (take-off) of the renal arteries. Aneurysms can grow, but they are asymptomatic until they begin to press on adjacent organs or tears develop within the blood vessel (dissection).**

## CAUSES/CONTRIBUTING FACTORS/RISK FACTORS
- Hereditary lack of elastin
- Vessel wall trauma
- Congenital defect
- Loss of vessel wall elasticity
- Atherosclerosis
- Elderly men with hypertension, coronary artery disease, or peripheral vascular disease

## SIGNS/SYMPTOMS
- Asymptomatic
- Painless, pulsating sensation or throbbing abdominal mass
- Chronic pain in middle or lower back
- With expansion or dissection: sudden onset of severe abdominal or back pain

## COMPLICATIONS
- Dissection
- Rupture
- Exsanguination
- Insufficient blood supply to the kidneys, bowels, and/or lower extremities
- Embolization (blood clots in the lower extremities)
- Heart attack (high incidence in older men)

## DIAGNOSTIC TESTS
- Describe each procedure, its purpose, and the normal feelings or sensations that are likely, as well as any preprocedural or postprocedural care.

- Abdominal ultrasonography: to determine the size and shape of the aneurysm
- Chest x-ray: to detect calcification and gauge the size of the aneurysm
- Computed tomography/magnetic resonance imaging: to locate an arterial tear and to determine the size of the aneurysm
- Aortography: to determine the condition of the vessel above and below the aneurysm

## TREATMENT

*Medical*
- Indications
  —Aneurysm <6 cm. The goal of medical treatment is to prevent enlargement of the aneurysm and to monitor its growth.
- Drugs
  —Antihypertensives: to lower and/or control blood pressure (BP)
  —Beta blockers: to reduce the force of the heart's pumping action and to decrease the pulsating feeling of the aneurysm
  —Analgesics: to relieve pain

*Surgical*
- Indications
  —Aneurysm >4-6 cm; emergence of symptoms (abdominal tenderness or pain); emergency procedure for dissection and rupture
- Procedure
  —Resection and grafting with autogenous graft (see Abdominal Surgery, p. 3)

## HOME CARE

- Give both patient and caregiver *verbal* and *written* instructions. Provide them with the name and telephone number of a physician or nurse to call if questions arise.
- *General information*
  —Describe and explain dissection and rupture.
- *Warning signs*
  —Stress the importance of seeking emergency care if the following occur:
      Sudden onset of severe pain (ripping or tearing) in the abdomen, back, or groin
      Pallor, sweating, and/or sudden loss of consciousness

A

• *Special instructions*
  —Stress the importance of adopting a life-style that prevents acceleration of the aneurysm's growth.
    Controlling weight to ease the work of the circulatory system
    Limiting fat to prevent progression of atherosclerosis
    Reducing or eliminating salt to control BP
  —Teach the patient how to care for the incision (review the signs of infection, thrombus, or embolism); instruct him or her to report any problems to a physician or nurse.
• *Medications*
  —Explain the purpose, dosage, schedule, and route of administration of the prescribed medications, as well as side effects to report to a physician or nurse.
  —Emphasize that the patient should not stop taking the medications without first checking with a physician or nurse.
• *Activity*
  —Advise the patient to alternate mild to moderate exercise with periods of rest; the patient should avoid vigorous exercise and heavy lifting.
  —Encourage the patient to discuss allowances or limitations related to occupation and to favorite recreational sports or activities.
• *Diet*
  —Encourage the patient to follow a low-fat, low-salt diet.

**FOLLOW-UP CARE**

• Stress the importance of regular follow-up visits. Make sure the patient has the necessary names and telephone numbers.
  —Medical patients: ultrasound scans to monitor the size of the aneurysm
  —Surgical patients: monitoring to ensure the patency of the graft and/or to detect a new aneurysm early

# Abdominal Surgery

—**Abdominal surgery: surgical incision into the abdomen. Abdominal surgery is performed for a number of reasons, such** as to treat gastrointestinal disorders, to remove parts of an organ (appendectomy) or a whole organ (gastrectomy), to transplant organs, or to monitor the progression of disease.

## PREPROCEDURAL TEACHING

- Using illustrations, review the physician's explanation of the procedure.
- Explain the need for written consent for surgery, anesthesia, and blood transfusions.
- Explain that the patient usually is admitted to the hospital the day of surgery, rather than before, unless extensive bowel preparation is needed.

### Review of Preprocedural Care

- The patient must not eat or drink anything after midnight the night before surgery.
- The patient may need to be shaved from the nipple line to the thigh (including the perineal area) to prevent infection of the surgical wound.
- A small cleansing enema, done at home, may be required the night before surgery.
- Before coming to the hospital, the patient may be instructed to shower with a bactericidal soap (e.g., Hibiclens).

### Review of Postprocedural Care

- Stress the importance of turning, coughing, and deep breathing.
- Discuss the purpose of the incentive spirometer, and demonstrate how to use it.
- Explain the importance of getting out of bed the first day after surgery.
- Explain the reason for wearing thigh-high elastic stockings and for alternating them with pressure stockings while in bed.
- Explain the importance of moving the arms and legs while in bed.
- Explain that pain is expected after surgery, but that analgesics are available to control it. Discuss the types of pain control:
    - Patient-controlled analgesia (PCA): the patient self-administers pain medication by pushing a button on a device regulated by a computerized time and dose schedule
    - Intramuscular injection: pain medication is injected as prescribed

**A**

- Explain that hydration is maintained by the IV line until the patient is allowed to eat and drink.
- Explain that a variety of tubes and suction systems may be used after surgery to drain excess blood and fluid around the incision. These may include: nasogastric (NG) tube, until bowel sounds return; urethral catheter; Penrose drain; Jackson-Pratt self-suction bulb drainage system; Hemovac self-suction drain.

## COMPLICATIONS

- Wound infection
- Wound dehiscence
- Deep vein thrombosis
- Paralytic ileus
- Fluid-electrolyte imbalance
- Bowel obstruction
- Urinary tract infection
- Pulmonary complications
- Hemorrhage
- Acute renal failure

## HOME CARE

- Give both patient and caregiver *verbal* and *written* instructions. Provide them with the name and telephone number of a physician or nurse to call if questions arise.
- *Wound/incision care*
  —Teach the patient how to change the dressings and how to care for the tubes and drains.
  —Help the patient obtain the necessary supplies, and make sure he or she knows what supplies to get and where to get them after discharge from the hospital.
- *Warning signs*
  —Review the signs and symptoms the patient should report to a physician or nurse.
    Wound infection: redness, tenderness, warmth, and swelling around the incision site; increased drainage
    Changes in bowel habits: diarrhea, constipation, flatulence
- *Medications*
  —Explain the purpose, dosage, schedule, and route of administration of the prescribed medications, as well as side effects to report to a physician or nurse.

- *Special instructions*
  —Review pain management techniques.
  —Instruct the patient to splint the abdomen when coughing.
  —Reassure the patient that as activity level increases, the pain and soreness will diminish.
- *Activity*
  —Explain the need for frequent rest periods.
  —Instruct the patient to increase activity gradually as tolerated.
  —Instruct the patient to avoid heavy lifting (>10 pounds) and strenuous work or sports for 4 to 6 weeks or longer, as the physician advises.
- *Diet*
  —Inform the patient that diet is as dictated by the underlying condition or diagnosis.

# Acquired Immune Deficiency Syndrome

—Acquired immune deficiency syndrome (AIDS): a progressive, incurable disease caused by the human immunodeficiency virus (HIV). AIDS destroys the CD4+ T cells, impairing the immune system and predisposing the individual to a number of opportunistic infections and cancers. HIV is transmitted through intimate sexual contact, use of contaminated needles, and exposure to HIV-tainted blood, body fluids that contain blood, and blood products. It also can be transmitted from mother to newborn.

## CDC CLASSIFICATION OF HIV INFECTION

Stage I: acute infection; a mononucleosis-like syndrome develops at the time of exposure; HIV-antibody seroconversion occurs about 3 months later

Stage II: no symptoms are present, but the individual tests positive for HIV antibody

Stage III: persistent, generalized lymphadenopathy appears; decrease in CD4T cells

Stage IV: HIV-related diseases develop

—Constitutional symptoms (persistent fever, weight loss, diarrhea)
—Neurologic disease
—Secondary infectious diseases
—Secondary cancers
—Associated conditions

## RISK FACTORS

- Homosexual/bisexual men
- Heterosexuals engaging in high-risk behavior (e.g., IV drug use; sharing of needles and syringes; unprotected sex with multiple partners)
- Neonates born to infected women
- Infants and children who receive HIV-contaminated blood or blood products (e.g., those with hemophilia)

## SIGNS/SYMPTOMS

- Prolonged period of silent infection, often lasting >10 years
- Viral syndrome resembling mononucleosis or influenza within a few days or weeks of infection
- Persistent, generalized swelling of the lymph nodes
- Skin disorders (e.g., seborrhea)
- Opportunistic infections
  —Bacterial (*Mycobacterium avium*)
  —Fungal (candidiasis, cryptococcosis, histoplasmosis)
  —Protozoal (cryptosporidiosis, pneumocystosis, toxoplasmosis)
  —Viral (cytomegalovirus, herpes simplex)
- Malignancies
  —Kaposi's sarcoma
  —Non-Hodgkin's lymphoma
  —Primary central nervous system lymphoma
  —Cervical cancer
  —Anal carcinoma
  —Malignant melanoma
  —Hepatocellular carcinoma

Metastasis to central nervous system, skin, mucous membranes, respiratory and gastrointestinal tracts. End-stage disease: unexplained weight loss, persistent fever, diarrhea, or night sweats

## DIAGNOSTIC TESTS

- Describe each procedure, its purpose, and the normal feelings

or sensations that are likely, as well as any preprocedural or post-procedural care.
- To confirm HIV infection
  —Enzyme-linked immunosorbent assay (ELISA)
  —Western blot
  —Polymerase chain reaction
- To measure severity of immunosuppression
  —T-cell count: <400,000 or depressed
  —WBCs: depressed
  —Lymphocytes: depressed
- To evaluate symptoms of opportunistic infection or malignancy

## TREATMENT

*Medical*
- Drugs
  —Antiretrovirals: to slow progression of the disease or inactivate HIV
    Azidothymidine
    Zidovudine (Retrovir)
  —Antiinfectives: as prophylaxis against opportunistic infections; also, to treat such infections as they arise

The treatment of AIDS is directed by the type of infection or malignancy that develops. It may include the following:
- Kaposi's sarcoma: chemotherapy, surgical excision, electrodesiccation, radiation therapy
- Non-Hodgkin's lymphoma: chemotherapy (mBACOD: methotrexate, bleomycin, doxorubicin, cyclophosphamide, vincristine, dexamethasone, folic acid); hematopoietic growth factors
- Primary CNS lymphoma: radiation therapy, corticosteroids
- Cervical cancer: radical hysterectomy, pelvic lymphadenectomy; chemotherapy, radiation therapy for advanced or systemic disease
- Anal carcinoma: fulguration or cryotherapy; chemotherapy; possibly radiation therapy

## HOME CARE

- Give both patient and caregiver *verbal* and *written* instructions. Provide them with the name and telephone number of a physician or nurse to call if questions arise.
- *General information for HIV-positive patients*
  —Explain how HIV is transmitted and the disease process.
- *Warning signs*
  —Review the signs and symptoms of infection (flulike symp-

toms, stiff neck) and cancers that should be reported to a physician or nurse.

- *Special instructions*
  —Stress the importance of preventing further exposure to or transmission of the virus by avoiding exchange of body fluids (e.g., vaginal or anal intercourse, oral sex) without using a latex condom, sharing of IV needles or sex toys, blood contact of any kind.
  —Discuss the importance of avoiding large crowds, as well as individuals who may be infectious or who have been vaccinated recently.
  —Teach the patient and caregiver the precautions they should take at home to prevent transmission of HIV.

  Wash hands meticulously before and after patient care.

  Use disposable gloves whenever contact with the patient's blood or body fluids is likely.

  Separate any bedding or clothing soiled by secretions or excretion, and wash it in a 10% bleach solution (¼ cup of bleach for each gallon of water).

  Wash dishes and eating utensils in hot, soapy water (no special handling is required).

  Dispose of dry waste (e.g., tissues, napkins) contaminated by blood or body fluids in a separate container and bag securely.

  Put all needles used to administer drugs in a sturdy, closed container before disposing of them.

  —See the specific malignancy for further care guidelines.

## FOLLOW-UP CARE

- Stress the importance of regular visits for medical care and laboratory tests. Make sure the patient has the necessary names and telephone numbers.
- Discuss the importance of informing health care providers about the HIV diagnosis.
- Explain the importance of refraining from donating blood or semen.

## REFERRALS

- Provide and assist with referrals as needed for financial help and for psychologic and community support (self-help support groups, home health services, hospice care).

# Adrenal Insufficiency
(Addison's Disease, Secondary Adrenocortical Insufficiency)

—**Adrenal insufficiency:** a chronic disorder of the adrenal glands. Hypofunctioning of the adrenal cortex leads to a deficiency of adrenocortical hormones (glucocorticoid, aldosterone) and androgens. These hormones regulate fluid blance, glucose formation, and secondary sex characteristics, particularly in women. *Addison's disease* is a primary adrenocortical insufficiency; *secondary adrenocortical insufficiency* is a consequence of other conditions.

## CAUSES

- Addison's disease: damage to the adrenal glands, which may result from an autoimmune factor, trauma, infection, or surgery
- Secondary adrenocortical insufficiency: reduced secretion of the pituitary adrenocorticotropic hormone (ACTH) caused by a pituitary tumor, head trauma, or optic gliomas

## SIGNS/SYMPTOMS

- Fatigue
- Weight loss
- Nausea, vomiting
- Postural hypotension
- Headache
- Salt craving
- Diarrhea
- Anorexia
- Abdominal pain
- Hyperpigmentation (bronze skin color)
- Loss of or decrease in body hair
- Muscle weakness that worsens through the day
- Women: amenorrhea, infertility, reduced libido

## COMPLICATIONS

- Addisonian (adrenal) crisis: a rapid drop in cortisol and aldosterone levels, which can result in shock, coma, and death. It can be precipitated by any stressor (e.g., emotion, infection, minor surgery, or trauma). *This is a medical emergency.*

## DIAGNOSTIC TESTS

- Describe each procedure, its purpose, and the normal feelings or sensations that are likely, as well as any preprocedural or postprocedural care.
    —Cortisol, ACTH levels; ACTH stimulation test: to confirm adrenocortical insufficiency and identify type
    —Blood chemistry, electrolytes (potassium, glucose, sodium, chloride)
    —Urinalysis: 24-hour urinalysis to detect sodium and/or free cortisol
    —Computed tomography/magnetic resonance imaging: to determine decrease in adrenal or pituitary size

## TREATMENT

*Medical*
- Diet
    —Diet high in calories, carbohydrates, protein, and vitamins
- Drugs
    —Corticosteroid replacement (e.g., cortisone, hydrocortisone)
    —Antibiotics for infection
    —Adrenal crisis
        IV hydrocortisone
        IV fluid replacement (with severe dehydration)
        Vasopressors to maintain blood pressure
        Cardiac monitoring

## HOME CARE

- Give both patient and caregiver *verbal* and *written* instructions. Provide them with the name and telephone number of a physician or nurse to call if questions arise.
- *General information*
    —Explain the underlying disorder, its cause, and contributing factors.
    —Discuss the effect stress can have on hormone levels.
    —Instruct the patient to notify the physician or a nurse during periods of heightened emotional stress, before elective surgery, or after a traumatic event so that drug dosages can be adjusted.

- *Warning signs of addisonian crisis*
  —Review the signs and symptoms of addisonian crisis (i.e., profound weakness, fatigue, dizziness, nausea, vomiting, abdominal pain, and cool, clammy skin).
  —Emphasize the importance of seeking immediate medical care if the above signs appear.
  —Make sure the patient and caregiver know the quickest way to an emergency department from home and from work.
  —Help the patient organize or obtain an emergency kit containing alcohol sponges and syringes with 100 mg of hydrocortisone.
  —Advise the patient to carry the emergency kit when traveling and to check the supplies regularly for expiration dates.
  —Teach the patient and caregiver how to prepare and administer a hydrocortisone injection in the event of adrenal crisis.
- *Special instructions*
  —Women: instruct the patient to report any changes in her menstrual pattern, such as amenorrhea.
  —Discuss other methods of dealing with stressful events (e.g., relaxation techniques, guided imagery, diversional activities).
- *Medications*
  —Explain the purpose, dosage, schedule, and route of administration of the prescribed medications, as well as side effects to report to a physician or nurse.
  —Emphasize that hormone replacement is a lifelong commitment.
- *Activity*
  —Instruct the patient to avoid strenuous exercise in hot, humid weather.
  —Advise the patient to increase intake of fluid and salt if he or she is sweating heavily.
- *Diet*
  —Caution the patient not to skip meals during periods of activity.
  —Urge the patient not to use salt-restricted foods or salt substitutes.
  —Advise an anorexic patient to eat small, frequent meals to enhance the nutritional condition.

## FOLLOW-UP CARE

- Stress the importance of regular follow-up visits. Make sure the patient has the necessary names and telephone numbers.

- Advise the patient to inform all physicians, dentists, and health care providers about the disease *before* a treatment or procedure.
- Help the patient obtain a Medic-Alert bracelet and identification card listing the diagnosis and medications and emergency treatment.

# Adrenalectomy

—**Adrenalectomy: surgical removal of one or both adrenal glands.**

## INDICATIONS

- Adrenal hyperfunction (Cushing's syndrome) and hyperaldosteronism
- Benign adrenal adenomas or malignant ACTH-producing tumors
- Secondary treatment of prostate and breast cancers dependent on adrenal hormone secretion

## PREPROCEDURAL TEACHING

- Review the physician's explanation of the procedure and the reason for surgery, the skin preparation process, and the location of the incision; encourage the patient to ask questions and to discuss any fears or anxieties.
- If both glands are to be removed, explain that the patient will need lifelong cortisone treatment; if only one gland is to be removed, the patient will take cortisone for 6 months to 2 years.
- Explain that the patient may be admitted to the hospital the day of surgery rather than before.
- Explain the need for written consent for surgery and anesthesia.

### Review of Preprocedural Care

- The patient should not eat or drink anything after midnight the night before surgery.
- The patient will be carefully monitored after surgery to prevent complications (e.g., adrenal crisis, infection, hypertension) that

may result from removal of one or both adrenals. (Refer to the primary disease for specific medications to be given, such as antihypertensives and glucose.)

**Review of Postprocedural Care**

- Stress the importance of turning, coughing, and deep breathing.
- Show the patient how to splint his or her side to reduce pain when coughing.
- Discuss the purpose of the incentive spirometer, and demonstrate how to use it.

**COMPLICATIONS**

- Adrenal crisis (see p. 10)
- Hemorrhage
- Infection
- Hypoglycemia
- Electrolyte imbalance
- Hypotension

**HOME CARE**

- Give both patient and caregiver *verbal* and *written* instructions. Provide them with the name and telephone number of a physician or nurse to call if questions arise.
- *Wound/incision care*
  —Teach the patient how to care for the incision.
  —Instruct the patient not to wear tight or restrictive clothing (e.g., belts, suspenders) over the incision because this may irritate the wound.
- *Warning signs*
  —Review the signs and symptoms that should be reported to a physician or nurse.
     Wound infection: redness, swelling, and increasing tenderness around the incision; increased drainage; fever
- *Special instructions*
  —Emphasize the importance of seeking immediate medical care if a crisis is suspected. Review the signs and symptoms of crisis: profound weakness, fatigue, dizziness, nausea, vomiting, abdominal pain, and cool, clammy skin. Make sure the patient and caregiver know the quickest way to an emergency department from home and from work.
  —Advise the patient to carry the emergency kit when traveling and to check the supplies regularly for expiration dates.

—Help the patient organize or obtain an emergency kit containing alcohol sponges and syringes with 100 mg of hydrocortisone.

—Teach the patient and caregiver how to prepare and administer a hydrocortisone injection in the event of crisis.

* *Medications*

—Explain the purpose, dosage, schedule, and route of administration of prescribed medications, as well as side effects to report to a physician or nurse.

—If the patient has had a unilateral adrenalectomy, explain that steroid replacement will be necessary until the remaining adrenal gland begins to function adequately. Steroid replacement will continue for a period ranging from a few months to a year.

—Patients who have a bilateral adrenalectomy require lifelong steroid replacement therapy; review the long-term management of adrenal insufficiency.

—Emphasize that hormone replacement is a lifelong commitment, and that discontinuing the drug suddenly can precipitate adrenal crisis.

—Stress the importance of not discontinuing the steroid medication suddenly.

* *Activity*

—Instruct the patient to allow for frequent rest periods, gradually increasing the activity level as tolerated.

—Tell the patient to avoid heavy lifting (>10 pounds) and strenuous work, exercise, and sports for 4 to 6 weeks or longer as the physician advises.

—Encourage the patient to discuss allowances and limitations regarding occupation and favorite recreational sports and activities.

* *Diet*

—Tell the patient to follow the diet prescribed by the primary/underlying disorder.

**FOLLOW-UP CARE**

* Stress the importance of regular follow-up visits. Make sure the patient has the necessary names and telephone numbers
* Help the patient obtain a Medic-Alert bracelet and identification card listing the surgery, medications, and emergency treatment.
* See Home Care under Adrenal Insufficiency (p. 11) for additional guidelines.

# Aldosteronism, Primary
(Hyperaldosteronism, Conn's Syndrome)

—Primary aldosteronism: overproduction of aldosterone by the adrenal glands, resulting in an excess of mineralocorticoids and, consequently, increases in sodium reabsorption and total body sodium. The most common cause is adrenal adenoma (60% of cases), but the disorder also may be caused by adrenal hyperplasia or adrenal carcinoma.

## SIGNS/SYMPTOMS

- Hypertension
- Postural hypotension
- Polydipsia, polyuria (especially nocturnal)
- Muscle weakness, fatigue
- Tetany

## COMPLICATIONS

- Heart failure
- Renal failure

## DIAGNOSTIC TESTS

- Describe each procedure, its purpose, and the normal feelings or sensations that are likely, as well as any preprocedural or postprocedural care.
  —Serum studies
     Electrolytes: sodium, potassium
     Aldosterone, plasma renin activity cortisol
  —Urine studies: 24-hour urinary aldosterone levels
  —Computed tomography: scans of the adrenal glands
  —Venous catheterization of the adrenal glands

## TREATMENT
*Medical*
- Therapy
  —Low-sodium, high-potassium diet
- Drugs
  —Spironolactone (Aldactone): to control blood pressure

*Surgical*
- Adrenalectomy: unilateral for adenoma, bilateral for hyperplasia

## HOME CARE

- Give both patient and caregiver *verbal* and *written* instructions. Provide them with the name and telephone number of a physician or nurse to call if questions arise.
- *General information*
  —Review the physician's explanation of the disease and its underlying causes. Explain adrenalectomy (see p. 13) if the procedure has been scheduled.
- *Warning signs*
  —Review the signs and symptoms that should be reported to a physician or nurse.
    Hyperaldosteronism: headache, fatigue, muscle weakness
    Hypokalemia: weakness, paresthesia, tetany, palpitation
- *Medications*
  —Explain the purpose, dosage, schedule, and route of administration of the prescribed medications, as well as side effects to report to a physician or nurse.
  —Emphasize that the patient should not stop taking the medications without first checking with a physician or nurse.
- *Activity*
  —Encourage the patient to discuss allowances and limitations regarding occupation and favorite recreational sports and activities.
  —Emphasize the importance of alternating exercise with rest periods.
- *Diet*
  —Stress the importance of following a low-sodium, high-potassium diet; the patient should avoid foods high in salt (most processed foods, luncheon meats, bacon, ham, and fast foods).
  —Encourage the patient to eat foods high in potassium (bananas, citrus fruit, tomatoes, dates).
  —Instruct the patient to read food labels for sodium content; suggest the use of herbs, spices, and sodium-free salt substitutes for flavoring.

## FOLLOW-UP CARE

- Stress the importance of regular follow-up visits. Make sure the patient has the necessary names and telephone numbers.

- Help the patient obtain a Medic-Alert bracelet and identification card listing the diagnosis and medications and emergency treatment.

# Allergy

—**Allergy: a hypersensitivity reaction to intrinsic antigens, most of which are environmental. It is estimated that 1 out of 6 Americans has a severe allergy and that more than 20 million have allergic reactions to airborne or inhaled allergens such as cigarette smoke, house dust, and pollen. Common allergies are divided into two types of reactions: immediate (or antibody-mediated) reactions, which occur within minutes of exposure as the result of release of a substance (e.g., histamine, bradykinin, or immunoglobulin) into the circulation (type I reactions); and delayed (or cell-mediated) reactions, which develop over 24 to 48 hours and are caused by antigens (type IV reactions).**

## COMMON ALLERGIES/REACTIONS

- Allergic conjunctivitis: hyperemia (reddening, warmth) of the conjunctivae, caused by allergens such as pollen, grass, topical medications, air pollutants, occupational irritants, and smoke
- Allergic dermatitis: an acute inflammation of the skin that occurs upon exposure to an allergen to which the individual is hypersensitive (e.g., poison ivy, nickel compounds)
- Allergic rhinitis: inflammation of the nasal passages, producing watery nasal discharge and itching of the nose and eyes, which is associated with airborne allergens such as house dust, animal dander, or an antigen (commonly pollen)

## SIGNS/SYMPTOMS

- Mild
  - —Conjunctivitis
  - —Urticaria
  - —Nasal congestion and drainage
  - —Bronchial congestion

—Erythema (redness), edema, scaling
—Vomiting
• Severe
—Anaphylaxis

## DIAGNOSTIC TESTS

• Describe each procedure, its purpose, and the normal feelings or sensations that are likely, as well as any preprocedural or post-procedural care.
—Allergy skin tests: to identify offending allergens
  Intradermal test
  Scratch test
  Patch text
—Blood tests: Complete blood count, eosinophil count, smear; serum IgE levels
—Radioallergosorbent test (RAST) to identify specific IgE antibodies

*For allergic rhinitis*
—Sinus x-ray: to rule out other disorders (e.g., nasal polyps), infection, and structural defects
—Computed tomography: scan of the sinuses to rule out other disorders and structural defects

## TREATMENT

*Medical*
• Therapy
—Immunotherapy (hyposensitization): for inhalant antigens (e.g., tree, grass, and weed pollens)
—Desensitization: to modify the hyperactivity of allergen
—Environmental control: to eliminate or modify offending allergens in the environment
• Drugs
—Antihistamines: via inhaler, nebulizer, or oral or nasal administration
—Sympathomimetic agents: oral or topical decongestants
—Corticosteroid: systemic, topical, or ocular
—Antiinfective agents
—Analgesics

## HOME CARE

• Give both patient and caregiver *verbal* and *written* instructions.

Provide them with the name and telephone number of a physician or nurse to call if questions arise.

- *General information*
  —Discuss the chronic nature of allergies; help the patient identify allergens that are a problem, and discuss ways to prevent symptoms through the use of medication and/or environmental control.
- *Specific instructions*
  —Explain environmental control as a means of preventing and treating symptoms.
  —Teach the patient how to assess home, work, and social environments for offending allergens; urge the patient to eliminate or avoid them if possible.
  —Explain that allergens may be seasonal (i.e., pollen counts are high in spring or after heavy rains) or may be more prominent in certain areas (e.g., open fields, woods, rural areas).
  —Review measures to eliminate or control common allergens:
    Trees, grass, weeds, and pollens: keep windows closed during the pollen season and use air conditioning.
    Mold spores: remove the source (e.g., plants, dirt); apply mold retardant solutions in damp areas such as the bathroom; use high-efficiency particulate-arresting (HEPA) air filters or electrostatic air cleaners.
    House dust, animal dander, mites: prevent household items from becoming "dust catchers": wash bedding frequently; encase mattresses in plastic; remove rugs and drapes, or vacuum them frequently; use damp dusting, and wear a face mask while dusting; use air filters; remove or avoid pets and other animals.
  —Instruct the patient to monitor response to treatments (medications, environmental control, immunotherapy, desensitization), to record any problems, new symptoms, or side effects, and to report them to the physician or a nurse.
- *Medications*
  —Explain the purpose, dosage, schedule, and route of administration of the prescribed medications, as well as side effects to report to a physician or nurse.
  —If an oral inhaler or nebulized drugs are prescribed, teach the patient how to use them (see Appendix I).
  —Stress the importance of not overusing or abusing prescribed or over-the-counter medications, since these drugs may have a cumulative effect.

- Activity
  —For allergic rhinitis, or conjunctivitis, instruct the patient to avoid or curtail strenuous work or exercise on days when the pollen count is high, especially if the allergens trigger an attack. If prescribed, medication may be taken before exercise or activity to prevent an attack.

**FOLLOW-UP CARE**

- Stress the importance of any prescribed follow-up care, including allergy testing and laboratory tests. Make sure the patient has the necessary names and telephone numbers.

# Alzheimer's Disease

—**Alzheimer's disease: progressive deterioration of the intellect, memory, and personality, leading to severe dementia. The specific cause is unknown, but the disorder is believed to arise from a deficiency in the brain's neurotransmitter. Immunologic, genetic, and environmental factors have been implicated. The onset of the disease is insidious, affecting people in their forties; the disease occurs in 10% to 15% of those over 65 years of age.**

**SIGNS/SYMPTOMS**

- Intellectual loss
  —Memory loss (initially the patient cannot remember recent events but can recall early life events)
  —Loss of sense of time
  —Poor decision-making ability
  —Loss of train of thought during conversations
  —Requires repetitive directions
  —Inability to perform arithmetic calculations
  —Shortened attention span
  —Inability to recognize family and friends
- Personality or affective loss
  —Personality changes
  —Apathy, loss of initiative

—Anxiety, fear, belligerence, stubbornness
—Suspicion, progressing to paranoia
—Loss of sense of humor
—Insensitivity to others
—Inattentiveness
—Conversation changes (slow speech, loss of words, use of clichés)
—Easily fatigued
—Reactive depression
—Crying spells
—Lethargy
—Neglect of self-care
—Nocturnal wandering
• Advanced stage
—Apathy, muteness
—Inability to recall recent or remote events
—Disorientation/confusion
—Inability to perform activities of daily living (ADLs)
—Incontinence

## COMPLICATIONS

• Physical and/or psychologic dependence
• Injury
• Bladder and bowel incontinence
• Dehydration/malnutrition
• Infection

## DIAGNOSTIC TESTS

• Describe each procedure, its purpose, and the normal feelings or sensations that are likely, as well as any preprocedural or postprocedural care.
—Positron emission tomography: to determine cerebral cortex metabolic activity
—Computed tomography: to detect progressive brain atrophy and ventricular enlargement and to rule out other neurologic problems
—Magnetic resonance imaging: used in early stage to detect any biochemical and anatomic changes
—Electroencephalography: to detect slowed brain wave activity
—Brain biopsy: to identify neurofibril tangles and neuritic plaques

**TREATMENT**

*Medical*

- No specific treatment is available; the prescribed treatment is directed toward controlling the symptoms and providing physiologic and psychologic support for the patient and family to enhance their ability to cope with the progressively deteriorating effects of the disease.
- Drugs
  —Ergoloid mesylate: to improve cognitive performance
  —Antidepressants: to relieve depression and elevate mood
  —Stimulants: for loss of spontaneity or inattention
  —Antipsychotic agents: to control severely agitated or combative patients
  —Tranquilizers, sedatives: to control restlessness, agitation, and sleep disturbances
  —Experimental drugs: choline derivatives; cholinergic therapy, anticholinesterase inhibitors, opioid antagonists

**HOME CARE**

- Give both patient and caregiver *verbal* and *written* instructions. Provide them with the name and telephone number of a physician or nurse to call if questions arise.
- *General information*
  —Discuss the disease and explain its progressive nature. To direct home care, help the caregiver identify the patient's functional stage (see box on p. 24).
- *Special instructions*
  —Teach the caregiver how to help the patient with reality orientation.
  > Introduce all caregivers by name each time, and have them wear name tags (encourage consistent use of caregivers).
  > Writing down instructions and directions may be helpful.
  > Put a clock with a large face and a calendar where the patient can see them; remind the patient of the time for a scheduled activity.
  > Be consistent and use repetition.
  > Give single-step, simple instructions.
  > Frequently remind the patient of the day, the hour, and where the patient is.

## STAGES OF FUNCTIONAL LOSS

*Stage I: Early confusion*
- Forgetful, loses things
- Expresses awareness of loss (depression not uncommon)

*Stage II: Late confusion*
- Increased difficulty with money management, work, driving, housekeeping, and shopping
- Social withdrawal from clubs, routine activities with friends
- Depression, increased fatigue
- Denies symptoms but may state "I feel like I'm losing my mind"
- May require placement in an adult care center or, if living alone, may need to move into a residential care center

*Stage III: Ambulatory dementia*
- Increased loss of ADLs
- Worsening of symptoms as day progresses
- Withdrawal from family and friends
- Appears unaware of losses
- Increased stress threshold behavior (nocturnal wakefulness; wandering, pacing; agitation, belligerence)
- Speech and writing difficult to understand

*Stage IV: Late-stage dementia*
- No longer ambulates; cannot remember to eat, swallow, or chew
- Little purposeful activity
- No recognition of caregivers or family
- Muteness or possibly spontaneous screaming
- Incontinent; may be totally dependent for physical hygiene
- Becoming increasingly vegetative

A

—Teach the caregiver how to deal with an agitated patient.

Speak in quiet tones

Maintain a quiet, calm environment and avoid rushing; reduce the amount and complexity of stimuli if the patient shows signs of frustration and agitation.

Be alert for factors that may precipitate agitation, so as to eliminate or modify them.

—Discuss the potential for injury as the patient's condition progressively deteriorates. Encourage the caregiver to establish home safety precautions.

Keep the patient's surroundings free of clutter and hazardous equipment.

Keep the area free of sharp objects and flammable items (e.g., lighter fluid).

Remove or dismantle door locks.

Have the patient use an electric razor, not a straight or safety razor.

Do not allow the patient to participate in potentially dangerous activities, such as smoking or cooking.

Put labels with the patient's name and telephone number in his or her clothing.

Provide assistance with daily routines (e.g., hygiene, diet, toileting). Medical supply stores carry special equipment for showers, bars for the toilet, and other devices.

Consider installing alarm systems.

—Discuss the patient's need for regular physical hygiene (i.e., bathing, shampooing, skin and oral care). Discuss the possibility of employing an attendant to help with daily care as dependency progresses.

—Explain that the patient needs to establish regular bowel and bladder habits.

—Discuss ways to prevent constipation.

Determine the patient's normal patterns

Remind the patient to go to the bathroom at scheduled times

Provide stool softeners and laxatives per prescription

Encourage the patient to drink fluids and eat high-fiber foods

Be alert for signs of impaction: no formed stool for 3 days; semiliquid stools, and restlessness (discuss the treatment for impaction: laxatives, suppositories, and enemas).

—Discuss ways to prevent urinary incontinence.
> Assess the patient's routine voiding patterns.
> Remind the patient to go to the bathroom q2h.
> Do not give the patient fluids before bedtime.
> Use disposable diapers and pads as indicated.

* *Medications*
  —Explain the purpose, dosage, schedule, and route of administration of the prescribed medication, as well as side effects to report to a physician or nurse.

* *Diet*
  —Alzheimer's patients need a properly balanced, high-fiber, high-calorie diet.
  —Present one course at a time (e.g., salad first, then entree); help the patient cut food as needed.
  —Use the following measures to prevent aspiration.
  > Evaluate the patient's alertness.
  > Monitor the patient's chewing and swallowing ability.
  > Remind the patient to eat slowly, take small bites, and swallow each bite before taking another.

**FOLLOW-UP CARE**

* Stress the importance of regular follow-up visits. Make sure the patient has the necessary names and telephone numbers.

**REFERRALS**

* Provide the names and telephone numbers of referral services, such as support groups for caregivers; social services for financial concerns and potential placement; home care services for possible in-home assistance and/or residential care centers.

# Amputation

—**Amputation: surgical removal of a body part (fingers, toes, upper extremity, or lower extremity). Most amputations are performed on the legs. The surgical goal in amputation is to**

A

**remove the least amount of tissue, leaving enough for a flap
with which to create a stump that will allow fitting of a prosthesis.**

## INDICATIONS

* Most common
  —Severe trauma
  —Crush injuries
  —Severe sepsis (e.g., gas gangrene)
  —Gangrene due to loss of arterial or venous circulation
* Less common
  —Severe or recurrent osteomyelitis
  —Musculoskeletal tumors
  —Intractable pain from limb paralysis

## TYPES OF AMPUTATION

* Forequarter: removal of the entire arm, forearm, and hand; the
  extremity is disarticulated at the shoulder joint
* Arm: amputation above the elbow or along the forearm
* Hemipelvectomy: removal of the entire thigh, leg, and foot (also
  called hindquarter amputation)
* Thigh: above-knee amputation (AKA)
* Lower leg: below-knee amputation (BKA)
* Foot: amputation of the toes and part of the foot at the metatar
  sal joints
* Finger or toe: amputation of part or all of one or more fingers
  or toes
* Disarticulation: amputation through a joint
* Closed amputation: creation of a weight-bearing stump, in
  which a flap composed of skin and soft tissues serves as padding over the bone end (also called definitive end-bearing amputation)
* Open (guillotine) amputation: creation of open stump surfaces
  as tissues are cut perpendicularly across with little initial incisional closure due to infection; the incision is closed later in
  another operation

## PREPROCEDURAL TEACHING

* Review the surgeon's explanation of the procedure and the reasons for it.
* Explain the need for written consent to surgery and anesthesia.

**Review of Preprocedural Care**

- Explain that the patient may be admitted to the hospital the day of surgery, rather than before.
- Explain that the patient must have nothing to eat or drink after midnight of the night before surgery.
  - —Explain that the patient's skin will be cleansed with a bactericidal soap or antiseptic solution to remove bacteria.
  - —Explain that a complete blood count and urinalysis will be done to check for infection and bleeding.
- If lower extremity amputation is involved, instruct the patient in proper crutch walking when possible.
- Encourage the patient to ask questions and discuss any fears, concerns, and grief over losing a limb.
- For psychologic support, try to arrange for a preoperative visit from a person who has adjusted well to a similar amputation.

**Review of Postprocedural Care**

- Explain the care of the stump area and dressing.
  - —The extremity will be elevated for 24 hours, then kept flat and extended (a longer period of elevation may be required, depending on the amount of swelling).
  - —The stump will be checked often to note color, drainage, swelling, bleeding, and wound, and to check the pulses proximal to the incision.
  - —The drainage around the incision may be scant or moderate; tubes and drains are used to drain fluid.
- Discuss the phenomenon of phantom pain, painful or irritating sensations that feel as if they arise from the amputated part. Explain that medications are available to control pain.
- Review the type of prosthesis prescribed by the surgeon.
  - —Delayed fitting: a dressing and an elastic bandage are applied to the stump after surgery, and a prosthesis is fitted in 2 to 3 months, once the swelling has diminished.

    Teach the patient and caregiver the proper method of wrapping the stump to help shape it for the prosthesis. Tell them that an orthotic technician will measure the stump to ensure a proper fit for the prosthesis.

    Immediate postsurgical fitting and immediate postoperative prosthesis: these are prescribed to allow immediate or early ambulation and weight bearing. A cast is applied to the stump, and the prosthesis is attached to the cast.

- Explain that the patient will be kept on bed rest with the stump elevated for the length of time prescribed by the surgeon. If the patient has had a lower extremity amputation, he or she then will be gotten up on crutches.
- Explain and demonstrate the adduction and extension exercises to be done on the amputated extremity to prevent contracture.
- For lower extremity amputations:
  —Stress the importance of range-of-motion exercises for the unaffected extremities.
  —Stress the importance of turning to the prone position to prevent contracture.
- For lower extremity amputations without a prosthesis:
  —Explain that the patient should avoid long periods of sitting in a chair; teach the patient how to use ambulation aids (e.g., crutches or a walker).
  —Encourage the patient to wear a good walking shoe and to keep the stump in a normal position (i.e., relaxed and in a downward position).
- For lower extremity amputations with a prosthesis:
  —Teach the patient how to use ambulation aids (e.g., crutches or a walker).
  —Explain that the periods of ambulation will be increased with the prescribed amount of weight bearing.
- Stress the importance of conditioning exercises (trunk flexion, sit-ups, hopping in place, hopping with the walker).
- Review medications, and discuss alternate methods to control phantom pain, such as distraction; behavior modification; relaxation; biofeedback; hypnosis; cutaneous stimulation with oil of wintergreen, heat, and massage; and transcutaneous electrical nerve stimulation.
- Instruct the patient to report prolonged or chronic phantom pain for possible exploration and resection of the stump of a neuroma at the site of resection.

## SIDE EFFECTS/COMPLICATIONS
- Hemorrhage, dehiscence
- Wound infection
- Phantom pain
- Contracture
- Abduction deformity

## HOME CARE

- Give both patient and caregiver *verbal* and *written* instructions; use visual aids to assist in explanations. Provide the patient and caregiver with the name and telephone number of a physician or nurse to call if other questions arise.
- *Warning signs*
  —Review the signs of infection to report to a physician or nurse: fever; chills; redness and swelling around the incision; drainage; or a foul odor from the incision or dressing.
  —Emphasize that prolonged phantom limb pain is unusual and should be reported to the physician or surgeon.
- *Special instructions*
  —Delayed fitting technique: teach the patient how to apply the elastic sleeve or wrap the stump for molding and shaping, and allow time for the patient to return the demonstration. Emphasize that the stump should not be wrapped too tightly, since this will impair circulation.
  —Teach and demonstrate stump care.
    Discuss the importance of daily hygiene to prevent infection and skin breakdown: wash the stump daily with soap and water and dry it well before applying the dressing, sleeve, or prosthesis.
    Stress the importance of inspecting and cleaning the stump daily; explain use of a hand-held mirror to check for signs of infection, pressure sores, skin irritation, or drainage. Advise the patient to report to the physician or surgeon any sign of skin irritation blisters (blebs), abrasions, or red or tender areas.
- *Medications*
  —Explain the purpose, dosage, schedule, and route of administration of prescribed drugs (antibiotics, analgesics, sedatives) and side effects to report to the physician or nurse.
- *Activity*
  —Stress the importance of participating in the prescribed rehabilitation program: physical therapy, daily conditioning, and stump-strengthening exercises.

## FOLLOW-UP CARE

- Discuss the importance of making and keeping follow-up appointments until recovery is complete. Make sure the patient has the necessary names and telephone numbers.

# Amyloidosis

—Amyloidosis: a rare, chronic disease characterized by accumulation of a proteinaceous material (amyloid) in the soft tissues. Amyloid can infiltrate one or more body organs, compromising organ function. Amyloidosis can occur as a primary disease, which may be familial, or as a secondary disorder stemming from a long-term, chronic inflammatory, infectious, or neoplastic disease. The cause of amyloidosis is unknown, but immunobiologic factors are believed to be involved.

## SIGNS/SYMPTOMS

The signs and symptoms of amyloidosis reflect organ system involvement and its complications.

- Neuropathy: decreased temperature, pain sensation; inability to sweat
- Gastrointestinal (GI) system: difficulty talking, swallowing, and eating due to macroglossia (swollen tongue); abdominal pain, constipation, diarrhea, GI bleeding
- Respiratory system: dyspnea, cough, wheezing, nasal lesions, vocal cord lesions
- Skin: waxy, indurated papules and purpura, thickening of the skin, alopecia
- Joints: early morning stiffness and fatigue

## COMPLICATIONS

- Cardiac system
  - —Restrictive cardiomyopathy
  - —Myocardial infarction
  - —Congestive heart failure
- Renal system
  - —Nephrotic syndrome
  - —Renal failure
- Gastrointestinal system
  - —Malabsorption syndrome
  - —Hemorrhage
  - —Protein-losing enteropathy
  - —Perforation, ischemic necrosis
  - —Hepatomegaly

- Neurologic system
  —Peripheral, sensorimotor neuropathy

## DIAGNOSTIC TESTS

- Describe each procedure, its purpose, and the normal feelings or sensations that are likely, as well as any preprocedural or postprocedural care.
  —Serum and urine electrophoresis
  —Tissue biopsy (sites may include gingiva, skin, abdominal fat pad, and rectal mucosa)

## TREATMENT

*Medical*

- Therapy
  —Plasmapheresis: to stop dissemination of amyloid chains
- Drugs
  —Antineoplastics: to reduce the concentration of amyloid
  —Colchicine, dimethyl sulfoxide (DMSO)
  —Corticosteroid: to treat underlying inflammatory disorder

## HOME CARE

- Give both patient and caregiver *verbal* and *written* instructions. Provide them with the name and telephone number of a physician or nurse to call if questions arise.
- *General information*
  —Review the physician's explanation of the disorder, its causes, and associated involvement of other body organs.
- *Warning signs*
  —Review the signs and symptoms of disease progression that should be reported to the physician or a nurse: chest pain, dyspnea, shortness of breath, peripheral edema, bleeding, abdominal pain, and diarrhea.
- *Special instructions*
  —Teach the patient how to care for skin lesions if present; stress the importance of reporting to the physician any signs of skin infection, such as reddened, warm, painful, draining lesions.
  —Discuss the need for safety measures at home if the patient has peripheral or sensory impairment:
  Test the temperature of the bathwater before getting into the tub.

Do not use heating pads.

Avoid wearing tight, constricting clothing (e.g., socks, stockings).

- *Medications*
  —Explain the purpose, dosage, schedule, and route of administration of the prescribed medication, as well as side effects to report to a physician or nurse.
  —If steroids are prescribed, emphasize that the patient should not abruptly stop taking the drugs without first checking with the physician.
- *Activity*
  —Encourage the patient to discuss allowances and limitations regarding occupation and favorite recreational sports and activities.
- *Diet*
  —Tell the patient to follow a regular diet or one ordered for the associated disease.
  —If the tongue is affected, instruct the patient to take small bites, to chew thoroughly, and to swallow each bite completely before taking another.
  —If the patient suffers from malnutrition, encourage the addition of high-calorie food supplements to the diet.

**FOLLOW-UP CARE**

- Stress the importance of regular follow-up visits. Make sure the patient has the necessary names and telephone numbers.
- Help the patient obtain a Medic-Alert bracelet and identification card listing the diagnosis and medications.

# Amyotrophic Lateral Sclerosis
("Lou Gehrig Disease")

—**Amyotrophic lateral sclerosis (ALS): a progressive lower motor neuron disorder that results in muscle wasting and weakness. The weakness begins in the upper extremities (upper arms and shoulders) and progressively involves the muscles of the neck and throat. The trunk and legs usually are not affected until late in the disease.**

## SIGNS/SYMPTOMS

- Irregular muscle fasciculations
- Cramping
- Incoordination of movement of the hands and fingers
- Muscle stiffness and wasting involving the hands, arms, and shoulders
- Spastic gait
- Slurred speech
- Progressive weakness, flaccidity, and atrophy of the legs
- Difficulty swallowing
- Dyspnea
- Excessive drooling
- Loss of reflexes

## COMPLICATIONS

- Neuromuscular deficit (mild to severe)
- Respiratory infection
- Aspiration
- Atelectasis
- Respiratory failure
- Injury

## DIAGNOSTIC TESTS

- Describe each procedure, its purpose, and the normal feelings or sensations that are likely, as well as any preprocedural or postprocedural care. Explain that the following diagnostic procedures help confirm the diagnosis.
  —Myelography
  —Computed tomography scan
  —Muscle biopsy
  —Electromyelography
  —Nerve conduction studies
  —Laboratory tests
  　　Creatinine phosphokinase (CPK): elevated
  　　Cerebrospinal fluid: elevated protein

## TREATMENT

*Medical*

- Therapy
  —Physical therapy
  —Occupational, speech therapy
  —Oxygen/ventilatory support

- Drugs
  —Anticholinesterase drugs
  —Steroids
  —Antibiotics
  —Muscle relaxants

*Surgical*

- Transtympanic neuroectomy
- Cricopharyngeal myotomy: to alleviate dysphagia
- Cervical esophagostomy

## HOME CARE

- Give both patient and caregiver *verbal* and *written* instructions. Provide them with the name and telephone number of a physician or nurse to call if questions arise. Use visual aids to assist in instruction.
- *General information*
  —Review the physician's explanation of the disorder, as well as the symptoms and the progression of the disease.
  —Discuss the importance of skin care to prevent skin breakdown (back rubs, frequent changes of position, use of air mattress, sheepskin, and footboard).
  —Explain the need to maintain good oral and eye hygiene. Explain the need for oral suctioning as the disease progresses, and demonstrate the procedure.
- *Warning signs*
  —Review the signs and symptoms of disease progression that should be reported to the physician or a nurse: excessive salivation, weakening voice, difficulty swallowing.
  —Explain to the patient and caregiver that cognitive processes are not affected. Emphasize the importance of expressing feelings about the progressive muscular wasting and weakness.
- *Special instructions*
  —Explain to the patient and caregiver the respiratory support equipment to be kept in the home (oxygen therapy, suction setup), and show household members how to use it. Ask the physician for a prescription, and help the patient and caregiver obtain equipment from a medical supply store or pharmacy.
  —Demonstrate how to use an electrolarynx to facilitate vocalization.

—Discuss the need to develop alternative methods of communication (using the eyes, blinking) when the voice no longer functions.

• *Medications*
  —Explain the purpose, dosage, schedule, and route of administration of the prescribed medication, as well as side effects to report to a physician or nurse.

• *Activity*
  —Teach the patient to balance passive or active range-of-motion activities with rest periods and to avoid strenuous exercise or activity; encourage participation in family activities.
  —Review the purpose of braces, splints, and cervical collars to support the hands, ankles, and neck, and demonstrate how to use them properly.

• *Diet*
  —Advise a high-calorie, high-protein soft diet as tolerated.
  —Teach the patient and caregiver how to manage problems with swallowing.
    Place pureed foods on the posterior aspect of the tongue.
    If solid foods are still possible, cut food into small pieces, chew thoroughly, and swallow each bite completely before taking another, to avoid aspiration.
  —Clean the corners of the patient's mouth after eating and prn.
  —Have the patient use a bib.
  —If nasogastric (NG) or gastrostomy feedings must be considered, demonstrate the procedure for NG tube feeding, as well as care of the equipment.
  —Explain the need to provide for and anticipate elimination; explain that the patient can prevent constipation by drinking fluids and using suppositories or stool softeners daily.

## FOLLOW-UP CARE

• Stress the importance of regular follow-up visits. Make sure the patient has the necessary names and telephone numbers.
• Encourage and help the patient obtain a Medic-Alert bracelet and identification card listing diagnosis and medications.

## REFERRALS

• Provide the patient and caregiver with the names and telephone numbers of referral services, such as home health care and physical and occupational therapy centers.
• Refer the patient and caregiver to an ALS support group.

# Anaphylaxis

—Anaphylaxis: a rapid, systemic, antigen-antibody hypersensitivity reaction that affects a number of organs throughout the body. It often is an immediate, life-threatening event that occurs with seconds to minutes of exposure to a causative allergen. The most common causes are insect venom (bees, wasps, hornets, yellow jackets), drugs (e.g., penicillin, iodine, and sulfonamides), blood products, and foods (e.g., shellfish and eggs).

## SIGNS/SYMPTOMS
- Early (within seconds of exposure)
  —Sweating
  —Weakness
  —Feeling of impending doom or fright
  —Shortness of breath
  —Pruritus, urticaria
  —Angioedema of the eyes, lips, and tongue
- Late (within minutes of exposure)
  —Respiratory
    Bronchospasm
    Dyspnea
    Wheezing
    Laryngeal edema
    Cyanosis
    Hypoxia
    Respiratory arrest
  —Cardiovascular
    Lightheadedness (due to hypotension)
    Rapid, weak pulse
    Arrhythmias
  —Neurologic
    Confusion
    Seizures
    Coma

## COMPLICATIONS

- Shock
- Respiratory failure
- Cardiac arrest
- Death

## DIAGNOSTIC TESTS

- No specific tests are used to diagnose anaphylaxis; the patient's history, signs, and symptoms direct the diagnosis and treatment (skin and scratch tests may be done to identify allergens in patients considered at risk for an anaphylactic reaction).

## TREATMENT

*Medical*

Anaphylaxis is *always* an emergency; treatment involves immediate, aggressive management of symptoms.

- Therapy
  —Intubation: to establish an airway
  —Admission to an intensive care unit for monitoring and management
- Drugs
  —Epinephrine: to counter the effects of the allergen
  —Vasopressors: to maintain blood pressure
  —Diphenhydramine (Benadryl): to treat angioedema and urticaria
  —Aminophylline: for bronchospasm

*Surgical*

- Tracheostomy: for severe airway obstruction

## HOME CARE

- Give both the patient and the caregiver *verbal* and *written* instructions. Provide them with the name and telephone number of a physician or nurse to call if questions arise.
- *General information*
  —Review the physician's explanation of the disorder, making sure the patient understands what caused the anaphylactic episode.
  —Stress the importance of avoiding known allergens in the future.
    If food was the allergen: help the patient list other foods that also may cause a reaction (e.g., if shrimp caused the

reaction, the patient should avoid all shellfish, such as oysters, lobster, and mussels).

If insect venom was the allergen: instruct the patient to avoid outdoor areas that may have a high concentration of insects during a particular season.

- *Warning signs*
  —See Signs/Symptoms above for early and late manifestations.
- *Special instructions*
  —Discuss with the patient the need to carry an anaphylaxis kit. If one is ordered, teach the patient and other family members how to administer the medication. Instruct the patient to check the kit regularly for expiration dates.

**FOLLOW-UP CARE**

- Discuss the need for any follow-up appointments, including future allergy testing when indicated. Be sure the patient has the necessary names and telephone numbers.
- Emphasize that the patient should inform health care providers about the allergy before any procedures are done.
- Explain the importance of obtaining a Medic-Alert bracelet and identification card listing the specific allergen.
- Advise the patient to identify the emergency department nearest home and work.

# Anorectal Abscess and Fistula

—**Anorectal abscess and fistula: a localized infection caused by inflammation of soft tissue of the anal canal, rectum, or perianal skin. Initially appearing as a collection of pus, an anorectal abscess may progress to a fistula in the soft tissues and perianal skin.**

## CAUSES/CONTRIBUTING FACTORS/RISK FACTORS

- Abrasion, trauma, or tearing of the lining of the anal canal, rectum, or perianal skin, with subsequent infection with *Escherichia coli,* staphylococci, or streptococci
- Infection of submucosal hematomas, sclerosed hemorrhoids, or anal fissures

- Obstruction of glands in the anal area
- Cryptitis
- Infection of apocrine glands
- Folliculitis in the perianal area
- Ulcerative colitis
- Crohn's disease

## SIGNS/SYMPTOMS

- Rectal pain (usually described as throbbing or dull and aching, depending on the abscess's location)
- Erythematous lump or swelling in the anal area
- Aggravation of pain with sitting, walking, or defecation
- Discharge or bleeding
- Anal pruritus
- Fever, chills, nausea, vomiting, malaise
- If fistula present: pink or red, elevated ulcer that produces a discharge on perianal skin

## COMPLICATIONS

- Perineal cellulitis
- Formation of scar tissue
- Anal stricture
- Peritonitis

## DIAGNOSTIC TESTS

- Describe each procedure, its purpose, and the normal feelings or sensations that are likely, as well as any preprocedural and postprocedural care.
  —Digital rectal examination
  —Proctoscopy: to visualize lesions
  —Additional procedures that may be performed to rule out other conditions
    Sigmoidoscopy
    Barium enema
    Colonoscopy

## TREATMENT

*Medical*
- Therapy
  —Diet high in fiber and fluids
- Drugs

　　—Stool softeners
　　—Antibiotics
　　—Analgesics
*Surgical*
* For anorectal abscess: surgical incision and drainage
* For fistulas: fistulotomy (removal of the fistula and granulated tissue) or fistulectomy (removal of the fistulous tract and drainage)

## HOME CARE

* Give both the patient and the caregiver *verbal* and *written* instructions. Provide them with the name and telephone number of a physician or nurse to call if questions arise.
* *General information*
　　—Explain how an anorectal abscess and fistula develop, and discuss the causes and contributing factors, diagnostic tests, care, and treatment.
* *Warning signs*
　　—Review the signs and symptoms that should be reported to a physician or nurse.
　　　　Infection (fever, purulent drainage from the incision, redness, swelling, tenderness)
　　—Instruct the patient to note the time of the first bowel movement after surgery, and to notify the physician or nurse if no bowel movement occurs or if constipation develops.
* *Special instructions*
　　—Help the patient obtain the appropriate supplies (dressings, perineal pads, mesh panties) to aid complete healing of the infected area after surgery.
　　—Demonstrate proper wound care and dressing changes (procedure, frequency, packing, irrigation). Show the patient how to use a mirror to inspect the area and to change the dressing.
　　—Instruct the patient to check the dressing after bowel or bladder elimination and to replace it if it becomes soiled. Advise the patient to dispose of soiled dressings in a plastic bag and to wash hands thoroughly.
　　—Advise the patient to shave the perianal area weekly to keep hair out of the affected area (a caregiver may need to help the patient with this).
　　—Encourage defecation to prevent fecal impaction.

—Teach the patient to avoid straining during a bowel movement, since this may increase discomfort and put pressure on the affected area.

—Stress the importance of perianal cleanliness at all times; explain that proper hygiene helps prevent infection.

—Provide warm sitz baths to cleanse the perianal region and to relieve the patient's discomfort; show the patient how to prepare one.

—Instruct the patient to use a thick pillow or pad when sitting.

—Explain that anorectal infections tend to recur and that anorectal sexual activities need to be modified to control recurrences or complications.

• *Medications*

—Explain the purpose, dosage, schedule, and route of administration of the prescribed drugs, as well as side effects to report to the physician or a nurse.

—Teach the patient that stool-softening laxatives, along with a high-fiber diet, will help prevent constipation.

• *Diet*

—Help the patient plan a diet high in fiber and fluids, which helps produce regular bowel movements.

**FOLLOW-UP CARE**

• Stress the importance of regular follow-up visits and make sure the patient has the necessary names and telephone numbers.

• Explain that follow-up visits are important because perianal fistulas can take 4-5 weeks to heal; deeper wounds may take 12-16 weeks.

# Anticoagulation Therapy

—Anticoagulation therapy: use of anticoagulant medications in the prevention or treatment of arterial or venous thrombosis (blood clots) for a number of medical diseases and disorders. The types of anticoagulants are warfarin, administered

**A**

**orally, and heparin, administered by subcutaneous injection.
The time a patient remains on anticoagulation therapy depends on the underlying condition for which it is prescribed;
it can be lifelong or of short duration.**

## INDICATIONS

- Pulmonary embolism
- Cerebral embolism
- Valvular heart disease
- Following placement of heart valve prosthesis
- Presence of mural thrombus
- Following myocardial infarction (heart attack)
- Use of vascular stents

## SIDE EFFECTS/COMPLICATIONS

- Bleeding
  —Nosebleeds
  —Bleeding gums
  —Hemoptysis (spitting up blood)
  —Hematemesis
  —Increased menstrual flow
  —Hemoccult positive
  —Hematoma, bruises, bleeding under the skin
- Pain in the abdomen, flank, or joints
- Symptoms of stroke or transient ischemic attacks, associated
  with noncompliance with medication

## HOME CARE

- Give both patient and caregiver *verbal* and *written* instructions.
  Provide them with the name and telephone number of a physician or nurse to call if questions arise. Use visual aids to assist
  in instruction.
- Initiate the teaching plan as soon as it is known that the patient
  will be discharged on anticoagulant therapy.
- *General information*
  —Review explanation of the condition that requires anticoagulation; the type of anticoagulant (warfarin or heparin) that is
  prescribed; the benefits, dosage, time of administration, and
  side effects; the importance of taking the medication at the
  prescribed time and never skipping a dose; and what to do if
  a dose is missed.

- *Warning signs*
    —Review signs and symptoms of bleeding the patient should report to a physician or nurse.
    > Spontaneous bleeding of nose or gums
    > Bleeding hemorrhoids
    > Bloody stools
    > Reddish or purplish spots on skin
    > Vomiting, diarrhea, and fever that last longer than 24 hours
- *Special instructions*
    —Instruct the patient to monitor all bruises by drawing a line around the margin of the bruise and notifying the physician or nurse if it begins to extend beyond the margins. For cuts, instruct the patient to apply firm pressure to the cut for 10 minutes; if the arm or leg is cut, elevate it above the level of the heart. If bleeding does not stop, seek immediate help.
    —Discuss safety precautions to prevent injury that might lead to bleeding.
    > Avoid vigorous nose blowing and toothbrushing. Avoid use of water-jet tooth cleaners. Use a soft-bristled toothbrush or electric toothbrush. Do not put a toothpick or sharp object in mouth.
    > Wear shoes and slippers at all times to prevent injury to the feet; see a podiatrist to trim calluses and corns.
    > Wear gloves while gardening.
    > Use an electric shaver instead of a safety blade or hair removal cream.
    > Avoid working or playing with sharp instruments or power tools.
    —For women:
    > Monitor menstrual flow if excessive (more than normal pattern) and notify physician or nurse of abnormally heavy flow.
    > Advise the patient to avoid pregnancy while taking warfarin, since it can cause serious birth defects. Stress the importance of consulting a physician or nurse if pregnancy is desired or suspected.
    > Consult with a physician or nurse as to appropriate type of contraception; avoid use of an intrauterine device.
    —Instruct the patient or caregiver in the procedure for administration of a subcutaneous injection.

Give the patient or caregiver sufficient time to practice the procedure.

Discuss the importance of rotating the injection site with every dose to prevent bleeding, infection, and soreness. If the site becomes sore, apply warm (not hot) dry heat.

Instruct the patient or caregiver to wash hands and use aseptic technique when handling the syringe and needle.

Demonstrate withdrawal of the correct amount of heparin.

Demonstrate and explain each step of the procedure.

○ Select injection site.

○ Use subcutaneous fatty tissue; avoid bruised areas, hematomas, incisions, or scarred tissue; and avoid area within 2 inches of the umbilicus.

○ Cleanse skin with alcohol.

○ Hold syringe filled with correct heparin dose like a pencil or dart.

○ Pinch up skin, forming a fat roll between fingers.

○ Insert needle at a 45-degree angle and quickly push into subcutaneous tissue up to hub or syringe; do not pull back on plunger. Inject medication, slowly withdraw needle, and press skin gently; avoid rubbing or massaging area.

○ Enter date, time, site, and dosage of each injection on home record.

Leave the equipment at bedside for practice. Arrange to have equipment that will be used at home available. Advise the patient where to purchase equipment.

—Instruct the patient or caregiver in the oral administration of warfarin.

Explain to the patient that the medication comes in different dosages and that each dose is a different color.

Review the prescribed dose and the schedule for administration.

Consistently large intakes of foods high in vitamin K, such as leafy green vegetables, tomatoes, bananas, and fish, can decrease the effect of warfarin.

Alcohol intake should be limited because alcohol can increase the effect of drugs.

• *Medications*

—Explain the purpose, dosage, schedule, and route of administration of the prescribed medications, as well as side effects to report to a physician or nurse.

—Discuss the importance of not taking over-the-counter medications that contain aspirin or salicylate. Instruct the patient to read labels of all medications and to check with a physician, nurse, or pharmacist for appropriate medications (e.g., cold remedies, vitamins, analgesics).

—Instruct the patient to refill medication 1-2 weeks before supply runs out; store medication in a cool place, avoiding extremes of hot and cold.

—Advise the patient to obtain extra medication before traveling and to arrange for laboratory tests at the place of the visit.

* *Activity*

—Tell the patient to refrain from dangerous hobbies or contact sports that can cause bodily trauma or injury. Encourage questions regarding activity allowances and limitations on occupational and leisure activities.

## FOLLOW-UP CARE

* Stress the importance of regular follow-up visits. Make sure the patient has the necessary names and telephone numbers.
* Stress the importance of having laboratory work done as ordered. Explain that frequent periodic blood tests will be required to monitor and adjust drug dosages. Once the desired level is reached, blood testing will decrease, although routine laboratory work will be needed for as long as anticoagulant therapy is prescribed.

—Therapeutic serum levels

Warfarin: prothrombin time 1.5 to 2 $\times$ control; International Ratio (INR) 1:3

Heparin: partial thromboplastin time 2 to 3 $\times$ control

* Help the patient obtain a Medic-Alert bracelet and identification card listing the diagnosis and medications.

---

# Aortic Aneurysm

---

—**Aortic aneurysm: an abnormal widening of the aorta, either at the beginning of the vessel (ascending) or after it curves toward the abdomen (descending). In a dissecting aneurysm, blood makes its way between the layers of the blood vessel, caus-**

**ing them to separate. An aneurysm can involve the full circum-ference of the vessel or only a weak patch on one side of the arte-rial wall. Blood pools in the pouch, causing blood clots.**

## CAUSES/CONTRIBUTING FACTORS/RISK FACTORS

- Atherosclerosis (ascending aorta)
- Infection (aortic arch and descending aorta)
- Coarctation of the aorta
- Trauma (descending aorta)
- Syphilis (ascending aorta)
- Hypertension (in dissecting aneurysm)
- Marfan's syndrome
- Men ages 50-70 years
- African-Americans

## SIGNS/SYMPTOMS

- Sudden onset of pain in anterior chest, extending to the neck, shoulder, lower back, or abdomen
- Syncope
- Pallor
- Sweating
- Shortness of breath
- Increased pulse rate
- Duskiness
- Leg weakness (involvement of the aortic valve, ascending an-eurysm)
- Wheezing
- Hoarseness
- Numbness (paresthesia)
- Neuralgia

## COMPLICATIONS

- Dissection, rupture
- Bleeding
- Embolization

## DIAGNOSTIC TESTS

- Explain that the following diagnostic procedures confirm the di-agnosis. Explain each procedure as it is ordered. Describe each procedure, its purpose, and the normal feelings or sensations that are likely, as well as any preprocedural or postprocedural care.

—Aortography: to show location of the aneurysm, its form, and whether the walls of the artery are separating (dissecting aneurysm)

—Electrocardiogram: to differentiate pain of thoracic aneurysm from that of a myocardial infarction

—Echocardiogram: to help identify dissecting aneurysm (separation of the arterial walls)

—Hemoglobin: to detect loss of blood

—Computed tomography: to locate and confirm the location of the aneurysm and monitor its progression

—Magnetic resonance imaging: to aid the diagnosis further

—Transesophageal echocardiogram: to locate the aneurysm from the back of the aorta

## TREATMENT

*Medical*

• Drugs

—Antihypertensive drugs; to keep blood pressure under control and alleviate undue pressure on the vessels, including the site of repair

*Surgical*

• Resection of the aneurysm and restoration of normal blood flow by using Dacron or Teflon graft replacement. If the aortic valve is involved or is insufficient, replacement is necessary (see Valve Replacement, p. 671).

## HOME CARE

• Give both patient and caregiver *verbal* and *written* instructions. Provide them with the name and telephone number of a physician or nurse to call if questions arise.

• *General information*

—Review the indications and causes of the patient's aneurysm. Discuss any factors that will help to prevent future aneurysms, such as controlling blood pressure and slowing the atherosclerotic process.

• *Specific instructions*

—Following surgery:

Instruct the patient in care of the incisional wound, reviewing signs of infection and thrombus formation within the graft.

A

Teach hypertensive patients how to monitor blood pressure and keep a record. Provide blood pressure parameters. Include information on where to obtain necessary equipment and supplies as indicated.

- *Medications*
  —Explain the purpose, dosage, schedule, and route of administration of the prescribed medications, as well as side effects to report to a physician or nurse.
- *Activity*
  —Advise the patient to alternate exercise with rest and avoid vigorous exercise or heavy lifting.
  —Encourage the patient to discuss allowances or limitations with respect to occupation, sports, and activities.
  —Caution the patient to avoid sudden outbursts of activity associated with stress.
  —Emphasize that the patient should not shovel snow, change a tire, or push a car.
- *Diet*
  —Advise the patient to follow a low-salt, low-fat diet.
  —Instruct the patient to limit alcohol consumption because of alcohol's effect on blood pressure.

**FOLLOW-UP CARE**

- Make sure that the patient has scheduled a follow-up visit. Check that the patient has the necessary names and telephone numbers.
- Stress the importance of not smoking because nicotine has negative effects on the blood vessels and blood pressure.

# Aortic Insufficiency
## (Incompetence, Regurgitation)

—**Aortic insufficiency: incompetence or insufficiency of the aortic valve, which permits blood to flow (leak) back into the left ventricle. This causes decreased flow of blood outward into** the tissues and increased volume in the left ventricle, adding to the work of the heart and resulting in a hypertrophic left ventricle. The cusps are unable to close because of the presence of lesions, perforations, or tears or the development of eroded or scarred tissue because of infection or fibrosis.

## CAUSES/CONTRIBUTING FACTORS

- Rheumatic fever
- Syphilis
- Hypertension
- Endocarditis
- Idiopathic
- Associated with Marfan's syndrome
- Dissection of aortic aneurysm
- Alkalizing spondylitis
- Congenital bicuspid aortic valve
- Chest trauma

## SIGNS/SYMPTOMS

- Palpitations
- Awareness of the heartbeat, especially when lying down
- Tachycardia
- Dyspnea
- Orthopnea
- Paroxysmal nocturnal dyspnea
- Fatigue
- Exertional angina

## COMPLICATIONS

- Heart rhythm abnormalities
- Congestive heart failure
- Ventricular hypertrophy
- Endocarditis
- Sudden death

## DIAGNOSTIC TESTS

- Describe each procedure, its purpose, and the normal feelings or sensations that are likely, as well as any preprocedural or postprocedural care.
  - —Electrocardiogram: to detect evidence of left ventricular hypertrophy

—Chest x-ray: to detect aortic valve calcification, left ventricle enlargement, and dilation of the ascending aorta
—Echocardiogram: to detect rhythm abnormalities, presence of left ventricle enlargement, and ischemic changes
—Radionuclide studies: to determine ejection fraction
—Cardiac catheterization: to determine severity of valve incompetence, assess ventricular function, and look for involvement of other valves

## TREATMENT

*Medical*
• Drugs
  —Inotropic drugs
  —Vasodilators
  —Antiarrhythmic agents
*Surgical*
• Aortic valve replacement

## HOME CARE

• Give both patient and caregiver *verbal* and *written* instructions. Provide them with the name and telephone number of a physician or nurse to call if questions arise.
• *General information*
  —Use heart models or diagram to assist in instruction. Show the patient location of the affected valve.
  —Discuss disease process and causes, explaining that appearance of signs and symptoms may reflect disease progression.
  —Explain the risk of endocarditis, discussing causes and means of prevention: alert dentist and other medical personnel (urologist, gynecologist) of valve disease. Explain importance of good oral hygiene and regular dental care. Stress importance of antibiotic prophylaxis before dental care or any invasive procedures (i.e., dilation and curettage, cystoscopy) for prevention.
  —Describe the need for valve replacement, if recommended (see p. 671).
• *Warning signs*
  —Review the signs and symptoms that should be reported to a physician or nurse.
      Exertional dyspnea
      Orthopnea

Paroxysmal nocturnal dyspnea

Fatigue

Palpitations

- *Specific instructions*
  —Provide female patients with instructions regarding pregnancy and appropriate forms of contraception. Emphasize the importance of planning all pregnancies.
- *Medications*
  —Explain the purpose, dosage, schedule, and route of administration of the prescribed medications, as well as side effects to report to a physician or nurse.
- *Activity*
  —Stress importance of avoiding strenuous activities. Encourage patient to discuss allowances and limitations with respect to occupation and recreational sports activities. Explain the need for moderate activity. Encourage frequent rest periods and avoid fatigue.
- *Diet*
  —Discuss need to restrict salt intake. Explain that further sodium restrictions may be necessary in the presence of heart failure.

**FOLLOW-UP CARE**

- Stress the importance of any prescribed follow-up care, including allergy testing and laboratory tests. Make sure the patient has the necessary names and telephone numbers.
- Stress the importance of not smoking or using tobacco products. Provide information and referrals to smoking cessation programs as necessary.

# Aortic Valve Stenosis

—**Aortic valve stenosis: narrowing of the three-leaflet aortic valve from the normal 2.6 to 3.5 cm opening to as little as 0.4 cm. The narrowing is due to the accumulation of plaque (calcification). This narrowing or obstruction restricts the flow of blood across the valve into the aorta, depriving the heart and**

**other organs of circulation and increasing the workload of the heart.**

## CAUSES/CONTRIBUTING FACTORS/RISK FACTORS

- Congenital bicuspid valve
- Rheumatic fever
- Males
- Persons over 60 years of age

## SIGNS/SYMPTOMS

- Symptoms appear late in the course of the illness
- Angina
- Syncope (faintness) with exertion
- Orthopnea, dyspnea, shortness of breath
- Fatigue
- Cool extremities
- Palpitations
- Dizziness

## COMPLICATIONS

- Arrhythmias
  —Atrial fibrillation
  —Conduction defects
- Heart failure
- Sudden cardiac death
- Ineffective endocarditis
- Embolization

## DIAGNOSTIC TESTS

- Describe each procedure, its purpose, and the normal feelings or sensations that are likely, as well as any preprocedural and postprocedural care.
  —Electrocardiogram: to detect rhythm abnormalities and identify left ventricular hypertrophy
  —Echocardiography: to determine severity of the obstruction and assess ventricular function
  —Cardiac catheterization and coronary angiography: to assess degree of obstruction across the valve, ventricular function, coronary blood flow
  —Chest x-ray: to detect valvular calcification, heart enlargement, and lung congestion

**TREATMENT**

*Medical*
- Therapy
  —Catheter balloon aortic valvuloplasty
- Drugs
  —Digitalis
  —Diuretics
  —Beta blockers
  —Vasodilator
  —Antiarrhythmic agents

*Surgical*
- Aortic valve replacement

**HOME CARE**

- Give both the patient and the caregiver verbal and written instruction. Provide them with the name and telephone number of a physician or nurse to call if questions arise.
- *General information*
  —Use heart models or diagrams to assist in instruction. Show the patient the location of the affected valve and explain its role in the arterial circulation.
  —If balloon angioplasty or surgery is recommended, help the patient understand why and explain what is involved in these procedures (see Valve Replacement, p. 671).
  —Discuss the disease process, contributing factors, the cause of obstruction, and the signs and symptoms of disease progression.
  —Explain the risk of endocarditis and discuss its causes and means of preventing it, including alerting the dentist and any other medical personnel (urologist, gynecologist) that the patient has valve disease, maintaining good oral hygiene, and receiving regular dental care. Explain the importance of antiobiotic prophylaxis before dental care and other invasive procedures (dilation and curettage, cystoscopy).
- *Warning signs*
  —Review the signs and symptoms that should be reported to a physician or nurse.
    Faintness
    Palpitations
    Shortness of breath

Dyspnea on exertion

Signs of systemic emboli: muscle weakness, paresthesias, confusion

- *Special instructions*
  —Provide female patients with instruction regarding contraception and risk of pregnancy. Stress the importance of pregnancy planning.
- *Medications*
  —Explain the purpose, dosage schedule, and route of administration of any prescribed drugs, as well as side effects to report to the physician or nurse.
- *Activity*
  —Emphasize the importance of avoiding strenuous activity, such as vacuuming, pushing a car, changing a tire, or engaging in competitive sports.
  —Encourage the patient to discuss limitations with respect to occupation and recreational activities.
  —Explain the need for moderate activity, such as walking for conditioning.
  —Encourage the patient to rest frequently and avoid fatigue.
- *Diet*
  —Discuss the need to restrict salt intake to 3000 mg per day. Explain that further sodium restrictions may be necessary in the presence of heart failure.

**FOLLOW-UP CARE**

- Stress the importance of regular follow-up visits. Make sure the patient has the necessary names and telephone numbers.
- Emphasize the importance of not smoking or using tobacco products. Provide information about and referrals to smoking cessation programs as necessary

# Aplastic Anemia
(Hypoplastic)

—Aplastic anemia: results from inability of the bone marrow to produce erythrocytes (RBCs). Usually the onset of aplastic anemia is insidious, but when it develops suddenly, it has a poor prognosis. **Hypoplastic anemia most often involves the depression of production of all three bone marrow elements: erythrocytes, platelets, and granulocytes (pancytopenia).**

## CAUSES

- Antineoplastic or antimicrobial agents
- Infectious processes
- Pregnancy
- Hepatitis
- Radiation

## SIGNS/SYMPTOMS

- Fatigue
- Shortness of breath
- Headache
- Weakness
- Pallor
- Dysphagia
- Numbness and tingling in extremities
- Easy bruising and bleeding
- Dizziness
- Fever
- Infection

## COMPLICATIONS

- Facial bleeding or infection

## DIAGNOSTIC TESTS

- Describe each procedure, its purpose, and the normal feelings or sensations that are likely, as well as any preprocedural and postprocedural care.
  —Complete blood count with differential
  —Platelet count
  —Bleeding time
  —Bone marrow aspiration
  —Reticulocyte count
  —Peripheral blood smear
  —Cultures (if infection is suspected)

A

## TREATMENT

*Medical*

- Therapy
  —Oxygen if anemia is severe
  —Transfusions
      RBCs, packed red cells
      Platelets
      Granulocytes
- Drugs
  —Steroids (see Steroid Therapy, p. 608)
  —Colony-stimulating factors
  —Antibiotics
  —Androgens

*Surgical*

- Bone marrow transplantation

## HOME CARE

- Give both the patient and the caregiver *verbal* and *written* instructions. Provide them with the name and telephone number of a physician or nurse to call if questions arise.
- *General information*
  —Explain aplastic anemia, its causes, and contributing factors to the patient.
- *Warning signs*
  —Review the signs and symptoms that should be reported to a physician or nurse.
      Infections: systemic: fever, malaise, fatigue; urinary tract: cloudy, malodorous urine; burning; frequency; urgency; upper respiratory: malodorous, purulent, colored, copious secretions; productive cough
      Bleeding/hemorrhage: melena, hematuria, epistaxis, ecchymosis, bleeding of gums
      Anemia: fatigue, weakness, paresthesias
- *Special instructions*
  —Teach the patient how to self-monitor laboratory values. Identify the patient's baseline levels to monitor further decreases or changes.
  —Stress the importance of avoiding exposure to individuals known to have acute infections.
  —Teach the patient to avoid trauma, abrasions, and breakdown of the skin, which could lead to infection.

—Discuss methods of preventing hemorrhage, such as using an electric razor and soft-bristled toothbrush and avoiding activities that might traumatize the tissues.

- *Medications*
  —Explain the purpose, dosage, schedule, and route of administration of any prescribed drugs, as well as side effects to report to the physician or nurse.
  —See Steroid Therapy (p. 608).
  —Explain that antibiotics must be taken for the entire period prescribed to prevent superinfection.
  —Advise the patient to avoid the use of aspirin, aspirin products, and ibuprofen products in the presence of a bleeding disorder.

- *Activity*
  —Encourage the patient to discuss limitations with respect to occupation, recreational sports, and activities.
  —Advise the patient to limit activities when fatigued and during episodes of infection.

- *Diet*
  —Discuss the need to maintain a well-balanced diet to enhance resistance to infection.
  —Discuss the need to increase dietary fiber (e.g., fresh fruit and vegetables) to prevent constipation and straining at stool.

**FOLLOW-UP CARE**

- Stress the importance of regular follow-up visits. Make sure the patient has the necessary names and telephone numbers.

# Appendicitis/Appendectomy

—**Appendicitis: obstruction of the appendix, a small, finger-like pouch attached to the cecum of the colon, causing inflammation, distention, decreased blood supply, necrosis, and sometimes perforation. If untreated, appendicitis causes generalized peritonitis or localized abscess.**

—**Appendectomy: surgical removal of the appendix.**

## RISK FACTORS

* Incidence highest in adolescent and young adult males
* Familial tendencies

## SIGNS/SYMPTOMS

* Early stage
  —Vague abdominal pain in periumbilical area
  —Nausea and vomiting
  —Fever
  —Sensitivity over appendix area (right lower abdomen)
* Intermediate or acute stage
  —Pain over right lower abdomen aggravated by walking or coughing
  —Feeling of constipation, urge to defecate
  —Loss of appetite
  —Malaise
  —Sometimes diarrhea
  —Decreased bowel sounds
  —Rapid pulse
  —Fever
  —Rigidity of abdomen when palpated

## COMPLICATIONS

* Perforated appendix
  —Sudden relief of pain with perforation, then development of peritonitis
* Peritonitis
  —Increased, generalized pain over abdomen
  —Recurrence of vomiting
  —Side-lying position with knees flexed
  —Rapid pulse, shallow respirations, low blood pressure
  —Chills, fever
  —Pallor or flushing
  —Irritability, restlessness, anxiety
  —Progressive abdominal distention and rigidity
  —Failure to pass flatus or stool
  —Decreased or absent bowel sounds
  —Loss of appetite
* Dehydration
* Sepsis
* Abdominal abscess
* Electrolyte imbalance

## DIAGNOSTIC TESTS

- Describe each procedure, its purpose, and the normal feelings or sensations that are likely, as well as any preprocedural and postprocedural care.
  - —Blood studies: increase in WBCs seen on differential
  - —X-ray of abdomen
  - —Intravenous pyelography: to eliminate kidney stones or pyelitis from the diagnosis (see Urolithiasis, p. 666)

## TREATMENT

*Medical (until taken to surgery)*

- Therapy
  - —Hydration, intravenous
  - —Comfort measures
  - —Nasogastric tube if excessive distention and vomiting
  - —Bed rest
- Drugs
  - —Antibiotics

*Surgical*

- Surgery within 24-48 hours of onset of symptoms or when patient is stabilized
- See Abdominal Surgery (p. 3) for preoperative and postoperative care.
- Appendectomy procedures
  - —Laparoscopic approach (used if appendix has not ruptured)
    
    Incision made below umbilius with three or four abdominal punctures to permit insertion of laparoscope for viewing and removal of appendix
    
    Procedure requires general anesthesia and overnight stay
  - —Abdominal surgical approach
    
    Right lower quadrant abdominal incision, performed under general anesthesia and requiring 2-day hospital stay
    
    If appendix is ruptured, drain remains in place and patient stays in hospital 5 days or more

## HOME CARE

- Give both the patient and the caregiver *verbal* and *written* instructions. Provide them with the name and telephone number of a physician or nurse to call if questions arise.
- *Warning signs*
  - —Review the postoperative signs and symptoms that should be reported to a physician or nurse.

      Redness

      Swelling

      Tenderness

      Skin warm to touch

      Drainage

- *Special instructions*
  - —Review any restrictions: avoid enemas until approved by physician, avoid tub baths, showers permitted.
  - —Advise patient on how and where to obtain supplies.
  - —Teach patient how to take care of wound and dressing changes. If appendix is ruptured, irrigation with sterile saline and sterile dressings may be required.
- *Medications*
  - —Explain the purpose, dosage, schedule, and route of administration of any prescribed drugs, as well as side effects to report to the physician or nurse.
- *Activity*
  - —Instruct the patient to avoid lifting anything over 10 pounds for the first 6 weeks (less time for laparoscopy), to rest when fatigued, and to increase activities as tolerated.
  - —Normal activities can usually be resumed within 4 weeks. Ask the patient to check with the physician or nurse before driving, returning to work, or engaging in recreational sports.

**FOLLOW-UP CARE**

- Stress the importance of regular follow-up visits. Make sure the patient has the necessary names and telephone numbers.

---

# Arterial Insufficiency

---

**—Arterial insufficiency: impaired arterial blood flow. Arterial insufficiency can occur in any part of the arterial system but generally affects the lower extremities (legs and feet). There are two forms: acute and chronic.** *Acute arterial insufficiency* **is a sudden decrease in arterial blood supply to an area, resulting in thrombus (clot), embolism, and trauma.** *Chronic arterial insufficiency* **is most commonly caused by arterio-**

sclerosis **(calcification of the arteries resulting from progressive narrowing, thickening, and loss of vessel elasticity) or atherosclerosis (gradual accumulation of plaque resulting from hardening of the arteries that occurs with age).**

## CONTRIBUTING FACTORS

- Atherosclerotic plaque
- Thrombus (blood clots)
- Aneurysms
- Trauma or fracture
- Embolism

## RISK FACTORS

- Familial tendency
- Diabetes
- Elevated cholesterol levels
- Diet high in animal fats
- Hypertension
- Sedentary life-style
- Tobacco use
- Age over 50 years
- Males

## SIGNS/SYMPTOMS

- Acute
  - —Sudden, severe pain
  - —Numbness, paralysis
  - —Pale yellow skin color
  - —Absence of pulse
- Chronic
  - —Intermittent claudication: severe cramps or burning sensation in calf (leg) muscle, buttock, or thigh that occurs with exercise and is relieved by rest; symptoms are constant and reproducible
  - —Sores and cuts that are slow to heal
  - —Discoloration and decreased sensation of the affected extremities
  - —Thickened nails
  - —Shiny skin
  - —Decreased temperature
  - —Absence of pulse

## COMPLICATIONS

- Leg ulcers
- Gangrene
- Thrombosis
- Limb amputation

## DIAGNOSTIC TESTS

- Describe each procedure, its purpose, and the normal feelings or sensations that are likely, as well as any preprocedural and postprocedural care.
  —Doppler ultrasound: identifies abnormal blood flow patterns proximal to occlusion
  —Plethysmography: records decrease in blood flow distal to occlusion
  —Echocardiography: determines whether an embolus from the heart is the source of obstruction
  —Arteriography: determines the location, type, and degree of obstruction; can be used to evaluate degree of collateral circulation
  —Duplex imaging: using ultrasound to assess arteries for plaque formation; measures flow and pressure
  —Digital subtraction angiography: visualizes arteries radiologically to determine presence and extent of occlusion
  —Exercise testing: to determine the level of exercise that precipitates the symptoms of lack of blood flow
  —Oscillometry: using a blood pressure cuff connected to a manometer to find occlusive sites, as evidenced by decreased pressure readings

## TREATMENT
### Chronic Obstruction

*Medical*

- Therapy
  —Risk reduction program: control of blood pressure, elimination of smoking, weight reduction, lowering of cholesterol and lipids
  —Program of daily walking
- Drugs
  —Antiplatelet therapy (dipyridamole and aspirin): to prevent arterial occlusion
  —Pentoxifylline (Trental): to improve blood flow through cap-

illaries; used to increase the distance patients with claudication can walk
—Aspirin: to relieve pain and prevent thromboembolism
—Calcium channel blockers: to reduce vasospasm
—Thrombolytic agents (urokinase, streptokinase, alteplase): to dissolve clots and relieve obstruction caused by thrombus

*Surgical*

- Amputation: surgical removal of limb if gangrene, uncontrollable infection, or intractable pain develops
- Atherectomy: shaving and removal of plaque from an artery by special catheters

**Acute Obstruction**

*Medical*

- Therapy
  —Percutaneous transluminal angioplasty: compression of the obstruction using balloon inflation catheter
  —Laser angioplasty: use of a hot-tip laser to vaporize (dissolve) the obstruction
  —Stents: insertion of a mesh wire that will stretch and mold to the arterial wall to prevent occlusion

*Surgical*

- Embolectomy: to remove clot from affected artery
- Thromboembolectomy: surgical opening of the artery to remove the athetotic plaque or thrombus
- Patch grafting: removal of the affected arterial segment with an autologous vein (i.e., saphenous vein) or with a Dacron graft
- Bypass graft: use of an autologous vein (i.e., saphenous vein) or a Dacron graft to bypass the affected arterial segment
- Lumbar sympathectomy

**HOME CARE**

- Give both patient and caregiver *verbal* and *written* instructions. Provide them with the name and telephone number of a physician or nurse to call if questions arise.
- *General information*
  —Discuss the arteriosclerotic and atherosclerotic process and its roles in producing arterial occlusive disease. Review causes and contributing factors. Show the patient the location of the suspected obstruction and describe collateral circulation. Explain intermittent claudication and how it develops.

- Teach the patient how to inspect the affected limb for color, warmth, and presence of pulses.
- *Warning signs*
  —Review the signs and symptoms that should be reported to a physician or nurse.
- *Special instructions*
  —Discuss skin care.
  —Inspect skin daily for redness, blistering, or cuts that are not healing.
  —Use mild, unperfumed lotions for dry skin.
  —Do not use heating pads or hot water bottles, which could burn the patient.
  —Avoid restrictive clothing that could interfere with circulation to the affected areas.
  —Keep skin warm and dry. Do not expose skin to cold. Avoid temperature extremes.
  —Avoid applying adhesive tape directly to the skin.
  —Demonstrate proper care of skin ulcerations; advise on how and where to obtain necessary supplies.
  —Discuss foot care.
      Inspect feet and toes daily for cuts, bruises, calluses, and corns.
      Wash with mild soap and warm water, rinse well, and pat dry. Check water temperature to avoid burns. Dry feet well, especially between toes.
      Apply mild, nonperfumed lotion for dry skin. Permit foot to dry completely before putting shoes and socks on.
      Cut toenails straight using clippers. If nails become thick or brittle, refer to podiatrist; instruct patient not to cut corns or calluses, but to rub gently or see podiatrist.
      Never go barefoot; wear comfortable, proper-fitting shoes.
  —Offer techniques for dealing with chronic pain, such as visualization, guided imagery, meditation, and biofeedback.
- *Medications*
  —Explain the purpose, dosage, schedule, and route of administration of any prescribed drugs, as well as side effects to report to the physician or nurse.
- *Activity*
  —Discuss planned exercise program.
      Explain importance of daily exercises to prevent further occlusion and to promote development of collateral circulation.

Review types of exercises permitted: walking, swimming, bicycling.

Explain that progressive exercise can reduce severity of claudication and increase distance that patient may walk. For example, the patient may begin by walking until claudication occurs, then stop and rest, then begin again when pain stops. Distance can be increased gradually.

Emphasize that for any type of exercise or activity, the patient should stop when pain occurs, rest, and resume activity when pain subsides.

—Instruct patient to avoid vigorous exercise of affected limb, since this can increase oxygen demand and increase pain.

—Instruct patient on techniques that can increase circulation to the lower extremities, such as sleeping in an upright position and dangling lower extremities over the side of the bed to relieve persistent leg pain.

—Instruct patient to avoid sitting or standing for prolonged periods, to keep legs elevated while sitting, and to avoid crossing the knees.

• *Diet*
—Stress the importance of developing a life-style that will decrease the risk of advancing the disease process: weight control, diet low in fats and cholesterol.

**FOLLOW-UP CARE**
• Stress the importance of regular follow-up visits. Make sure the patient has the necessary names and telephone numbers.
• Stress the importance of not smoking. Provide information on and referral to smoking cessation programs as necessary; provide literature and discuss nicotine's effect on circulation.

# Arterial Revascularization

**—Arterial revascularization: surgical procedure that increases arterial blood flow by bypassing a stenosed or occluded**

artery. **Grafting material for bypass surgeries may be constructed from an autologous vein (i.e., saphenous vein) or a
synthetic graft (Dacron).**

## TYPES OF BYPASS PROCEDURE

- Aortofemoral bypass graft: graft runs from the abdominal aorta
  to the external iliac or femoral arteries, increasing arterial blood
  flow to the lower extremities
- Aortoiliac bypass graft: graft runs from the abdominal aorta
  down to the iliac or femoral artery(ies)
- Axillofemoral bypass: graft runs from the axillary artery down
  alongside the artery in a tunnel created under the skin to the
  femoral artery(ies)
- Femoropopliteal bypass
- Femorotibial bypass

## INDICATIONS

- Arterial insufficiency
  —Acute
    Embolism
    Thrombosis
    Trauma
  —Chronic
    Arteriosclerosis obliterans
    Arterial insufficiency
    Buerger's disease

## PREPROCEDURAL TEACHING

- Review the physician's explanation of the procedure and the reason for it; encourage the patient to ask questions and to discuss
  fears or anxieties.

### Review of Preprocedural Care

- Discuss the number of incisions that will be performed (e.g.,
  for aortofemoral bypass there may be two or three incisions:
  one midline abdominal and one groin site for each femoral graft
  done) and the type of anesthesia to be used.
- Instruct the patient to discontinue any anticoagulant or antiplatelet medications 1 week before surgery; ask the patient to check
  with the physician or nurse about any other medications, including cardiac, birth control, and hormone drugs.

**Review of Postprocedural Care**

- Axillofemoral bypass
  —Instruct the patient not to lie on the same side as the graft, since this could cause graft occlusion, and to avoid reaching high overhead or lifting anything heavy, which could dislodge the graft from the donor site.
  —Discuss and demonstrate passive range-of-motion exercises to the affected limb.
- Femoral-popliteal-tibial grafts
  —Explain that the patient may have an indwelling catheter and that surgery will be done under general anesthesia.
  —Inform the patient that walking will be permitted 1-3 days after surgery, that ambulation will progress gradually, and that a cane or walker may be required for a few days.
  —Discuss the importance of not bending the knee and hip of the affected limb and of not sitting or standing for prolonged periods, which could lead to graft occlusion.
  —Inform the patient that a heat cradle may be used to avoid pressure on the affected limb.
- Review postoperative medications.
  —Anticoagulants or aspirin: to keep graft open
  —Antibiotics: to prevent infection
  —Vasodilator: to promote circulation to the lower extremities

**COMPLICATIONS**

- Hematoma
- Graft thrombosis
- Infection of the entire graft
- Embolization to kidneys and bowel
  —Renal failure
  —Bowel ischemia

**HOME CARE**

- Give both the patient and the caregiver verbal and written instructions. Provide them with the name and telephone number of a physician or nurse to call if questions arise.
- *Warning signs*
  —Review the signs and symptoms that should be reported to a physician or nurse.
    Infection: fever; incision sites that drain, are warm or hot to touch, or become red or more painful

Thrombosis: pain in the surgical area or legs when the patient is at rest; abdominal bloating or tenderness

Intermittent claudication: muscle cramping or burning that occurs with exercise and is relieved by rest

- *Special instructions*
  - —Teach the patient to use antiembolic stockings, if prescribed.
  - —For axillofemoral bypass graft: instruct the patient to avoid forceful use of the affected side, not to wear tight or restrictive garments (belt, suspenders) over graft site, to check graft pulse and notify physician or nurse if pulse is not felt.
- *Medications*
  - —Explain the purpose, dosage, schedule, and route of administration of any prescribed drugs, as well as side effects to report to the physician or nurse.
- *Activity*
  - —During the 6- to 8-week healing period:
    Patient should avoid sitting for prolonged periods, keep legs elevated while sitting, avoid crossing knees, and avoid vacuuming, lawn mowing, or lifting >25 pounds.
    Patient should walk every day, in a progressive program that begins slowly and increases in distance as directed.
    Rest periods should be scheduled during the day.
  - —Long-term: To preserve the benefits of the surgery, the patient should follow habits that improve circulation and prevent further acceleration of atherosclerosis: careful diabetic control, control of blood pressure, regular exercise to promote circulation, avoidance of prolonged squatting.
  - —Discuss effects of stress on circulation. Review stress reduction (e.g., by relaxation, exercise).
- *Diet*
  - —The patient should eat a balanced low-fat diet that includes protein to help tissues heal and fruits and vegetables to prevent constipation.
  - —Alcohol use should be limited or avoided completely if the patient is taking medications that enhance its effects.

## FOLLOW-UP CARE

- Stress the importance of regular follow-up visits. Make sure the patient has the necessary names and telephone numbers.
- Emphasize the importance of not smoking. Refer the patient to smoking cessation programs, if necessary. Provide literature on smoking and discuss the effect nicotine has on circulation.

# Arthritis

—**Rheumatoid arthritis (RA):** a chronic, systemic, autoimmune disease of unknown origin affecting primarily the synovial joints. RA is characterized by remissions and exacerbations of inflammation of the connective tissues throughout the body, leading eventually to destruction of joint cartilage and subsequent deformities. The most commonly affected joints are the hands, wrists, shoulders, elbows, feet, ankles, hips, and knees. Susceptibility is genetically determined. RA is a common condition with a prevalence of 1% to 2% in the general population. Females outnumber males 3:1. RA usually develops between 25 and 55 years of age, although juvenile RA or Sill's disease develops between 8 and 15 years of age.

—**Osteoarthritis (degenerative joint disease):** a chronic, progressive disease characterized by increasing pain, deformity, and loss of function caused by degenerative changes in the cartilage covering the ends of bones, primarily in the major weight-bearing joints: hip, knee, and spinal column. The joints of the fingers, elbows, wrists, and ankles are affected to a lesser degree. Osteoarthritis is a disease of older persons, affecting nearly everyone over 75 years of age. Women are affected more often than men, and the incidence increases after menopause. More than 50 million Americans have osteoarthritis.

## CONTRIBUTING FACTORS

- For osteoarthritis (secondary osteoarthritis)
  —Obesity
  —Overuse of joints
  —Trauma

## SIGNS/SYMPTOMS

- General
  —Joint involvement
      Stiffness, especially early morning)
      Pain (worsens with activity and is relieved by rest)
      Swelling and deformity

Instability and impaired function
Decreased range of motion
Bony enlargements in affected joints
• Rheumatoid arthritis
—Local warmth, redness
—Anemia
—Malaise, weight loss, fever
—Red, blue, or white color of fingers and toes
—Multiple joint involvement
—Subcutaneous rheumatoid nodules over bony prominences (hands, elbows, knees)
—Shiny, taut skin over impaired joint
—Numbness, tingling in hands and feet

## COMPLICATIONS

• General
—Avascular necrosis of hip joint
—Contractures
—Loss of range of motion of joints (ankylosing of joints)
—Muscle wasting
—Loss of sensation and decreased mobility
• Rheumatoid arthritis
—Cardiac degenerative conditions: cardiomyopathy, congestive heart failure, pericarditis
—Chronic renal failure
—Chronic obstructive pulmonary disease
—Septic arthritis
—Tenosynovitis

## DIAGNOSTIC TESTS

• Describe each procedure, its purpose, and the normal feelings or sensations that are likely, as well as any preprocedural and postprocedural care.
—Laboratory tests
Complete blood cell count
White blood cell count
Erythrocyte sedimentation rate
Synovial fluid analysis and tissue biopsy
For RA:
○ Antistreptolysin O (ASO) titer
○ Rheumatoid factor: positive in RA
○ C-reactive protein: present in acute episode of RA

○ Serum complement: decreased in acute episodes of RA
—Radiologic studies: to confirm diagnosis by showing narrowing of joint spaces
—Magnetic resonance imaging/computed tomography: to show changes before x-ray studies detect them
—Gait analysis: to show leg length discrepancy
—Muscle testing: to detect weakness of muscles supporting joints
—Bone scan

**TREATMENT**

*Medical*

• Therapy
—Physical therapy
Paraffin glow: to provide heat to affected small joints (hands and feet)
Whirlpool
Thermotherapy: moist heat, application of cold or heat to relieve pain and improve joint flexibility
Joint exercise: passive and active range-of-motion exercises to strenthen the muscles and tissues supporting the joint and to maintain as much joint mobility as possible
—Orthotics: splints, braces, etc. to maintain proper joint position and support and to rest the joint
—Use of ambulatory adjuncts: crutches, cane, walker, wheelchair, etc. to protect joints from stress
—Assistive devices
Stocking helpers
Builtup eating utensils
Pick-up sticks
Raised toilet seats
• Drugs
—General
Salicylate medications, usually aspirin
Nonsteroidal antiinflammatory agents
Tranquilizers, antidepressants
Analgesics
Muscle relaxants
Intraarticular steroid injections
—Rheumatoid arthritis
Antirheumatic agents
Corticosteroids

Immunosuppressive agents
Antimalarials

*Surgical*
- Synovectomy: removal of the inflamed synovium
- Athroplasty: repair of weakened joint
- Osteotomy: to correct bony malalignments
- Implant arthroplasty: repair of joint with prosthesis to increase functional capability
- Arthroscopy: for diagnosis and treatment (removal of foreign bodies, redundant tissue, and cartilage abraded through arthroscope)
- Arthodesis: joint fusion to produce stability and reduce pain in severely affected joints
- Total joint replacement: see Hip Replacement (p. 373), Replacement of Knee or Shoulder (p. 573)

## HOME CARE

- Give both the patient and the caregiver *verbal* and *written* instructions. Provide them with the name and telephone number of a physician or nurse to call if questions arise.
- *General information*
  —Explain and discuss type of arthritis, contributing factors, and signs and symptoms associated with the disease process. Discuss the progressive nature of the disease, explaining that effects of arthritis can change daily and that the patient will have good and bad days. Discuss the importance of maintaining the prescribed medication and activity program to slow disease progression.
- *Warning signs*
  —Review the signs and symptoms that should be reported to a physician or nurse.
      Exacerbation ("flare-up") of symptoms
      Increased pain
      Fatigue
- *Special instructions*
  —Discuss the importance of maintaining a safe home environment.
      Handrails in shower, tub, or toilet
      Raised toilet seat
      Rubber-tipped walker, cane, crutches
      Raised chair
      Wheelchair in locked position when stationary

—Discuss the role that emotions such as stress and depression play in disease progression. Encourage participation in support groups as needed; provide phone numbers for referral.

—Discuss pain management: applying heat or cold to a painful joint for temporary relief; avoiding temperature extremes, since decreased sensitivity to temperature can result in injury; maintaining proper body alignment to reduce pain.

Extend joints as tolerated.

Avoid external rotation of extremities.

Avoid use of pillow under knee.

Avoid flexion of neck.

Avoid sitting for extended periods.

- *Medications*
  —Explain the purpose, dosage, schedule, and route of administration of any prescribed drugs, as well as side effects to report to the physician or nurse.

  Aspirin, NSAIDS: nausea, vomiting, gastrointestinal burning, blood in stool or sputum, headache, bleeding gums, ringing in ears

- *Activity*
  —Discuss the importance of alternating activities with rest periods and of getting 8-10 hours of sleep at night.

  —Emphasize that the patient should maintain a regular exercise program that includes such activities as walking and swimming to provide stretching and joint mobility. Daily exercise can relieve soreness caused by stiff, unused muscles and helps maintain joint range of motion.

  —Reinforce the need for range-of-motion exercises to prevent stiffening of joints.

  —Discuss the importance of using splints and braces to support affected joints.

  —Explain the use of ambulatory aids such as crutches or a cane to lessen joint stress. Assist the patient in obtaining such equipment.

  —Discuss the importance of physical therapy exercises to maintain strength and function.

  —Encourage the patient to discuss allowances and limitations with respect to occupation, recreational sports, and activities.

  —Remind the patient to dress warmly and wear gloves in cold, damp weather.

A

- *Diet*
  —Encourage the intake of iron-rich foods (dried fruits, green vegetables) to combat anemia.
  —Stress the importance of a well-balanced diet.
  —Instruct the patient to reduce caloric and fat intake for weight reduction because increased weight or obesity increases joint stress.

## FOLLOW-UP CARE

- Stress the importance of regular follow-up visits, including laboratory examinations and physical therapy. Make sure the patient has the necessary names and telephone numbers.

## REFERRALS

- Advise the patient on community resources and support programs.

# Arthroscopy

—Arthroscopy: the examination of joint tissues with a fiber-optic endoscope (arthroscope), which allows direct visualization of the interior of a joint. Arthroscopy can be performed on any joint (wrist, elbow, shoulder, ankle, hip), but it is most frequently done for the diagnosis and treatment of knee injuries.

—Diagnostic arthropathy: reveals the condition of internal joint tissues, the existence of loose bodies, the presence of tears in cartilage or ligaments, or the condition of synovial tissues.

—Therapeutic, surgical arthropathy: removal (excision), repair, or reconstruction of loose bodies and torn cartilage; biopsy of tissues through an arthroscope.

## INDICATIONS

- Meniscus injuries: removal or repair of meniscus
- Ligament tears: reconstruction

- Damage to cartilage: removal or shaving of rough cartilage
- Patella injury: realignment or shaving

## PREPROCEDURAL TEACHING

- Review the physician's explanation of the procedure and the reason for it; encourage the patient to ask questions and to discuss any fears or anxieties.
- Explain that the procedure may take anywhere from ½ hour to several hours.
- Discuss the need for written consent for surgery and anesthesia.
- Explain that hospital admission may be on the day of surgery but that an overnight hospital stay may be necessary.

### Review of Preprocedural Care

- The patient is NPO from midnight of the night before surgery.
- Skin preparation includes a shower with bactericidal soap and shaving of the incision site.
- Routine preoperative blood and urine tests will be conducted.
- Describe the procedure.
  —Depending on the joint, the procedure will be done under local anesthesia, regional block, or general anesthesia.
  —Tell the patient that the scope may be inserted in more than one area to visualize all areas of the joint and that two or three incisions (portals) may be needed.

### Review of Postprocedural Care

- If surgery is done on an outpatient basis, the patient is discharged in the evening.
- The joint will be elevated with a compression dressing and ice bags to lessen swelling and pain.
- Vital signs and neurovascular status are checked every 15 minutes for the first hour, then with decreasing frequency.
- Bed rest is needed until the patient is fully alert; then the patient can be up as tolerated.
- Moving the extremities is important to improve circulation and keep the joint mobile (e.g., move the feet after knee arthroscopy).
- After knee arthroscopy the patient will need external knee support by an elastic wrap or a knee immobilizer. Crutches may be ordered.

## SIDE EFFECTS/COMPLICATIONS

- Infection
- Bleeding/hemorrhage
- Phlebitis/thrombus formation
- Posttraumatic degeneration and arthritis
- Instrument breakage in joint
- Effects of anesthesia

## HOME CARE

- Give both the patient and the caregiver verbal and written instructions. Provide them with the name and telephone number of a physician or nurse to call if questions arise.
- *Wound/incision care*
  —Keep the dressing clean and dry.
  —Serosanguineous drainage should be scant; report any increase in drainage or signs of new bleeding to the physician or nurse.
  —Do not remove dressing until directed by the physician.
  —Avoid bathing until able to stand for 10 to 15 minutes; then showering with the extremity covered by a plastic bag may be permitted. Check with the physician or nurse before resuming showers.
- *Warning signs*
  —Review the signs and symptoms that should be reported to a physician or nurse.
     Excess bleeding
     Infection: persistent or worsening pain, swelling, discoloration of skin at incision site, fever, joint immobility, purulent discharge
     Neurovascular impairment of joint and extremity: fingers and toes cold and discolored; increasing pain with joint movement; numbness or tingling of extremity (stress the importance of reporting these symptoms immediately)
     Phlebitis: swollen, painful, reddened, warm extremity
- *Special instructions*
  —Discuss the importance of keeping the extremity elevated above heart level on firm pillows and the need for applying ice bags to the surgical site to control swelling and relieve pain. Caution the patient not to apply the ice pack directly to the skin, but to wrap the ice bag in a small towel. The use of hot tubs, whirlpool baths, and heating pads should be avoided.

—Discuss the importance of moving the extremities (fingers, toes, feet) to improve circulation and prevent blood clots. For example, after knee arthroscopy the patient should wiggle the toes every few minutes for the first week.

• *Medications*
—Explain the purpose, dosage, schedule, and route of administration of any prescribed drugs, as well as side effects to report to a physician or nurse.

• *Activity*
—The patient may ambulate as tolerated with an assistive device. Refer to physical therapy as indicated.
—Following knee arthroscopy, instruct the patient in the proper use of crutches. Review physical therapy exercises needed for a gradual increase in strength and mobility.
—Encourage the patient to discuss allowances and limitations with respect to occupation and resumption of recreational sports and activities.

• *Diet*
—Encourage a light diet and fluids, progressing to a regular diet as ordered.

**FOLLOW-UP CARE**
• Stress the importance of regular follow-up visits. Make sure the patient has the necessary names and telephone numbers.

# Asthma

—**Asthma: a chronic respiratory disorder characterized by episodes of sudden, acute attacks of dyspnea, wheezing caused by airway narrowing (bronchospasm), and mucosal swelling that leads to mucus production. An attack may last minutes to hours and may resolve spontaneously or in response to medication and treatment. Although the exact cause is unknown, obstruction of the airways may occur as a result of spasms of the bronchial muscles caused by an irritant or by inflammation of the airways, which causes swelling of the mucous membranes.**

## CONTRIBUTING FACTORS

Bronchial irritants that can trigger asthmatic attacks include:

- Environmental allergens
    —Foods: shellfish, eggs, nuts, chocolate
    —Pollens: trees, flowers and ragweed, spores
    —Feathers: pillows, down comforters, wool
    —Animal dander: dogs, cats, rabbits, chickens
    —Dust: from carpets, brooms, dusters, dirty filters on furnaces and air conditioners
    —Household cleaners: polishes, cleaning solvents, paint thinners
    —Weather and temperature: air pollution, extreme heat or cold, seasonal changes, excessive humidity or dryness
    —Industrial pollutants: wood vapors, dust, or fumes; metals; cotton
    —Other: powders, perfumes, tobacco smoking (cgarettes, cigars, pipes)
- Intrinsic factors
    —Respiratory infections: cold, flu, viruses
    —Fatigue, overexertion
    —Emotions: anxiety, stress

## SIGNS/SYMPTOMS

- Wheezing
- Prolonged expiration
- Dyspnea; feeling of not being able to catch one's breath
- Physical exhaustion
- Anxiety
- Thick, tenacious mucus

## COMPLICATIONS

- Status asthmaticus
- Pneumonia
- Respiratory arrest

## DIAGNOSTIC TESTS

- Describe each procedure, its purpose, and the normal feelings or sensations that are likely, as well as any preprocedural and postprocedural care.
    —Serum studies: white blood cell count to identify infections, arterial blood gases to determine oxygen content of blood and evaluate acid-base status (elimination of carbon dioxide); the-

ophylline blood levels drawn until therapeutic levels (10-29 g/ml) are achieved
—Sputum studies: to evaluate increase in viscosity or presence of mucus plugs; culture and sensitivity to detect infection
—Pulmonary function: to evaluate degree of obstruction and narrowing of the airways
—Chest x-ray

## TREATMENT

*Medical*
- Therapy
  —Oxygen therapy
  —Nebulizer
  —Nutritious, well-balanced diet
  —Oral or parenteral fluids to maintain adequate dehydration
- Drugs
  —Bronchodilator: to relieve bronchospasm
  —Steroids: to relieve inflammatory response
  —Aminophylline: to relax smooth muscle
  —Antibiotics: for infection

## HOME CARE

- Review the disease process. Give both the patient and the care-giver *verbal* and *written* instructions. Provide them with the name and telephone number of a physician or nurse to call if questions arise. Use visual aids to assist in instruction.
- *General information*
  —Help the patient identify irritants that trigger an asthmatic attack and discuss the importance of avoiding them or removing them from the patient's environment. Advise keeping a diary of activities, foods, or irritants present before attacks.
- *Warning signs*
  —Review the signs and symptoms that should be reported to a physician or nurse.
- *Special instructions*
  —Review the purpose and demonstrate proper use of an oral inhaler, home nebulizer, humidifier, or incentive spirometer as ordered.
  —Discuss the importance of avoiding smoking or being in a smoke-filled room. Refer the patient to smoking cessation programs as needed.

—Discuss the importance of emotions and their role in triggering attacks. Review the need to learn to modify or deal with stressful events using deep muscle relaxation techniques or pursed-lip breathing techniques to prevent an attack.

—Discuss the importance of preventing respiratory infections; avoid persons with infections and check with the physician about annual flu and pneumococcal vaccinations.

• *Medications*

—Explain the purpose, dosage, schedule, and route of administration of any prescribed drugs, as well as side effects to report to the physician or nurse.

—Warn against stopping or decreasing medication dose when feeling better without checking with physician.

—Discuss the importance of not using over-the-counter allergy drugs when taking prescribed drugs.

• *Activity*

—Emphasize the importance of regular exercise to tolerance and of avoiding or curtailing activities when fatigued, during extremes of weather, and on smoggy days.

• *Diet*

—Instruct the patient to maintain a well-balanced diet, eat small frequent meals during and after attacks, and drink plenty of fluids (2 3 liters per day) to keep mucus thin.

## FOLLOW-UP CARE

• Stress the importance of regular follow up visits. Make sure the patient has the necessary names and telephone numbers.

• Encourage or assist patient to obtain a Medic-Alert bracelet listing diagnosis and medications.

## REFERRALS

• Refer the patient to the American Lung Association for a support group and further information.

# Atelectasis

—**Atelectasis: collapse of alveoli or airless condition of lung.**

## CAUSES/CONTRIBUTING FACTORS

- Mucus plugs
- Excessive secretions
- Compression of lung tissue by tumors, effusions, pneumothorax, or shallow breathing

## SIGNS/SYMPTOMS

- Elevated temperature
- Labored breathing
- Shortness of breath
- Nasal flaring
- Tachypnea
- Anxiety
- Restlessness
- Tachycardia
- Absent or decreased breath sounds over affected area

## COMPLICATIONS

- Pneumonia
- Pneumothorax

## DIAGNOSTIC TESTS

- Describe each procedure, its purpose, and the normal feelings or sensations that are likely, as well as any preprocedural and postprocedural care.
  —Chest x-ray: to define collapsed areas of the lung
  —Arterial blood gases: to detect hypoxia
  —Bronchoscopy: insertion of a fiberoptic scope into the airways for direct visualization and possible obtaining of specimens

## TREATMENT

*Medical*
- Therapy
  —Oxygen therapy
  —Chest physiotherapy
  —Intermittent positive-pressure breathing (IPPB)/incentive spirometry
  —Bronchoscopy

## HOME CARE

- Give both the patient and the caregiver *verbal* and *written* instructions. Provide them with the name and telephone number of a physician or nurse to call if questions arise.

- *General information*
  —Explain the underlying cause or contributing factors.
- *Warning signs*
  —Review the signs and symptoms that should be reported to a physician or nurse.
  > Upper respiratory infection
  > Flu
  > Difficulty breathing
  > Persistent cough
  > Elevated temperature
- *Special instructions*
  —Discuss the importance of preventing respiratory infections by avoiding persons with infections.
  —Demonstrate the use of an incentive spirometer and discuss how frequently to use it.
  —Instruct the patient in coughing and deep breathing techniques. Demonstrate how to splint the chest when coughing.
- *Medications*
  —Explain the purpose, dosage, schedule, and route of administration of any prescribed drugs, as well as side effects to report to the physician or nurse.
  > Explain the need to avoid taking over-the-counter medications without checking with a physician.
  > Caution the patient to avoid the use of respiratory depressants.
- *Activity*
  —Emphasize the importance of exercising to tolerance. Stress the need to avoid fatigue and to plan rest periods.
- *Diet*
  —Regular diet. Encourage the intake of fluids unless contraindicated by underlying condition.

## FOLLOW-UP CARE

- Stress the importance of regular follow-up visits. Make sure the patient has the necessary names and telephone numbers.
- Stress the importance of not smoking or using tobacco products. Tobacco smoking increases the risk of respiratory infection because of cumulative damage to lung structures. Provide information about smoking cessation programs and offer a referral.

# Back Pain

—Back pain: one of the most common health problems in the United States, affecting people of all ages and from all walks of life, from heavy laborers to those who lead sedentary lives. Persons with back pain may be in good health or have significant disease. The majority of back injuries occur in the lumbar (L) and lumbosacral spine, a portion of the spinal column that provides the flexibility necessary for movement and thus is especially vulnerable to strain and injury. The most commonly affected areas are the cervical spine (neck), C5-6 and C6-7, in which osteophyte formation causes nerve compression. Low back pain (LBP) is caused by a herniated nucleus pulposus, also known as a slipped disk or a herniated disk.

## CAUSES/CONTRIBUTING FACTORS

- Ligament strain and fatigue
- Muscle strain or spasm
- Disk injury/trauma
- Disease: arthritis, ruptured disk, osteoporosis, congenital deformities
- Intervertebral degeneration (in elderly)
- Poor posture: slouching, swayback
- Lack of exercise: weak abdominal and back muscles
- Obesity, especially abdominal obesity
- Infection
- Spinal tumors

## SIGNS/SYMPTOMS

- Muscle spasm
- Pain radiating down arm or leg
- Tenderness of back and involved extremity
- Lumbago: painful catches in lower back
- Sciatica: sharp pain in back of leg and buttocks
- Soreness, stiffness, achiness
- Neck stiffness, headache, dizziness, shoulder and arm pain (with cervical involvement)
- Paresthesia, numbness

**COMPLICATIONS**

- Paresis
- Motor weakness
- Sensory changes
- Footdrop
- Loss of bowel or bladder control

**DIAGNOSTIC TESTS**

- Describe each procedure, its purpose, and the normal feelings or sensations that are likely, as well as any preprocedural and postprocedural care.
  - —Back x-rays: may show narrowing of intervertebral spaces, loss of curvature of the spine
  - —Myelogram: to document level of disk involvement
  - —Computed tomography: to identify disk protrusion or evaluate any bone or soft tissue involvement
  - —Magnetic resonance imaging: to confirm rupture of disk and identify any disk compression on the spinal column
  - —Electromyography: to determine level of spinal injury

**TREATMENT**

*Medical*

- Therapy
  - —Lower back

      Bed rest in position of comfort during acute pain: side-lying or recumbent position with pillow under knees

      Ice massage to lumbosacral area

      Back support or brace

      Exercise regimen to strengthen back and abdominal muscles (see Back Exercises, p. 89)

      Traction: skin traction with pelvic belt, bilateral Buck's traction, hanging traction
  - —Cervical spine

      Head Holter traction

      Skeletal (halo) traction
  - —General

      Ultrasound diathermy with back massage

      Heating pad to back to relieve stiffness; use for short intervals only (15-30 minutes)

      Transcutaneous electrical nerve stimulation

- Drugs
  —Analgesic-antipyretic agents
  —Muscle relaxants
  —Nonsteroidal antiinflammatory agents
  —Narcotic analgesics for severe pain uncontrolled by the above medications
  —Corticosteroids to reduce edema
  —Laxatives/stool softeners to prevent constipation or straining that can aggravate pain

*Surgical*

- Surgery is considered only after conservative management has failed to relieve symptoms or if there are signs of spinal cord compression such as motor or sensory loss or loss of sphincter control.
- Laminectomy
  —Diskectomy: to remove one or more vertebrae
  —Spinal fusion: to stabilize spine
- Microdiskectomy: removal of affected disk using microscopic surgery performed through a 1-inch incision
- Percutaneous lateral diskectomy: removal of disk performed by insertion of metal cannula under fluoroscopy; requires 2 or 3 days in hospital
- Chemonucleolysis: injection of enzymes directly into affected disk to dissolve fibrocartilage causing compression on the spinal cord; rarely done

## HOME CARE

- Give both the paient and the caregiver *verbal* and *written* instructions. Provide them with the name and telephone number of a physician or nurse to call if questions arise.
- *General information*
  —Discuss the disorder and contributing factors.
- *Warning signs*
  —Review the signs and symptoms that should be reported to a physician or nurse.
      Increased sensory loss (numbness, tingling)
      Increased motor loss/weakness (paralysis)
      Loss of bowel and bladder function
- *Medications*
  —Explain the purpose, dosage, schedule, and route of adminis-

tration of any prescribed drugs, as well as side effects to report to the physician or nurse.

B

Nonsteroidal antiinflammatory agents: warn the patient not to take over-the-counter analgesics or muscle relaxants without checking with a physician.

- *Activity*
  —Advise the patient to avoid factors that enhance muscle spasm, such as staying in one position too long, fatigue, chilling, and anxiety.
  —Explain the importance of resting when tired or stressed and of not exercising when in pain.
  —Discuss the importance of maintaining good body mechanics to relieve back strain.

  Standing
  - ○ Explain that standing erect or bent over for long periods increases pressure on the spine and causes lower back and hips to sag forward. Therefore instruct the patient to stand with hips flexed and with one foot on a stool or a step.
  - ○ Women should avoid wearing high heels, which can lead to swayback.

  Sitting: to avoid increasing the sway in the lower back, teach the patient to sit in the correct position:
  - ○ Do not slouch.
  - ○ Sit in a relaxed position.
  - ○ Do not twist in the chair.
  - ○ The back of the chair should support the back.
  - ○ Feet should be firmly on the floor.
  - ○ Make sure the chair is firm, not soft.
  - ○ Do not sit with head and neck thrust forward.
  - ○ When driving, so not sit with the car seat too far back.

  Sleeping: explain that serious strains to the back occur during sleeping. To avoid this strain, advise the patient to:
  - ○ Sleep on a firm mattress.
  - ○ Place a piece of plywood between the mattress and springs.
  - ○ Sleep on the floor if away from home or in a motel where the mattress is too soft.
  - ○ Never sleep on the abdomen.

Lifting, stooping, stretching: straining or injuring the back is common when performing ordinary activities. To minimize the chance of this:
○ Never lean forward without bending the knees.
○ Always bend the knees when lifting an object.
○ Always carry objects close to the body. Never lift anything above the level of the elbows.
○ When reaching or stretching upward, make sure there is a wide base of support and do not twist or rotate the body.
○ Never lie flat on the back with legs and hips stretched straight out.
○ Do not lie on back with high pillow under head or neck.
○ Lie on side with hips and knees bent.
○ Lie on back with a lift under legs to relieve swayback.
○ Place an 8- to 10-inch support under the knees to relieve swayback and prevent sleeping on the abdomen.
At rest: maintain a position that will relieve back tension and pain (by straightening the spine):
○ Assume a squatting position.
○ Sit in a chair, lean forward, and lower the head to the knees.
○ Lie with back flat on floor and place legs on a chair.
○ Stand upright and place hands in the small of the back; bend forward slowly.
—Encourage general exercise such as daily walks, which provide strengthening and stretching of back and thigh muscles and help with weight control.
—Remind patient to wear comfortable, well-cushioned support shoes and to avoid shoes with more than half-inch heels.
• *Diet*
—Advise the patient to maintain a weight appropriate for age, sex, and height. If the patient is overweight, explain that excess body weight aggravates the strain on the spine. Refer the patient to a dietitian for a weight reduction diet.

## FOLLOW-UP CARE

• Stress the importance of regular follow-up visits. Make sure the patient has the necessary names and telephone numbers.

B

## BACK EXERCISES

Explain that to strengthen the back, the patient must have strong abdominal muscles to support the spinal column. Weak abdominal muscles allow the spinal column to sag forward, causing swayback. This places pressure on the cartilage disks between the vertebrae and on the nerves. Explain that the only way to build strength in the back is through regular exercise.

Stress the importance of obtaining the advice of the physician before beginning any exercise program.

Discuss the importance of doing all exercises slowly, faithfully, and exactly as directed by the physician or physical therapist. Remind the patient that exercises done occasionally will not help at all.

The following exercises should be done by those who have just recovered from a period of severe back pain. Review them with the patient and provide a demonstration.

*Knee-to-chest lift (to stretch hip, buttocks, lower back muscles)*
* Lie on back on the floor with knees bent and feet flat on floor.
* Draw both knees up to chest
* Place both hands around knees and pull them firmly against chest. Hold for 30 seconds.
* Lower legs and return to starting position.
* Repeat 5-10 times.

*Simple leg lift*
* Lie flat on back on floor with left knee bent and left foot flat on floor.
* Raise right leg as high as comfortably possible.
* Hold for 5 counts.
* Slowly return leg to floor.
* Bend right knee and put right foot flat on floor.
* Raise left leg and hold for 5 counts.
* Repeat 5-10 times for each leg.

*Continued.*

## BACK EXERCISES—cont'd

*Double leg lift*
- Lie flat on back.
- Slowly lift legs until feet are 12 inches from the floor.
- Keep legs straight and hold this position for 10 counts.
- Lower legs to floor.
- Repeat 5 times.

*Pelvic tilt*
- Lie flat on back on floor with knees bent and feet flat on the floor.
- Firmly tighten your buttock muscles.
- Hold for 5 counts.
- Relax buttocks.
- Repeat 5-10 times.
- Be sure to keep lower back flat against floor.

*Half sit-ups (to strengthen abdominal muscles)*
- Lie flat on floor on back with knees bent, feet flat on floor, and hands on chest.
- Slowly raise head and neck to top of chest.
- Reach both hands forward and place them on knees.
- Hold for 5 counts.
- Return to starting position.
- Repeat 5-10 times.

*Elbow props (to extend lower back)*
- Lie face down with your arms beside your body and your head turned to one side.
- Stay in this position for 2-5 minutes, making sure that you relax completely.
- Remain face down and prop yourself on your elbows.
- Hold this position for 2-3 minutes.
- Return to starting position and relax for 1 minute.
- Repeat 5-10 times.

*Hip tilts*
- Lie flat on back with knees bent.
- Slowly bend legs and hips to one side as far as possible.
- Bend to other side.
- Repeat 5 times.

*Continued.*

B

---

### BACK EXERCISES—cont'd

***Toe touches***
- Stand straight and relaxed.
- Lower head and body and try to touch floor with fingertips.
- Keep knees straight.
- Do not jerk or lunge toward floor.
- Bend only as far as you can.
- Repeat 5 times.

---

# Bladder Cancer

—Bladder cancer: the bladder is the most common site of urinary tract cancer. Types of cancer include transitional cell carcinomas, squamous cell carcinomas, and adenocarcinomas. The cancer spreads by local invasion into the bladder muscle, by regional spread into surrounding lymph nodes, the pelvis, and other pelvic structures, and via the blood to the lungs, bones, and liver. The bladder may also be invaded by cancer from other structures, such as the uterine body and cervix, prostate, sigmoid colon, and rectum.

### RISK FACTORS
- Occupational exposure to dust or fume of dyes, rubber, leather and its products, paint, and such organic chemicals as benzidine
- Cigarette smoking

### SIGNS/SYMPTOMS
- Hematuria
- Marked urgency, dysuria, and frequency with small volumes of urine
- Low back pain, which may indicate sacral or lumbar metastases
- Pelvic pain or leg edema related to lymphatic or venous obstruction

**DIAGNOSTIC TESTS**

- Describe each procedure, its purpose, and the normal feelings or sensations that are likely, as well as any preprocedural and postprocedural care.
  —Urine culture: to determine presence of infection
  —Excretory urography: to detect ureteral or urethral obstruction
  —Cystoscopy with biopsy and cytology: to see tumor and determine presence of malignant cells
  —Cystoscopic retrograde ureteropyelography: to see tumor and determine presence of obstruction
  —Renal arteriography and ultrasound: to determine extent of tumor, vessels, obstruction
  —Computed tomography and magnetic resonance imaging of abdomen and pelvis: to determine extent of lymph node involvement
  —Chest and skeletal x-rays, bone scan, liver function studies: to determine extent of metastatic disease

**TREATMENT**

*Medical*

- Therapy
  —Radiation therapy: external beam for palliation of hemorrhage and bony metastases
  —Photodynamic therapy
  —Chemotherapy
      For noninvasive bladder cancer: intravesical instillation with bacille Calmette-Guerin (BCG), thiotepa, doxorubicin, mitomycin-C, interferons
      For invasive bladder cancer: CMDV (cisplatin, methotrexate, doxorubicin, vinblastine); MVC (methotrexate, vinblastine, cisplatin); single agents (methotrexate with or without leucovorin, doxorubicin, vinblastine)

*Surgical*

- For noninvasive bladder cancer: endoscopic resection and fulguration; laser therapy
- For invasive bladder cancer: radical cystectomy with urinary diversion
  —Complications: ureterocutaneous fistula, wound dehiscence, partial small bowel obstruction, wound infection, small bowel fistula

**B**

## HOME CARE

- Give both the patient and the caregiver *verbal* and *written* instructions. Provide them with the name and telephone number of a physician or nurse to call if questions arise.
- *General information*
  —Discuss the disease, causes, and contributing factors.
- *Warning signs*
  —Review the signs and symptoms that should be reported to a physician or nurse.

    Infection: cloudy, odorous urine; frequency, urgency, burning

    Ileal conduit complications: stomal stenosis with pain, stones; ureteral reflux

    Kock pouch complications: leakage at stoma, difficult catheterization, stones
- *Special instructions*
  —Assist the patient to obtain appropriate and adequate supplies for care of a urinary diversion (see Care of a Urinary Diversion, p. 696).
  —Teach female patient to reduce the incidence of urinary tract infections by voiding after sexual intercourse, avoiding bubble baths, and wearing cotton undergarments.
  —Provide information about pain management as needed (see Pain Management, p. 501).
- *Activity*
  —Emphasize the importance of exercise and adequate rest.
- *Diet*
  —Stress the importance of adequate fluid intake.
  —Advise the patient to choose fluids and foods that cause alkaline urine, such as fruits, vegetables, and milk.
  —Advise the patient to avoid fluids and foods that irritate the bladder, such as alcohol, tea, and spices.

## FOLLOW-UP CARE

- Stress the importance of regular follow-up visits. Make sure the patient has the necessary names and telephone numbers.
- Advise the patient to avoid using tobacco.

## REFERRALS

- Assist the patient to obtain referral services such as sperm banking, sexual counseling, and reconstructive or implant surgery.

# Blindness
## (Visual Impairment)

—Blindness: diminished visual acuity ranging from low vision (partial vision) to total blindness; may involve one or both eyes. Types of blindness include color blindness (inability to distinguish certain colors), legal blindness (maximum acuity 20/200 with optimum correction and or visual field reduced to range of 20 degrees [normal is 180 degrees]), loss of peripheral vision, and loss of central vision.

### CAUSES/CONTRIBUTING FACTORS

- Retinal detachment/degeneration
- Glaucoma
- Cataract
- Amblyopia
- Diabetes
- Stroke
- Aneurysm
- Brain tumor
- Trachoma (chronic conjunctivitis)
- Leprosy
- Onchocerciasis (river blindness caused by black fly bites)
- Xerophthalmia
- Corneal diseases
- Herpes simplex virus
- Trauma

### SIGNS/SYMPTOMS

- The following signs and symptoms necessitate evaluation to prevent permanent visual loss.
  —Blurred vision
  —Double vision
  —Sudden loss of vision
  —Alternating dimming and clearing of vision
  —Eye pain
  —Loss of side vision
  —Haloes (colored rays or circles around lights)

—Twitching or shaking eye
—Floaters (dots, streaks, or strands)
—Pressure or pulling within the eye
—Discharge, crusting, excessive tearing
—Swelling in eye
—Bulging or one or both eyes
—Unequal pupil size

## HOME CARE

* Give both the patient and the caregiver *verbal* and *written* instructions. Provide them with the name and telephone number of a physician or nurse to call if questions arise.
* *General information*
  —Reinforce the physician's explanation for the type and cause of blindness (disease process or trauma). Stress the importance of notifying the physician of any changes in the condition.
  —Clarify the prognosis, explaining whether the visual impairment is temporary or progressive.
* *Warning signs*
  —Review the signs and symptoms that should be reported to a physician or nurse.
    Itching
    Redness
    Swelling
    Discharge
* *Special instructions*
  —Provide instruction and assist patient to develop skills needed to maximize self-care and promote independence.
    Explore and map out furniture, steps, and doorways in the home through guidance and touch.
    Use another's arm as guide when walking.
    Trace the wall or rail with hand to orient to perimeters of room when walking.
    When walking alone, use cane or walking stick to identify obstacles.
    Touch food, containers, liquids, and utensils before eating.
    Feel chairs, toilet before turning to sit.
    Organize clothing and shoes to facilitate selection.
    Place articles for grooming and hygiene in same position.

—Discuss home care with patient and caregiver, stressing need to avoid hazards.

Living quarters should not be rearranged once the patient is familiar with the placement of furniture and furnishings.

Encourage the patient to move slowly and to have assistance when exploring living arrangements.

Ensure that living quarters are free of clutter (remove loose throw rugs, articles on floor or stairs, electrical cords).

Encourage the patient to explore outdoors slowly and with assistance to avoid falls on uneven ground, steps, loose gravel, and icy patches.

Encourage the patient to explore the community slowly and with assistance.

Encourage self-care, discussing the need to avoid being overprotective.

—Provide instruction on caring for the eyes.

Review the method for administering eyedrops or ointment.

Advise the patient of the importance of keeping eyes free of infection: keeping eye dropper clean, using clean tissue or cloth to wipe eyes, wiping eyes from inner to outer lid.

- *Medications*
  —Explain the purpose, dosage, schedule, and route of administration of any prescribed drugs, as well as side effects to report to the physician or nurse.
  —Avoid over-the-counter medications, eyedrops, or ointments unless their use has been discussed with the physician.

## FOLLOW-UP CARE

- Stress the importance of regular follow-up visits. Make sure the patient has the necessary names and telephone numbers.
- Encourage or assist the patient to obtain a Medic-Alert bracelet and identification card listing the diagnosis and medication.

## REFERRALS

- Encourage or assist the patient and family to seek additional support from community and health agencies for the visually impaired (e.g., state agency for the blind), which can provide early assistance with computer-assisted reading, talking books, time and temperature devices, rehabilitation for future employment, and acquisition of new skills.

# Bone Cancer

—Bone cancer: primary bone cancers are uncommon, accounting for 0.2% of all malignancies in the United States. Peak incidence is between 15 and 19 years of age and after 65 years. Types include osseous (classic or periosteal osteosarcoma), cartilaginous (primary or secondary chondrosarcoma), fibrous (fibrosarcoma, malignant fibrous histiocytoma), and reticuloendothelial (Ewing's sarcoma, multiple myeloma).

## RISK FACTORS

- Paget's disease
- Fibrous dysplasia
- Enchondromatosis
- Bone infarction
- Prior exposure to radiation

## SIGNS/SYMPTOMS

- Osteosarcoma: complaints of pain or swelling in affected extremity, usually worse at night and increasing as tumor expands; severe, unremitting pain and pathologic fracture seen in presence of Paget's disease
- Chondrosarcoma: persistent, dull, aching pain; firm, swollen area over tumor site
- Fibrosarcoma: pain and swelling of affected area
- Ewing's sarcoma: pain and swelling of affected area; anemia; leukocytosis; elevated erythrocyte sedimentation rate

## DIAGNOSTIC TESTS

- Describe each procedure, its purpose, and the normal feelings or sensations that are likely, as well as any preprocedural and postprocedural care.
    —Computed tomography and magnetic resonance imaging: to define location and extent of tumor
    —X-ray: to define location, extent, and type of destruction and amount of reactive bone formed
    —Bone scans: to detect multiple areas of disease, extent of local disease, tumor activity, skeletal metastases

—Biopsy: to determine type, stage, and grade of tumor
—Chest x-ray: to detect pulmonary metastases

## TREATMENT

*Medical*

- Therapy
  —Radiation therapy: external beam
  —Chemotherapy
    For osteogenic sarcoma
    ○ Doxorubicin
    ○ Cisplatin
    ○ High-dose methotrexate
    ○ Ifosfamide
    ○ Dactinomycin
    ○ Cyclophosphamide
    For Ewing's sarcoma
    ○ Combinations of vincristine, actinomycin D, doxorubicin, and cyclophosphamide; ifosfamide and etoposide

*Surgical*

- Wide excision with limb salvage
- En bloc resection: wide excision of normal tissue around tumor, removal of entire muscle bundles at points of origin and insertion, resection of involved bone as well as vascular structures
  —Complications: long operating time, lengthy anesthesia, extensive blood loss
- Amputation (see Amputation, p. 26)
- Reconstruction: allograft, autograft, vascularized graft
- Prosthesis

## HOME CARE

- Give both the patient and the caregiver *verbal* and *written* instructions. Provide them with the name and telephone number of a physician or nurse to call if questions arise.
- *General information*
  —Explain to a patient who has undergone limb salvage that he or she will not regain preoperative gait and will be partially disabled.
  —Reinforce the physician's explanation of type of cancer and prescribed treatment (see Chemotherapy, p. 178; Radiation Therapy, p. 559; Amputation, p. 26).

# Bone Marrow Harvest

**B**

—**Bone marrow harvest: removal of bone marrow from a donor for purposes of transplanting into a patient.**

## PREPROCEDURAL TEACHING

- Review the physician's explanation of the procedure and the reason for it; encourage the patient to ask questions and to discuss any fears or anxieties.

### Review of Preprocedural Care

- Review the need for written consent and explain that the hospital stay will be from 1 to 3 days.
- Review preprocedural tests: blood tests to ensure the donor's bone marrow matches the recipient's, physical examination, chest x-ray, electrocardiogram, urinalysis.
- Explain that the evening before the harvest the donor will take a shower with an antiseptic solution and will be NPO from midnight on.
- Describe what will happen on the day of the procedure.
  - —A nurse will insert an IV line and administer a sedative and anesthetic agents to make the donor relaxed and drowsy.
  - —The bone marrow will be harvested from the donor's hip. The physician will insert a needle several times into the rear portion of the hip bones and withdraw a total of 1-2 quarts of bone marrow and blood.
  - —A pressure dressing will be applied over the harvest sites to prevent bleeding.
  - —The entire procedure will take about 2-3 hours.

### Review of Postprocedural Care

- The patient will awaken in the recovery room after the anesthetic has worn off.
- A nurse will check on the donor every 15 minutes to record vital signs (pulse, blood pressure, temperature, and respirations) and ensure that no bleeding is occurring from the harvest sites. Blood transfusions may be given to make up for the loss of blood.
- Explain that if the marrow is for the donor's future use, it will

be frozen until needed. If it is for another recipient, it will be given immediately to the recipient through an IV transfusion.

- Within a day the donor will be able to eat solid food and begin walking around. The pressure dressing will be removed and replaced by a bandage. If the donor has pain, the physician can prescribe medication to relieve it.
- The donor will be able to leave the hospital after 1 or 2 days and to resume normal activities soon after.

## HOME CARE

- Give both the patient and the caregiver *verbal* and *written* instructions. Provide them with the name and telephone number of a physician or nurse to call if questions arise.
- *General information*
  —Explain the need to keep the harvest sites clean and covered with a bandage for 3 days.
- *Warning signs*
  —Review the signs and symptoms that should be reported to a physician or nurse.
    Bleeding
    Pain
    Swelling at site

# Bone Marrow Suppression

—Bone marrow suppression: depression of the immune system caused by cancer and cancer treatment. As a result, the patient is made more susceptible to infection, bleeding, and anemia.

## INFECTION

- The sites of infection most commonly associated with bone marrow suppression are the bladder and urinary tract, skin, lungs, and blood.

### Signs/Symptoms

- Fever over 100°
- Redness, swelling, or pain around or in any wound

- Coughing, sore throat, stuffy or runny nose
- Nausea, vomiting, or diarrhea
- Chest pain or shortness of breath
- Burning or frequency of urination; change in color or odor of urine
- Sores or white patches in mouth

**Prevention**

- Advise the patient of ways to prevent infection.
  —Eat healthy meals, drink plenty of fluids, get enough rest, and avoid stress as much as possible.
  —Keep mouth, teeth, and gums clean; use a soft-bristled toothbrush and saltwater rinse.
  —Wash hands often with soap and water, especially before eating and after using the toilet.
  —Shower rather than taking a bath.
  —Cleanse perianal area after each bowel movement.
  —For women, avoid bubble baths, douches, and feminine hygiene products such as tampons. Change sanitary napkins frequently.
  —Use a commercial lubricant during sexual intercourse.
  —Urinate before and after intercourse.
  —Avoid the following.
      People who are sick
      People recently vaccinated with a live virus
      Crowded places (waiting rooms, malls)
      Raw fruits and vegetables, raw eggs, and raw milk; eat only cooked food and pasteurized milk and milk products
      Sources of stagnant water (water in flower vases, pitchers, denture cups, humidifiers, and breathing equipment); water in these containers should be changed daily; preferably such items should not be in patient's room
      Dog, cat, and bird feces; bird cages or litter boxes should not be in patient's room; if they are, someone else should change them

**BLEEDING**

- Bleeding, especially from the skin or mucous membranes or internally, occurs because the bone marrow is not producing enough platelets (special blood cells that cause the blood to clot) or because the platelets already in the blood are being destroyed.

The cancer, allergic reactions to medications, radiation therapy, or chemotherapy can cause bleeding.

## Prevention

- Check the skin each day for bruises and call the physician if bruises get larger after first being noticed.
- Report to a physician any bleeding that does not stop after 5 minutes.
- Bleeding from the skin
  —Avoid physical activities that could cause injury, such as contact sports.
  —Shave with an electric razor.
  —Keep nails short; file rough edges.
  —Draw a circle around the perimeter of a bruise to measure increase in size.
- Bleeding from the mucous membranes of the mouth, nose, gastrointestinal system, and genitourinary tract
  —Brush with a soft-bristled toothbrush. If gums still bleed, use sponge-tipped applicators or a Water-Pik. Do not floss. Keep lips moist with petroleum jelly. Check with physician before having dental work done.
  —Avoid hot foods that might burn mouth.
  —Blow nose gently. Humidify house if the air is too dry. If nose bleeds, pinch nostrils shut for a few minutes. If bleeding persists, put an ice bag on back of neck.
  —Use stool softeners and drink plenty of water if constipated. Do not use enemas or suppositories. Take acetaminophen (e.g., Tylenol) or ibuprofen rather than aspirin, which can cause stomach bleeding. Avoid douches and vaginal suppositories. Use a lubricating jelly before sexual intercourse.
- Internal bleeding
  —Arrange furniture to avoid bumping into it. Keep clutter and loose rugs off floor.
  —Avoid tight-fitting clothing and any buttons or ornaments that could bruise or chafe skin.
  —Do not lift heavy objects.

## ANEMIA

- Anemia is caused by not having enough red blood cells to carry oxygen to the cells and take away carbon dioxide. Patients may tire easily and need to rest more often.

**Signs/Symptoms to Report**

- Pallor
- Dizziness
- Ringing in the ears
- Chest pain
- Shortness of breath

**Special Instructions**

- Schedule frequent rest periods during activities.
- Eat a high-protein diet.
- Take a multivitamin supplement with minerals.

# Bone Marrow Transplantation

—Bone marrow transplantation (BMT): destruction of the patient's bone marrow with high doses of cancer chemotherapy or radiation and replacement with healthy bone marrow. The transplanted marrow begins making new blood cells within 10 to 14 days after the transplantation. BMT is a treatment for some cancers. The procedure involves intravenous infusion of bone marrow into the patient to replace the defective hematopoietic system with healthy stem cells. Types of BMT include autologous (harvesting of patient's marrow after treatment with cytoreductive therapy and sometimes cancer chemotherapy), syngeneic (using an identical twin as donor), and allogeneic (donation by a family member, usually a sibling, or by an unrelated donor with compatible human leukocyte antigen [HLA] and mixed lymphocyte culture [MLC]). The type selected depends on the disease or disorder, the availability of histocompatible donors, and the health status of potential donors.

## INDICATIONS

- Leukemias
- Non-Hodgkin's lymphoma
- Burkitt's lymphoma

- Multiple myeloma
- Osteosarcoma
- Breast cancer

## PREPROCEDURAL TEACHING

- Review the physician's explanation of the procedure and the reason for it; encourage the patient to ask questions and to discuss any fears or anxieties.

### Review of Preprocedural Care

- For donor selection and bone marrow harvest, see Bone Marrow Harvest, p. 99.
- Explain that the hospital stay will last from 1½ to 2 months if there are no serious complications.
- Discuss the use of high-dose chemotherapy, either alone or with total body irradiation, as preparation for transplantation.
  —May take as long as 10 days
  —Common side effects: nausea, vomiting, anorexia, mucositis, parotitis, xerostomia, excessive salivation, diarrhea, low-grade fever, alopecia, electrolyte imbalance, aplasia
  —Life-threatening effects: severe thrombocytopenia, syndrome of inappropriate antidiuretic hormone, renal failure, sepsis, venous occlusive disease, capillary leak syndrome
- Describe the BMT procedure.
  —The patient is alone in a room with constant monitoring.
  —The patient is hydrated with bicarbonate solution to force brisk alkaline urine flow to prevent RBC hemolysis.
  —Emergency drugs for anaphylactic reactions are kept at bedside.
  —Bone marrow is infused via central line without a filter over a 1- to 4-hour period.

### Review of Postprocedural Care

- Explain that after BMT the recipient progresses through stages of aplasia, lingering side effects of preparatory therapy, and finally engraftment of the donor marrow.
- Review self-care procedures that patient will need to do while in the hospital: handwashing techniques, mouth care, skin care, measuring intake and output, use of incentive spirometer.
- Discuss activity allowances, limitations, use of exercycle.

B

- Explain dietary procedures, use of total parenteral nutrition, and restrictions, such as food allowances.
- Explain posttransplant medications, their expected side effects, and use of indwelling catheter for administration.
- Discuss complications and measures that will be taken to prevent or treat them.
  —Infection: patient will be placed in protective isolation or laminar airflow rooms; prophylactic systemic antibiotics and antiviral agents; routine cultures of blood, urine, throat, stool
  —Acute graft versus host disease: usually appears within 2 weeks to 3 months after BMT; may cause erythema, maculopapular rash, blistering and desquamation, liver failure, diarrhea, abdominal pain, denuding of gastrointestinal tract; mild cases usually self-limiting; severe cases require such agents as high-dose steroids, antithymocyte globulin, monoclonal antibody, OKT-3
  —Chronic graft versus host disease: occurs 3 months to 1 year after BMT; manifested as scleroderma-like changes in skin, GI tract, and liver; immune deficiency; marrow suppression; changes in respiratory and musculoskeletal function; treated with prednisone and azathioprine
  —Potential long-term problems: neurologic damage; cataract formation; endocrine problems; changes in skin, eyes, mouth, and GI tract

## SIDE EFFECTS/COMPLICATIONS

- Acute
  —Mucositis
  —Viral infection
  —Bacterial and fungal sepsis
  —Renal failure
  —Interstitial pneumonia
  —Venoocclusive disease
  —Graft versus host disease
- Common
  —Anemia
  —Bleeding stomatitis
  —Skin changes
  —Nausea
  —Vomiting
  —Diarrhea

## HOME CARE

- Give both the patient and the caregiver *verbal* and *written* instructions. Provide them with the name and telephone number of a physician or nurse to call if questions arise.
- *General information*
  —Explain measures for preventing complications (see also Bone Marrow Suppression, p. 100).

    Infection

    ○ Precautions are more rigid during the first 3 months after BMT and become more relaxed as the year progresses.
    ○ Wear a face mask when outside the home in public.
    ○ Avoid contact with persons who may be infectious, young children attending school, or persons recently vaccinated.
    ○ Avoid crowds and trips to grocery stores, theaters, and restaurants.
    ○ Avoid having multiple sexual partners.
    ○ Wash hands before eating and after using the toilet.
    ○ Avoid contact with pets for the first 3 months after BMT. Do not clean litter boxes or come in contact with animal feces.
    ○ Avoid contact with plants and flowers.
    ○ Do not swim in private or public pools.

    Bleeding

    ○ Discuss emergency procedures to follow if spontaneous hemorrhage occurs. The patient or caregiver should have emergency numbers on hand. Teach methods for applying pressure to the bleeding site.
    ○ Review measures to prevent bleeding: maintain a safe, clutter-free environment; remove loose scatter rugs; avoid using sharp objects; use electric razors; wear protective gloves when gardening; avoid going barefoot; use soft-bristled toothbrush; use soft sponge with mouthwash if gums are sensitive and bleeding.
    ○ Inform dentist and other medical personnel about BMT before any procedures are performed.

    Stomatitis

    ○ Discuss the importance of routine oral hygiene in the morning, after meals, and at bedtime.
    ○ Discuss the need to avoid putting objects into the mouth.
    ○ Instruct the patient to avoid using mouthwash containing alcohol.

B

○ Discuss the need to avoid irritating foods such as citrus fruits and spicy or hard fruits and vegetables.

○ Instruct the patient on the use of any prescribed mouthwashes, sprays, or anesthetics.

○ Plan with the patient or caregiver for necessary changes in activities of daily living (see Bone Marrow Suppression, p. 100).

- *Warning signs*
  —Review the signs and symptoms that should be reported to a physician or nurse.
  
  Fever

  Rash

  Change in color or consistency of stool, urine

  Nausea or vomiting

  Pain

  Dryness of mouth, difficulty swallowing

  Change in skin color

  Cough or shortness of breath

- *Special instructions*
  —Teach self-care procedures as indicated.
  
  Central venous access device (see External Venous Catheter, p. 163)

  Administration of total parenteral nutrition

  Use of volumetric pump

  Use of incentive spirometer

  Taking and recording of temperature; intake and output; urine and stool testing for blood

  —Discuss preparation of home environment.

  Advise patient on obtaining necessary equipment and supplies.

  Instruct patient's caregiver to have house cleaned and dusted before arrival of patient, to remove all plants and flowers, and to board pet away from home for the first 100 days or as ordered.

- *Medications*
  —Explain the purpose, dosage, schedule, and route of administration of any prescribed drugs, as well as side effects to report to the physician or nurse.
  —Emphasize the importance of not taking over-the-counter medications without checking with a physician or nurse.

- *Diet*
  —Explain need to maintain diet as ordered.

—Suggest high-protein, high-caloric diet.
—Encourage frequent small, light meals.

## FOLLOW-UP CARE

• Stress the importance of regular medical and laboratory follow-up visits. Make sure the patient has the necessary names and telephone numbers.

## REFERRALS

• Assist the patient to obtain referral services for psychologic support.

# Bowel Obstruction and Resection with Anastomosis

**—Bowel obstruction and resection with anastomosis: surgical resection of diseased intestinal tissue and anastomosis of the remaining healthy bowel segments. The surgical incision site depends on the location of the diseased intestinal tissue. The bowel resection may result in an end-to-end anastomosis or a side-to-side anastomosis. (If temporary ostomy is required, see Urinary Diversion, p. 650)**

## INDICATIONS

• Localized obstructive intestinal disorders, such as diverticulitis, intestinal polyps, adhesions, malignant or benign intestinal lesions
• Localized bowel cancer

## PREPROCEDURAL TEACHING

• Review the physician's explanation of the procedure and the reason for it; encourage the patient to ask questions and to discuss any fears or anxieties.

### Review of Preprocedural Care

• Review the need for informed consent and anesthesia.
• Discuss the administration of antibiotics, laxatives, and enemas.

**Review of Postprocedural Care**

- Discuss anticipated postoperative care, including nasogastric tube, IVs for fluid replacement, abdominal drains, and ambulation.
- Warn patient against manipulating or repositioning the nasogastric tube.
- Stress the importance of turning, coughing, deep breathing, and incisional splinting.
- Discuss the purpose of the incentive spirometer and demonstrate its use.

## SIDE EFFECTS/COMPLICATIONS

- Bleeding
- Leakage from the anastomosis site
- Peritonitis
- Sepsis
- Postresection obstruction

## HOME CARE

- Give both the patient and the caregiver *verbal* and *written* instructions. Provide them with the name and telephone number of a physician or nurse to call if questions arise.
- *General information*
  —Review any explanation about the surgery and follow-up care.
  —Demonstrate proper wound management and dressing changes: procedure and frequency of dressing changes and inspection of the incision with each dressing change.
  —Advise the patient to dispose of soiled dressings in a plastic bag and thoroughly wash hands.
  —Instruct the patient to note and record the frequency and amount of bowel movements and the characteristics of the stool.
- *Warning signs*
  —Review the signs and symptoms that should be reported to a physician or nurse.
    Infection: fever, malase, leakage of bowel contents, purulent drainage, foul odor, redness, tenderness at incision
    Abdominal distention, increased abdominal pain, bloody stools, leakage of bowel contents, abdominal rigidity
    Changes in frequency and amount of bowel movements or the characteristics of the stool

- *Special instructions*
  —Advise the patient where to obtain appropriate supplies, such as sterile dressings.
- *Medications*
  —Explain the purpose, dosage, schedule, and route of administration of stool softeners and analgesics, as well as side effects to report to the physician or nurse.
  —Advise the patient against using laxatives without consulting the physician.
- *Activity*
  —Encourage the patient to discuss allowances and limitations with respect to occupation, recreation, or activities.
  —Instruct the patient to avoid abdominal straining, such as during defecation, and heavy lifting until the sutures are completely healed or until advised by a physician.
- *Diet*
  —Advise a semibland diet until the bowel is completely healed, usually 4-8 weeks.
  —Advise the patient to drink plenty of fluids.
  —Advise the patient to avoid carbonated beverages and gas-producing foods.
  —Provide the patient with a list of specific gas-producing foods.

**FOLLOW-UP CARE**

- Stress the importance of regular follow-up visits. Make sure the patient has the necessary names and telephone numbers.

**REFERRALS**

- If appropriate, assist the patient to obtain a referral to the American Cancer Society, support groups, and home health support services.

# Brain Tumors

—Brain tumors: space-occupying lesions that compress, invade, or destroy surrounding brain tissue and nerve structures. Brain tumors can occur at any age. In adults the inci-

**B**

dence is highest between 40 and 60 years of age. In children most brain tumors occur before age 1 or between ages 2 and 12. Tumors are classified by histologic geatures and grade of malignancy. Tumors may have primary, metastatic, or developmental origins.

## CAUSES/CONTRIBUTING FACTORS

- The cause of brain tumors is unknown. Some theories include genetic, hormonal, or angiogenesis factors, chemicals, radiation, trauma, viruses, or diet.

## SIGNS/SYMPTOMS

The onset of signs and symptoms is insidious. Findings are specific to the type of tumor, its location, and the degree of invasion.

- Headache: localized or generalized
- Seizures
- Mental, behavioral, and personality changes: disorientation; inability to follow commands; irritability; forgetfulness; memory loss; impaired judgment
- Decreased level of consciousness, stupor, or coma
- Vomiting with or without nausea
- Dizziness occurring with position changes; vertigo
- Visual changes: double vision, decreased visual acuity; visual field defects
- Decreased motor strength; hemiparesis; hemiplegia
- Aphasia
- Gait disturbances; impaired balance; incoordination
- Auditory disturbances
- Sensory disturbances: hyperesthesia, paresthesia, astereognosis, agnosia, apraxia, agraphia
- Cranial nerve dysfunction

## COMPLICATIONS

- Cerebral edema
- Compression of the brain, cranial nerves, and cerebral vessels
- Intracranial hypertension
- Seizures
- Neurologic defects: mild to severe
- Hydrocephalus
- Hormonal changes
- Altered level of consciousness

- Alteration in respiratory function
- Brain herniation

## DIAGNOSTIC TESTS

- Describe each procedure, its purpose, and the normal feelings or sensations that are likely, as well as any preprocedural and postprocedural care.
  —Skull x-rays: to locate the tumor and any calcified areas
  —Computed tomography brain scan: to locate the tumor, determine its size, and detect the presence of cerebral edema
  —Cerebral angiography: to assess the vascularity of tumor and the surrounding vessels
  —Magnetic resonance imaging: to assess tumor location, size, vascularity, and cerebral edema
  —Tumor biopsy: to assess histologic type and grading of tumors
  —Intracranial pressure monitoring

## TREATMENT

- Specific treatments vary with tumor histologic type, location, accessibility, and radiosensitivity.

*Medical*

- Therapy
  —Radiation therapy
  —Chemotherapy
- Drugs
  —Corticosteroids such as dexamethasone (Decadron): to control cerebral edema and decrease intracranial pressure
  —Osmotic diuretics: to decrease cerebral edema
  —Anticonvulsants such as phenytoin (Dilantin): to prevent seizures
  —$H_2$ blockers such as cimetidine (Tagamet) or ranitidine (Zantac): to prevent stress ulcers
  —Antacids
  —Analgesics: to relieve headaches
  —Antiemetics: to minimize nausea and vomiting

*Surgical*

- Surgical resection
- Laser surgery
- Microsurgery
- Ventriculoatrial or ventriculoperitoneal shunting of cerebrospinal fluid

**HOME CARE**

- Give both the patient and the caregiver *verbal* and *written* instructions. Provide them with the name and telephone number of a physician or nurse to call if questions arise.
- *General information*
  —Reinforce the explanation of brain tumor type, its causes, and contributing factors.
  —Patient education is individualized, depending on the location and the type of tumor and its malignancy.
- *Warning signs*
  —Review the signs and symptoms that should be reported to a physician or nurse.
      Seizure activity
      Behavioral or neurologic changes
      Altered level of consciousness
      Changes in respiration
      Infection, including fever
      Bleeding
      Stress ulcers: abdominal distention, pain, vomiting, tarry stools
- *Special instructions*
  —Assist the patient in obtaining appropriate adaptive devices for self-care, rehabilitation, mobilization, and sensory function, such as hearing aids or eyeglasses.
  —Assist the caregiver in identifying and correcting hazards in the home if the patient develops deficits.
  —Teach the patient and caregiver seizure precautions.
- *Medications*
  —Explain the purpose, dosage, schedule, and route of administration of any prescribed drugs, as well as side effects to report to the physician or nurse.
  —Explain the adverse effects of chemotherapy and radiation therapy, if appropriate. Explain actions the patient can take to alleviate them.
- *Activity*
  —Identify and discuss limitations imposed by changes in neurologic function.
- *Diet*
  —Explain that the diet should be regular or as prescribed by a physician.

**FOLLOW-UP CARE**

- Stress the importance of regular follow-up visits. Make sure the patient has the necessary names and telephone numbers.

**PSYCHOSOCIAL CARE**

- Encourage the patient to continue to function in usual roles (occupational and social) as much as possible and to avoid sensory deprivation and social isolation.
- Encourage the patient to seek assistance to perform activities as needed.

**REFERRALS**

- Refer the patient to occupational and physical therapists to begin a rehabilitation program. If appropriate, refer the patient to a speech pathologist.
- Refer the patient for a dietary consultation to ensure adequate nutrition during chemotherapy and radiation therapy.
- Refer the patient to support groups, the American Cancer Society, and home health support services.

# Breast Cancer

—Breast cancer: cancer of the breast, the most common malignancy among American women. One in nine women will be diagnosed with breast cancer in her lifetime. Breast cancer is believed to be a systemic disease, with the possibility of occult distant metastases occurring early in the disease with or without lymph node involvement.

**RISK FACTORS**

- Family history of breast cancer: sister, mother, grandmother, aunt
- Menarche before age 12
- Menopause after 55 years
- No children, or first child after 30 years of age

- Exposure to excessive radiation, especially before age 35
- Fibrocystic change (atypical epithelial hyperplasia)
- Previous history of breast cancer
- Personal history of other cancers (endometrial, ovarian, colon, or thyroid types)

## SIGNS/SYMPTOMS

- Painless mass or thickening in breast most common
- Nipple discharge: spontaneous, unilateral, from single duct, watery and clear, serosanguineous, bloody in color
- Advanced disease: skin or nipple dimpling; puckering or retraction; changes in breast size, shape, or contour; skin edema; discoloration; dilated superficial blood vessels; frank skin ulcerations; hard, fixed mass in axilla

## COMPLICATIONS

- Metastases, most commonly to lungs, liver, bone
- Hypercalcemia
- Spinal cord compression
- Brachial plexopathy
- Pleural effusion
- Pathologic fracture

## DIAGNOSTIC TESTS

- Describe each procedure, its purpose, and the normal feelings or sensations that are likely, as well as any preprocedural and postprocedural care.
    —Clinical examination: palpation of breasts and axillae
    —Mammogram: to determine shape, size, and location of tumor
    —Biopsy: to identify type of malignant cells
    —Estrogen and progestin receptors: to determine tumor response to hormones

## TREATMENT

*Medical*
- Therapy
    —Radiation therapy
    —Bradytherapy
    —External beam
    —Regional node irradiation

- Drugs (as adjuvant therapy for radiation)
  —Combination chemotherapy: CMF (cyclophosphamide, methorexate, 5-fluorouracil); CMFVP (CMF with vincristine and prednisone); CA (cyclophosphamide and doxorubicin); CAF (cyclophosphamide, doxorubicin, 5-fluorouracil)
  —Antiestrogen therapy (ablative): tamoxifen citrate
  —Estrogens (additive): diethylstilbestrol, ethinyl estradiol
  —Androgens (additive): fluoxymesterone, testosterone, methyl-testosterone
  —Progestins (additive): megestrol acetate, medroxyprogester-one

*Surgical*
- Lumpectomy: wide excision and removal of tumor and margin of healthy tissue
- Partial mastectomy: simple excision of tumor and wider margin of healthy tissue
- Quadrantectomy: removal of one quarter of breast
- Mastectomy
  —Subcutaneous: removal of all breast tissue, preserving over-lying skin and nipple-areolar complex
  —Total (simple): complete removal of breast tissue and skin from clavicle to costal margin and from midline to the latis-simus dorsi; axillary nodes not removed
  —Modified radical: removal of breast and axillary lymph nodes
  —Radical: removal of breast underlying pectoral muscles and of axillary nodes
  —Extended or super radical: removal of internal mammary lym-phatic chain with breast, pectoral muscles, and axillary nodes
- Breast reconstruction
- Bone marrow transplantation (see Bone Marrow Transplanta-tion, p. 103)

## HOME CARE

- Give both the patient and the caregiver *verbal* and *written* in-structions. Provide them with the name and telephone number of a physician or nurse to call if questions arise.
- *General information*
  —Review explanation of the disease, the prescribed surgical procedure, and adjuvant therapy to be carried out. Explain that the decision is based on the stage of breast cancer, age, meno-pausal state, hormonal receptor status, and patient preference.

- *Special instructions*
  —Encourage discussion of feelings and emotions regarding impending surgery, adjuvant therapies, and prognosis. Clarify any misconceptions.

## FOLLOW-UP CARE

- Stress the importance of regular follow-up visits. Make sure the patient has the necessary names and telephone numbers.

## PSYCHOSOCIAL CARE

- Stress the importance of verbalizing feelings about the impact losing a body part will have on life-style, sexuality, and relationships.

## REFERRALS

- Encourage the patient to visit or talk with another cancer survivor; contact Reach for Recovery for volunteer.

# Breast Surgery

—Breast surgery: surgical treatment for breast cancer, determined by the size of the tumor, whether it has spread, the woman's age and physical condition, and her preference. Types of breast surgery include lumpectomy (the removal of the lump and a margin or healthy tissue surrounding it) and mastectomy, which may be as simple as removing all breast tissue while preserving the overlying skin and nipple-areolar complex or may involve radical removal of the internal mammary lymphatic chain with the breast, pectoral muscles, and axillary lymph nodes.

## PREPROCEDURAL TEACHING

- Review the physician's explanation of the procedure and the reason for it; encourage the patient to ask questions and to discuss any fears or anxieties.

### Review of Preprocedural Care

- Review the need for written consent for surgery and anesthesia.
- Explain that the skin will be cleansed with bactericidal soap or antiseptic solutions to remove bacteria.
- Discuss the complete blood count and urinalysis to check for infection and bleeding.
- Explain that the patient will be NPO from midnight of the evening before surgery.
- Describe the types of dressings and equipment that will be used postoperatively.
- Instruct the patient in exercises, hand and arm care, and drainage tube management.
- Encourage questions and the verbalization of fears, anxieties, and grieving for a change in body image.
- Encourage a preoperative visit by a Reach to Recovery volunteer for psychologic support when possible.

### Review of Postprocedural Care

- Instruct the patient to report any unusual pain or swelling in the operative area or the arm on the operative side, as well as signs of infection (redness, pain, swelling, feeling of tenderness, fever, nonserous drainage or odor).
- For modified radical or partial mastectomy with axillary node dissection, explain that the patient may be discharged with one or more drains in place.
- Review hand and arm care instructions (see box opposite).
- Teach arm exercises as prescribed.
- Alert the patient to possible phantom breast experience; sensation is usually twinges or itching of the total breast or nipple.

### SIDE EFFECTS/COMPLICATIONS

- Side effects are uncommon in all but radical procedures, which are done less frequently.
  - —Infection in the incision line
  - —Seroma
  - —Lymphedema
  - —Impaired shoulder mobility
  - —Nerve injury

### HOME CARE

- Give both the patient and the caregiver *verbal* and *written* instructions. Provide them with the name and telephone number

B

of a physician or nurse to call if questions arise. Use visual aids to assist in instruction.

• *General information*

—Review explanation of the disease, the prescribed surgical procedure, and adjuvant therapy to be carried out.

—Explain that if the axillary nodes are removed, the affected arm may swell and is less able to fight infection.

• *Wound/incision care*

—Teach the patient how to care for the skin at the site of surgery, as well as the arm on the affected side.

—For modified radical or partial mastectomy:

Teach the patient to change the dressing, assess appearance of the incision and drain site, empty the drainage container, and record the amount and character of drainage.

Caution the patient not to abduct the affected arm or raise the arm or elbow above the shoulder until drains are removed.

Instruct the patient to report any redness or drainage around the drain.

—Instruct the patient to avoid use of deodorants or antiperspirant until stitches and drains have been removed from the ax-

---

### HAND AND ARM CARE INSTRUCTIONS

• While the patient is in bed, position the affected arm on one small and one large pillow so that the wrist is slightly higher than the elbow, and the elbow is slightly higher than the shoulder.
• The patient should get out of bed on the unaffected side.
• Encourage the patient to perform ball-squeezing and range-of-motion exercises as instructed by the physical therapist.
• Have the patient avoid using deodorants or antiperspirants until the stitches have been removed from the axilla and the wound has healed.

---

*Continued.*

### HAND AND ARM CARE INSTRUCTIONS
### —cont'd

- Encourage the patient to perform activities of daily living (ADLs) as tolerated with the following precautions:

  —Wear canvas gloves when gardening.

  —Wear a long, padded glove on the affected arm when reaching into an oven.

  —Wear a thimble when sewing.

  —Wear rubber gloves when using harsh detergents or steel wool.

  —Apply hand lotion to prevent dry skin.

  —Use an electric razor for underarm shaving to avoid nicking the skin.

  —Do not allow injections, intravenous lines, blood to be drawn, or blood pressure to be taken on the affected arm.

  —Use insect repellent to avoid insect bites.

  —Avoid using constricting jewelry or clothing on the affected arm.

  —Use a sunscreen (SPF of 15 or greater), and avoid overexposure to the sun.

  —Use cuticle cream and a nail file to trim fingernails.

  —If the affected arm is burned, apply ice and leave it exposed to the air until the blister breaks. Then wash with soap and water, apply antiseptic solution (e.g., iodine), and cover the area with a bandage. Notify the health care provider if the area does not heal.

  —If the affected arm is cut, wash the area with soap and water, apply an antiseptic (e.g., iodine), and cover the area with a bandage. Notify the health care provider if the area does not heal.

  —Call the health care provider if redness, pain, or increased swelling develops.

From Brown M et al: *Standards of oncology nursing practice,* New York, 1986, John Wiley & Sons.

illa and the wound has healed. If no drain is present, the patient may shower.

—Caution the patient not to allow injections, intravenous lines, drawing of blood, or taking of blood pressure in the affected arm.

—Instruct the patient to avoid wearing constricting clothing or jewely on the affected arm and to carry her handbag on the unaffected arm.

—Discuss the types of temporary and permanent prostheses available; assist with referral as needed. Advise the patient not to use an external prosthesis or bra pad until swelling has subsided and healing of the incision is complete. Tell her to check with a physician or nurse before using a prosthesis.

—Discuss types of reconstruction available.

—Stress the importance of continuing breast self-examination and mammography of the unaffected breast.

• *Warning signs*

—Review the signs and symptoms that should be reported to a physician or nurse.

> Swelling of arm
>
> Drainage from incision, excessive drainage or blood in Hemovac, difficulty keeping container flat
>
> Infection: redness, purulent drainage, pain, incision warm to touch

• *Medications*

—Explain the purpose, dosage, schedule, and route of administration of any prescribed drugs, as well as side effects to report to a physician or nurse.

—Provide pain management, offering alternative methods to deal with postoperative pain: visualization, guided imagery, meditation, relaxation, biofeedback.

• *Activity*

—Discuss the need to continue postmastectomy exercises to regain full range of motion.

—Encourage discussion of allowances and limitations with respect to occupation, recreational sports, or activities.

—Encourage resumption of self-care activities (feeding, combing hair) and activities of daily living as tolerated.

—Explain that sexual activity may be resumed when desired. The partner should use a position that does not place pressure on the chest wall.

**FOLLOW-UP CARE**

- Stress the importance of regular follow-up visits. Make sure the patient has the necessary names and telephone numbers.
- Prepare the patient for adjuvant therapies: hormone therapy, chemotherapy, radiation therapy.

**REFERRALS**

- Assist the patient to obtain referral services and contact support groups such as the American Cancer Society's Reach to Recovery program to cope with alterations in body image and other concerns.

# Bronchitis

**—Bronchitis: inflammation of the large airways (bronchi) and their branches (tracheobronchial tree) that results in production of mucus. Chronic bronchitis results from repeated exposure of irritants that cause tissue irritation, swelling (hypertrophy) of mucus-producing cells in bronchi, and mucus secretion. Long-term exposure to irritants such as cigarette smoking, air pollutants, and toxic industrial gases or fumes is known to cause hypertrophy of mucus-producing cells.**

**SIGNS/SYMPTOMS**

- Cough that is persistent and productive
- Sputum: clear and copious in the morning; thick, tenacious, and purulent during acute attack
- Wheezing and bronchospasm
- Duskiness or cyanosis
- Fever

**COMPLICATIONS**

- Emphysema
- Respiratory infections
- Respiratory failure

**B**

## DIAGNOSTIC TESTS

- Describe each procedure, its purpose, and the normal feelings or sensations that are likely, as well as any preprocedural and postprocedural care.
    - —Serum studies: complete blood count: to evaluate presence of elevated hemoglobin (polycythemia), presence of infections with increased WBCs
    - —Arterial blood gases: to evaluate presence of hypoxemia and acid-base abnormalities
    - —Chest x-ray: to detect changes in chest (anterior-posterior) diameter
    - —Sputum culture: to detect presence of infection
    - —Pulmonary function: to evaluate degree of impaired respiratory function (reduced vital capacity, increased residual volume due to air trapping)

## TREATMENT

*Medical*
- Therapy
    - —Chest physiotherapy: to loosen and mobilize secretions
    - —Oxygen therapy: low flow rate (1-2 liters) to treat hypoxemia
    - —Well-balanced diet; increased caloric intake if the patient begins to experience weight loss due to anorexia
    - —Oral or IV fluids: to maintain adequate hydration
- Drugs
    - —Bronchodilators: to relieve bronchospasm
    - —Sympathomimetics
    - —Antibiotics: for infections
    - —Diuretics: to reduce fluid retention in the presence of cardiac complications such as heart failure

## HOME CARE

- Give both the patient and the caregiver *verbal* and *written* instructions. Provide them with the name and telephone number of a physician or nurse to call if questions arise. Use visual aids to assist in instruction.
- *Warning signs*
    - —Review the signs and symptoms that should be reported to a physician or nurse.

- *Special instructions*
  —Review the purpose and demonstrate the proper use of all equipment to be used at home, including the oral inhaler and oxygen therapy equipment. For the latter, include discussion of when to use it, the importance of not increasing the flow rate without checking with a physician or home health nurse, and the procedure for ordering replacements.
- *Medications*
  —Explain the purpose, dosage, schedule, and route of administration of any prescribed drugs, as well as side effects to report to a physician or nurse.
- *Activity*
  —Encourage regular exercise to tolerance; avoid or curtail activities when fatigued, during weather extremes, or on smoggy days.
- *Diet*
  —Instruct the patient to eat a well-balanced diet. As the patient becomes more dyspneic, frequent small feedings may be needed to maintain adequate caloric intake.
  —Encourage fluid intake to keep secretions moist (1 liter per day unless contraindicated).

# Bronchoscopy

—**Bronchoscopy: direct visual examination of the trachea and tracheobronchial tree with a flexible fiberoptic tube.**

## INDICATIONS

- To determine the cause of respiratory symptoms
- To obtain a tissue specimen for analysis of lung diseases, infections, and bronchogenic cancers
- To remove foreign bodies, mucus plugs, or excessive secretions from the airway
- To prevent or treat collapsed lung tissue

**B**

## PREPROCEDURAL TEACHING

- Review the physician's explanation of the procedure and the reason for it; encourage the patient to ask questions and to discuss any fears or anxieties.

### Review of Preprocedural Care

- Discuss who will perform the procedure and where it will take place.
- Instruct the patient to have someone available after the procedure to drive the patient home.
- Instruct the patient not to eat or drink fluids for 6 to 12 hours before the test.
- Describe the procedure.
  —It is usually done on an outpatient basis and takes 45 to 60 minutes.
  —The patient is given medications before the procedure: atropine to decrease secretions and a barbiturate or narcotic for sedation.
  —The patient is usually placed in a supine position (alternative position is sitting upright) with the neck hyperextended. The patient is instructed to breathe through the nose.
  —The physician sprays a local anesthetic in the patient's throat and nasal cavity to anesthetize the vocal cords and suppress the gag reflex. The anesthetic may cause a cold, unpleasant sensation in the throat.
  —The lubricated bronchoscope is inserted through the nose or mouth. Explain that the patient will be able to breathe through and around the tube. The tube is advanced into the trachea and bronchi.
  —Once the examination is completed and/or the specimens are obtained, the bronchoscope is removed.

### Review of Postprocedural Care

- After the procedure the patient is moved to a recovery area where vital signs are monitored frequently. The patient remains NPO until the gag reflex returns.
- Explain that the patient may experience temporary hoarseness and a sore throat. Lozenges and throat gargles can be provided after the gag reflex returns.

**HOME CARE**

- Give both the patient and the caregiver *verbal* and *written* instructions. Provide them with the name and telephone number of a physician or nurse to call if questions arise.
- *Warning signs*
  —Review the signs and symptoms that should be reported to a physician or nurse.
  - Difficulty breathing
  - Chest pain
  - Inability to swallow
  - Bloody mucus
- *Medications*
  —Explain the purpose, dosage, schedule, and route of administration of any prescribed drugs, as well as side effects to report to a physician or nurse.
- *Diet*
  —Inform the patient that a soft or liquid diet is needed for the first day or until throat pain disappears.
  —Explain that extremely hot foods or liquids should be avoided.
  —Encourage fluid intake unless contraindicated.

**FOLLOW-UP CARE**

- Stress the importance of regular follow-up visits. Make sure the patient has the necessary names and telephone numbers.
- Discuss the importance of not smoking.

# Buerger's Disease

—**Buerger's disease: a rare arterial vascular disease characterized by acute inflammatory lesions and occlusive thrombosis of the small and medium arteries and veins. The legs, feet, upper limbs, and viscera are most frequently affected. The arteries most commonly involved are the anterior and posterior tibial, plantar, digital, radial, ulnar, and palmar.**

## CAUSES/CONTRIBUTING FACTORS

- Hypersensitivity to nicotine
- Autoimmune disorder

- Male, age 20 to 40 years
- Heavy smokers
- Genetic predisposition
- Jewish ancestry
- Persons living in India and other Asian countries

## SIGNS/SYMPTOMS

- Pain
- Intermittent claudication of the instep of the foot, cyanosis, and numbness of feet when exposed to cold, changing later to red, hot, tingly feet
- Ulcerated, painful fingertips, with associated impairment of peripheral pulses and thrombophlebitis
- Changes in the appearance of the nails or skin
- Edema of the legs
- Gangrene with involvement of the lower leg and in patients with diabetes

## COMPLICATIONS

- Ulcerations
- Gangrene
- Muscle atrophy
- Infection

## DIAGNOSTIC TESTS

- Describe each procedure, its purpose, and the normal feelings or sensations that are likely, as well as any preprocedural and postprocedural care.
    —Arteriography: to locate lesions and rule out atherosclerosis
    —Skin temperature determination
    —Blood studies
    —Chest x-rays
    —Doppler ultrasound: to show diminished circulation in the peripheral vessels
    —Plethysmography: to help detect decreased circulation in the peripheral vessels

## TREATMENT

*Medical*

- The goal of medical treatment is to arrest the progress of the disease.

- Drugs
  —Vasodilators: to promote circulation, relieve pain, and provide emotional support

*Surgical*
- Regional sympathetic ganglionectomy: to produce vasodilation
- Amputation: for cases of severe infection or toxicity and to relieve extreme pain in severe cases of gangrene

## HOME CARE

- Give both the patient and the caregiver *verbal* and *written* instructions. Provide them with the name and telephone number of a physician or nurse to call if questions arise.
- *General information*
  —Review explanation of the disease, underlying causes, and precipitating factors.
  —Discuss the role nicotine plays in advancing the disease; stress the importance of not smoking or using tobacco.
- *Warning signs*
  —Review the signs and symptoms that should be reported to a physician or nurse.
    - Intermittent claudication
    - Coldness and numbness of extremities
    - Ulcerations or sores that will not heal
- *Special instructions*
  —Caution the patient to avoid precipitating factors.
    - Extreme temperatures or prolonged exposure
    - Injuries to the feet
    - Emotional stress
  —Discuss measures to prevent complications.
  —Provide instruction on daily foot care.
    - Wear well-fitted shoes; avoid going barefoot.
    - Use cotton or wool socks.
    - Inspect feet daily for cuts, abrasions, and sores and report any found to the physician or nurse.
    - Keep feet clean and dry.
  —Instruct the patient on treating ulcers or gangrene.
    - Maintain bed rest, using a padded footboard or heat cradle to avoid pressure from bed linens.
    - Wash ulcers with mild soap and tepid water; avoid vigorous rubbing. Rinse thoroughly and dry well.
    - Apply cotton padding over the area for protection or as directed.

B

>     If there are sores between the toes, separate the toes with
>       cotton to promote healing.
>   —Caution the patient to avoid use of heating pads and hot wa-
>     ter bottles.
> • *Medications*
>   —Explain the purpose, dosage, schedule, and route of adminis-
>     tration of any prescribed drugs, as well as side effects to re-
>     port to a physician or nurse.
> • *Activity*
>   —Encourage the discussion of allowances and limitations with
>     regard to exercise and activities.

**FOLLOW-UP CARE**

- Stress the importance of regular follow-up visits. Make sure the
  patient has the necessary names and telephone numbers.
- Provide information about smoking cessation programs.

---

# Bunion
## (Hallux Valgus)

—**Bunion: bony prominence of the first metatarsal head and
enlarged bursa that develops secondary to the hallux valgus
deformity. Bunions form because of pressure and inflammation in almost all cases of hallux valgus.**

—**Hallux valgus: lateral deviation (outward bending) of the
great toe, away from the midline.**

—**Hallux valgus deformity: angulation of the great toe away
from the midline toward the second and other toes. In some
cases the great toe deviates over or under one or more of the
toes. The deformity is common in women in their sixties with
a strong familial tendency and in adolescent girls.**

**CAUSES/CONTRIBUTING FACTORS**

- Prolonged pressure aggravated by wearing narrow-toed shoes
  that do not fit properly, are high heeled, or do not adequately
  support the feet

- Degenerative conditions: rheumatoid arthritis, osteoarthritis, diabetes mellitus
- Congenital hallux valgus

## SIGNS/SYMPTOMS

- Valgus (away from midline) deformity with altered gait
- Inflammation of the bursa (bunion): redness, swelling, warmth, tenderness, pain
- Great difficulty in fitting shoes
- Deformity and crowding of second toe
- Splayfoot (spreading out of foot)

## COMPLICATIONS

- Development of bunion
- Stress fracture
- Degenerative joint disease

## DIAGNOSTIC TESTS

- Describe each procedure, its purpose, and the normal feelings or sensations that are likely, as well as any preprocedural and postprocedural care.
    —X-rays: to show displacement of the great toe, degenerative arthritic joint changes

## TREATMENT

*Medical*
- Therapy
    —Appropriately fitted or molded footwear to accommodate the deformity
    —Night splints to decrease discomfort
    —Felt ring pads or covering cap around bunion to relieve pressure
    —Application of moist compresses to bursitis area
    —Application of ice to site of bunion to lessen pain and inflammation
    —Foot exercises to lessen splayfoot
*Surgical*
- Bunionectomy and arthroplasty

## HOME CARE

- Give both the patient and the caregiver *verbal* and *written* instructions. Provide them with the name and telephone number of a physician or nurse to call if questions arise.

B

- *General information*
  —Review explanation of the disease and contributing factors.
- *Special instructions*
  —Discuss the importance of and give examples of proper footware and its role in prevention and progression of bunion formation.
  —Provide instruction in the proper application of felt rings or pads and other orthoses to prevent the progression of deformities.
- *Medications*
  —Explain the purpose, dosage, schedule, and route of administration of any prescribed drugs, as well as side effects to report to a physician or nurse.
    Analgesics
    Antipyretics
    Antiinflammatory medications
- *Activity*
  —Instruct the patient in exercises to strengthen foot muscles, such as standing at the edge of a step on the heel and then raising and inverting the top of the foot.

# Bunionectomy

—**Bunionectomy: surgical procedure to correct hallux valgus, performed when the patient has significant pain and alterations in ambulation. This surgery involves removal of the projecting metatarsal head as well as excision of the proximal part of the proximal phalanx. Depending on the extent of involvement of the joint and surrounding soft tissues, a number of other procedures may be included in the operative procedure. The addition of these procedures will affect the length of recovery and rehabilitation:**

- **Arthroplasty: removal of part of the bone and realignment to permit rebuilding of the joints**
- **Osteotomy: cutting of the bone and resetting it using a pin or pins to maintain proper alignment**

- **Soft tissue reconstruction: realignment of the toes where the soft tissue, tendons, and muscles of the foot have become stretched or contracted**
- **Prosthetic implant: removal of part of the joint and replacement with an implant**

## INDICATIONS

- Severe deformity and pain of hallux valgus

## PREPROCEDURAL TEACHING

- Review the physician's explanation of the procedure and the reason for it; encourage the patient to ask questions and to discuss any fears or anxieties.

### Review of Preprocedural Care

- Explain that the procedure is usually done on an outpatient basis.
- Discuss preoperative tests: blood tests, chest x-ray, electrocardiogram.
- Discuss skin preparation: the patient should shower with bactericidal soap the night before; the skin at the operative site will be shaved.
- Explain that the patient is NPO from midnight of the night before surgery.

### Review of Postprocedural Care

- Discuss the need to immobilize the affected foot with a short leg cast, slipper cast, or bunion boot (to immobilize the great toe).
- Discuss the need to maintain complete bed rest for 24-48 hours, then up with crutches without weight bearing as prescribed by the physician.
- Explain the need to elevate the extremity on firm pillows to lessen swelling.
- Explain that ice bags will be placed on the operative site to reduce swelling for 24-72 hours.
- Inform the patient that vital signs and neurovascular status will be checked every 15 minutes for the first hour and then with decreasing frequency.

## SIDE EFFECTS/COMPLICATIONS

- Excessive scarring or recurrence of bunion
- Weakening of foot joint

B

- Infection
- Neurovascular damage

## HOME CARE

- Give both the patient and the caregiver *verbal* and *written* instructions. Provide them with the name and telephone number of a physician or nurse to call if questions arise.
- *Warning signs*
  —Review the signs and symptoms that should be reported to a physician or nurse.
     Neurovascular impairment of affected extremity: persistent changes in color (pallor, cyanosis, redness), coolness, paresthesias (numbness, tingling)
     Infection: increased redness, swelling at incision, purulent drainage from wound, foul odor from cast or dressing, fever, increasing pain
- *Special instructions*
  —Discuss the importance of wearing an immobilization device (cast or bunion boot) for 3-6 weeks after surgery.
  —Instruct the patient on caring for the casted extremity (or dressed foot) (see Cast Care, p. 155).
  —Advise the patient to wear flat, wide-toed shoes and sandals after the dressing or cast is removed.
  — Instruct the patient to elevate the feet whenever experiencing pain or swelling of the feet and to report to the physician if pain and swelling do not subside.
- *Medications*
  —Explain the purpose, dosage, schedule, and route of administration of any prescribed drugs, as well as side effects to report to a physician or nurse.
- *Activity*
  —Inform the patient of the importance of limiting activity and resting frequently with feet elevated.
  —Discuss the importance of using crutches without weight bearing as prescribed by the physician. Refer the patient to physical therapy for instruction.
  —Review safety precautions to be taken when ambulating with crutches (see Crutch Walking, p. 219).

## FOLLOW-UP CARE

- Stress the importance of regular follow-up visits. Make sure the patient has the necessary names and telephone numbers.

# Burns

—**Burn: injury to the skin and epithelial tissues that results from direct contact or exposure to temperature extremes or electrical, chemical, or radiation sources.**

## CLASSIFICATION OF BURNS

- Superficial (first degree): epidermis is red with no blister formation
  —Signs/symptoms
     Pain
     Redness
     Blanching with pressure
     Normal texture
- Partial thickness (second degree): epidermal and dermal layers are blistered, with subcutaneous edema and pain
  —Signs/symptoms
     Pain
     Blisters
     Redness
     Blanching with pressure
     Firm texture
- Full thickness (third and fourth degree): all layers of skin involved; fat, muscle, nerves, blood supply, and bone may be affected
  —Signs/symptoms
     Dryness
     Pale, white, brown, or red color
     Charring
     No capillary refill
     No pain
     Firm, leathery skin texture

## CAUSES

- Thermal burns: exposure to flames, hot liquids, radiation
- Chemical burns: contact, ingestion, inhalation, or injection of acids, alkalies, or vesicants
- Electrical burns: electrical current passing through the body to the ground

**COMPLICATIONS**

- Dehydration
- Hypoxia
- Circulatory collapse
- Hematuria, oliguria
- Anemia
- Adult respiratory distress syndrome
- Septic shock
- Emotional shock
- Curling's ulcer
- Gastric atony
- Disseminated intravascular coagulation
- Disuse atrophy, contractures
- Infection

**DIAGNOSTIC TESTS**

- Describe each procedure, its purpose, and the normal feelings or sensations that are likely, as well as any preprocedural and postprocedural care.
  —Laboratory studies
      Complete blood count
      Electrolytes
      Blood urea nitrogen, creatinine
      Arterial carboxyhemoglobin
      Arterial blood gases
      Bilirubin
      Phosphorus
      Alkaline phosphatase
      Urine for myoglobin and hemoglobin tests
  —Bronchoscopy: to determine upper airway injury
  —Lung scan: to determine small airway burns

**TREATMENT**
**Immediate Treatment of Major Burns**

*Medical*

- Therapy
  —NPO for first 12-24 hours; total parenteral nutrition
  —Airway maintenance
  —Fluid replacement
  —Urethral catheterization

—Nasogastric tube insertion
—Wound cleansing with bactericidal solution
• Drugs
  —Narcotic analgesics
  —Sedatives
  —Tetanus immunization
  —Diphtheria-tetanus vaccine

*Surgical*
• Escharotomy
• Fasciotomy

## Long-term Treatment of Major Burns

*Medical*
• Therapy
  —Hydrotherapy: 1-2 times daily to remove dressings and debride wounds
  —Dressings: wet to dry or dry
  —Hyperalimentation if necessary; high-calorie, high-protein diet with vitamin and iron supplement
• Drugs
  —Antibiotics: topical sterile application
  —Narcotic analgesics

*Surgical*
• Skin grafts
• Amputation if limb severely injured
• Wound debridement

## Minor burns

*Medical*
• Therapy
  —Wound cleansing with bactericidal solution
  —Wound debridement
  —Dressing changes: nonadherent multilayered dressings changed 1-2 times daily; polyurethane, hydrocolloid, silver sulfadiazine dressings left on for several days to 1 week
• Drugs
  —Tetanus vaccine
  —Diphtheria-tetanus vaccine
  —Topical antibiotics
  —Narcotic analgesics
  —Analgesic-antipyretics

## HOME CARE

- Give both the patient and the caregiver *verbal* and *written* instructions. Provide them with the name and telephone number of a physician or nurse to call if questions arise.
- *General information*
  —Review the explanation of the type of burn and the extent of damage.
  —Discuss and prepare the patient for transfer to rehabilitation or long-term facility as ordered.
- *Wound/incision care*
  —Instruct the patient in wound care and dressing changes (for minor burns).
    Inspect wound for signs of infection.
    Cleanse wound with half-strength Betadine using sterile gauze; rub gently to remove existing topical agent.
    Apply topical antibiotic thickly enough to cover wound to provide healing and prevent dressing from adhering.
    Apply nonadherent fine-mesh gauze, then fluffed bulky coarse gauze to absorb drainage. Hold in place with semielastic net to exert even pressure.
  —Discuss the importance of avoiding contamination. Explain how to dispose of soiled dressings.
  —Review the care of healed burns.
    Wash skin gently, rinse well, dry thoroughly, and apply cream.
    Avoid exposure to sunlight, harsh detergent, fabric softeners, and irritation by rubbing of clothing.
    Use moisturizers and sunscreens to decrease irritation.
- *Warning signs*
  —Review the signs and symptoms that should be reported to a physician or nurse.
    Fever, malaise
    Bleeding, odor, drainage from burn area
- *Special instructions*
  —Advise the patient to avoid contact with persons with infections, especially upper respiratory infections.
  —Advise and assist the patient in obtaining medical supplies for dressings and any special assistive devices for home care management.
- *Medications*
  —Explain the purpose, dosage, schedule, and route of adminis-

tration of any prescribed drugs, as well as side effects to report to a physician or nurse.

—Caution the patient to avoid using over-the-counter medications unless approved by a physician.

* *Activity*
  —Explain the importance of planning rest periods.
  —Discuss maintaining normal activity as tolerated.
  —Encourage active and passive range-of-motion exercises of affected limbs to prevent muscle wasting and contractures.
  —Instruct the patient on the use of any assistive-adaptive or positioning devices as ordered.
  —Explain the importance of physiotherapy to assist in the exercise regimen.
  —Encourage water exercises to maintain limb mobility.
  —Encourage discussion of allowances and limitations with regard to occupation, recreational sports, and activities.
* *Diet*
  —Emphasize the importance of a diet high in calories, protein, and vitamins to maintain weight and aid in healing. Refer the patient to the dietary department for assistance in meal planning.
  —Encourage adequate fluid intake.

**FOLLOW-UP CARE**

* Stress the importance of regular follow-up visits with physician, laboratory, and physical therapy until recovery is complete. Make sure the patient has the necessary names and telephone numbers.

**REFERRALS**

* Advise about and refer the patient to support groups and community resources to assist in the resumption of usual activities and relationships.

# Cancer

—Cancer: the most common cause of death in the United States, cancer is a universal disease that affects people without regard to race, gender, socioeconomic status, or culture. However, different forms of cancer strike specific age, ethnic, and gender groups with varying frequency and severity. The most common sites of fatal cancer in men are the lungs, prostate, colon, and rectum; in women they are the lungs, breasts, colon, and rectum. Some cancers, such as those of the stomach, breast, colon, rectum, uterus, and lung, occur in a familial pattern. Certain diseases, such as multiple familial polyposis and Gardner's syndrome, are premalignant. Other possible causes of cancer include immunosuppressive drugs and viruses (adenoviruses, papovaviruses, herpes viruses, human T-cell lymphoma-leukemia virus, Epstein-Barr virus, and hepatitis B virus).

## PREVENTION

- Assess the patient's level of knowledge about risk factors, preventive measures, and signs and symptoms of specific types of cancer that should be reported to a physician or nurse. Clarify any fears or misconceptions.
- Review primary prevention guidelines.
  —Smoking: do not smoke; stop smoking if already a habit; avoid use of tobacco products such as cigarettes, cigars, snuff, chewing tobacco, and pipe tobacco.
  —Sunlight: avoid exposure to sunlight; use a sunscreen if being in the sun is necessary; wear protective clothing, especially a cover for the face and head.
  —Radiation: avoid excessive exposure to ionizing radiation and radon.
  —Occupational hazards: avoid exposure to industrial agents such as asbestos.
  —Alcohol: limit consumption of alcohol.
  —Nutrition: eat high-fiber foods, low-fat foods, and vegetables and fruits rich in vitamins A and C; avoid salt-cured, smoked, and nitrite-cured foods; maintain proper weight for age, sex, and body frame.
- Inform female patients of specific preventive measures for women:
  —Perform monthly breast examinations, preferably after the menstrual period.
  —Have regular breast examinations: every 3 years from women ages 20-39, every year for women 40 and older.

—Have mammography: baseline examination between the ages of 35 and 39, every 1-2 years for ages 40-49, every year for ages 50 and older.

—Have a Papanicolaou (Pap) test and pelvic examination every year if sexually active or age 18 and over.

—Use caution with estrogen replacement therapy to control symptoms of menopause.

—Avoid prolonged use of estrogen birth control pills.

• Inform male patients of specific preventive measures for men.

—Perform testicular self-examination every month after age 15.

—Have regular physical examinations for prostate cancer: yearly for men less than 50 years, every 6 months for men 50 years and older.

## STAGING AND GRADING OF CANCER

The purpose of cancer staging and grading is to describe the extent of the malignant tumor so that the physician can plan treatment, determine the prognosis, and evaluate the results. Staging should be done during the pretreatment phase of disease and after surgery if that is one of the prescribed treatments. It is also done if the disease recurs after a disease-free interval.

Clinical staging includes physical examination and evaluation of biopsy specimens (tumor and lymph nodes). The generally used staging system (TNM) is based on measurement of primary tumor (size, depth of penetration, invasion of adjacent structures); lymph node involvement (presence, extent, and location); and metastatic spread (presence of distant metastases) (see table on opposite page).

Grading is histologic classification of tumor, which is useful in determining prognosis. Cancers are usually classified as 1 (well differentiated) to 4 (poorly differentiated). The more poorly differentiated a tumor is, the less it looks like normal cells and the poorer the prognosis.

## GENERAL CARE

The patient may experience loss of appetite, nausea and vomiting, or stomatitis as a result of cancer or its treatment. Both the patient and caregiver should know what problems may develop and how to manage them.

Cancer staging using TNM classification*

| Stage | T | N | M | Survival | Comments |
|-------|---|---|---|----------|----------|
| I | 1 | 0 | 0 | 70%-90% | Operable and resectable |
| II | 2 | 1 | 0 | 50%± | Operable but uncertainty of total resection |
| III | 3 | 2 | 0 | 20%± | Operable but not resectable |
| IV | 4 | 3 | + | <5% | Distant metastases; inoperable |

*T*, Primary tumor; $T_1$, $T_2$, $T_3$, $T_4$, progressive increase in tumor size or involvement; *N*, regional lymph modes; $N_1$, $N_2$, $N_3$, increasing degree of abnormal regional lymph nodes; *M*, metastasis present; $M_0$, absence; $M_+$, presence.

*Survival rates and comments may vary with type and location of primary tumor, nodes, and metastases.

### Loss of Appetite

Loss of appetite can be a serious problem, leading to malnutrition and severe weight loss. Eating enough of the right kinds of food can be difficult when the patient has little or no appetite.

- Take a walk before mealtime; mild exercise can stimulate appetite.
- Avoid drinking liquids before meals, since fluids are filling. If drink is desired, drink something nutritious such as juice or milk.
- Eat with family or friends if possible. Eating will seem less of a chore if it is a social event.
- Eat a variety of foods. Make food more appealing with herbs, spices, and sauces. Use butter, bacon bits, croutons, wine sauces, and marinades.
- Do not fill up on salads or "diet" foods. Eat vegetables and fruits with meat, poultry, and fish to ensure enough calories and proper nutrition.
- Eat smaller meals more often.
- The physican may recommend dietary supplements that can be added to milk, soup, or pudding.

### Nausea and Vomiting

Nausea and vomiting are common side effects of cancer chemotherapy and radiation therapy. Physicians often prescribe an antiemetic a few hours before treatment and every 3 or 4 hours after treatment for 1 or 2 days.

- Eat soda crackers and suck on sour candy balls during the day to relieve queasiness.
- Choose cold or room-temperature foods instead of hot ones, since hot and warm foods seem to cause nausea.
- Avoid salt, fatty and sweet foods, or any food with a strong odor. Choose bland, creamy foods such as cottage cheese, toast, and mashed potatoes.
- Stay away from nauseating odors, sights, and sounds. Get as much fresh air as possible; a leisurely walk can help relieve nausea.
- Do not eat just before a cancer treatment. Eat lightly for a few hours after treatment.
- Try relaxation therapy, self-hypnosis, or imagery to relieve nausea-inducing tension.
- Encourage distraction with a book, television, or activity.
- Sleep during episodes of nausea, if possible.
- If vomiting occurs, eat or drink nothing until the stomach is settled, usually a few hours after the last vomiting episode. Then begin sipping clear liquids or sucking on ice cubes. If liquids are tolerated, begin eating bland foods a few hours after starting liquids.

**Stomatitis**

Inflammation of the lining of the mouth may occur 7-14 days after the beginning of cancer chemotherapy or radiation therapy to the mouth, or may begin earlier if other problems are present. A dentist should assess the status of the mouth and teeth before treatment begins.

- Stomatitis can be prevented or alleviated by using a soft-bristled toothbrush and rinsing with a solution of 1 pint of water with ½ teaspoon of salt and ½ teaspoon of baking soda after meals and at bedtime. Flossing with unwaxed dental floss, drinking water or nonacidic juice, eating artificially sweetened candy, chewing artificially sweetened gum, and using artificial saliva sprays for dry mouth may also help.
- Watch for signs and symptoms of stomatitis: burning feeling in mouth; red, irritated oral lining; swollen, inflamed tongue; sores in mouth.
- Treatment is based on the extent and seriousness of the stomatitis. Measures include rinsing with the solution described above; loosening thick mucus and crusted drainage with Milk

of Magnesia, Maalox, or another antacid; or using an analgesic rinse before meals to lessen pain of swallowing.
- Wear dentures only during meals.
- Avoid spicy, acidic, and crusty or rough foods and hot or cold foods and beverages.
- Report signs of infection to the physician or nurse: soft, white patches; dry, brownish yellow ulcers with well-defined edges; or open areas on the lips or mouth.

**TERMINOLOGY**

Benign versus malignant: see table below

Doubling time: mean length of time for division of all tumor cells present; it has been calculated that approximately 30 doubling times are required for a tumor to reach 1 centimeter in diameter

Direct invasion of contiguous organs or local spread: tumor cells can invade a structure such as the uterus; spread from one organ to another, such as from the colon to the liver; or implant in surrounding serous cavities such as cancer of the ovary that spreads to the peritoneal surface (also called seeding)

Differences between benign and malignant tumors

| Characteristic | Benign tumor | Malignant tumor |
| --- | --- | --- |
| Structure and differentiation | Typical of tissue origin | Atypical of tissue origin |
| Rate of growth | Usually slow | May be slow, rapid, or very rapid |
| Progression | Slowly progressive (may remain stationary; may regress); rarely fatal if treated | Usually progressive; almost always fatal if untreated |
| Mode of growth | Expansion (encapsulated) | Infiltration and/or metastasis |
| Tissue destruction | No | Common (ulceration and necrosis) |
| Recurrence | Rare | Common |
| Prognosis | May be fatal if inaccessible | Fatal if uncontrolled |

From Belcher AE: *Cancer nursing*, St Louis, 1992, Mosby.

Metastasis: spread of cancer from a primary site of origin to distant organs by lymphatics or blood vessels, for example, the spread of lung cancer to the brain; common sites of metastasis are the lungs, liver, bones, and brain

Types of cancer:

Carcinomas: cancers of epithelial cells

Sarcomas: cancers of bone, muscle, or connective tissue

Leukemias: cancers of blood-forming organs

Lymphomas: cancers of infection-fighting organs

# Cardiac Catheterization

—**Cardiac catheterization: an invasive procedure used to visualize the heart's chambers, valves, great vessels, and coronary arteries.**

## INDICATIONS

- To evaluate heart muscle and valve function
- To evaluate coronary arteries
- To diagnose valve abnormalities (insufficiency and stenosis)
- To identify and diagnose congenital heart anomalies
- Used in diagnostic and therapeutic procedures: electrophysiologic studies, hemodynamic monitoring, percutaneous transluminal angioplasty (PTA), palliative procedures for congenital heart defects

## PROCEDURE

The procedure, which uses a flexible radiopaque catheter, may involve one or all of the following:

- Right-sided catheterization: performed to evaluate the function of the right side of the heart, including pressures and cardiac output. This technique is also used for continuous hemodynamic monitoring at the bedside. Catheter insertion is through the arm, neck (basilic or subclavian vein), or leg (femoral vein). The catheter is then guided into the chambers of the right side of the heart and the pulmonary artery.

- Left-sided catheterization: performed to evaluate function and pressures of the aorta and left side of the heart. Information about muscle function and the mitral and aortic valves can be obtained. Catheter insertion is usually via an artery in the arm (brachial) or leg (femoral). The catheter is guided up to the aorta and then into the left ventricle across the aortic valve. The route of entry for either left or right catheterization is by cut-down or more commonly percutaneously.

- Angiography: performed during left-sided catheterization, angiography involves injection of radiopaque contrast material through a cardiac catheter to obtain sequential films that selectively visualize the coronary blood vessels or heart chambers. There are two filming methods: cineangiography, a technique that produces a motion picture film of the fluoroscopic images, and serial angiography, which produces a series of x-ray (roentgenographic) films.

Other techniques that are available to evaluate heart function include the following:

- Coronary arteriography: shows abnormalities in the coronary arteries
- Ventriculography of the right or left ventricle: demonstrates chamber volume, wall thickness, and wall motion and detects abnormalities of contraction and atrioventricular valve regurgitation

**PREPROCEDURAL TEACHING**

- Review the physician's explanation of the procedure and the reason for it; encourage the patient to ask questions and to discuss any fears or anxieties. Explain the need to obtain informed consent.

**Review of Preprocedural Care**

- Determine whether the patient has any allergies to shellfish or iodine.
- Explain that the procedure is usually done on an outpatient basis and that no food or fluids are permitted for 6-12 hours beforehand.
- Inform the patient that routine medications must be withheld as directed by the physician.
- Explain that the skin at the insertion site will be shaved and cleansed.

- Describe the procedure.
  - —The patient is taken to a special laboratory room and placed on a padded surgical table.
  - —Depending on the type of catheterization to be performed, the procedure takes 1-3 hours.
  - —The selected site is again cleansed and sterilized.
  - —A local anesthetic is injected into a selected site (groin, inside of right arm, right side of neck).
  - —A catheter is inserted and threaded up through the vein or artery. Once it is in place, the physician injects a contrast dye through it.
- Review sensations likely to be experienced during the procedure: palpitations; warm, flushed feeling; nausea or chest pain during insertion of the dye. Assure the patient that the sensations will pass quickly. Instruct the patient to follow directions to cough or breathe deeply.

**Review of Postprocedural Care**

- Explain that after the procedure is completed, the catheter is removed and a pressure dressing is applied to the site to control bleeding. The site is checked frequently for bleeding. For certain procedures (e.g., PTA), the catheter may be left in place. If the procedure is being done for diagnostic reasons, the patient is returned to a recovery room. If it is done for therapeutic reasons, the patient may be transferred to a special care unit.
- Discuss the sensations that may be felt: soreness at the insertion site, possible backache from lying on a table for 1-3 hours.
- Inform the patient of the need to maintain complete bed rest with the head slightly (20-30 degrees) elevated.
- Stress the importance of keeping the extremity straight and immobile for 2-4 hours after the procedure or as ordered.
- Inform the patient that vital signs, including peripheral pulses, will be checked every 15 minutes for the first hour, then with decreasing frequency.
- Tell the patient that diet and fluids will be resumed after return to the recovery area. Fluids are encouraged.

**SIDE EFFECTS/COMPLICATIONS**

- Ventricular dysrhythmias
- Allergic reaction to dye
- Nausea and vomiting

- Hypotension
- Thrombus (pain) at insertion site
- Local infection
- Cardiac perforation
- Myocardial ischemia
- Cardiac tamponade

## HOME CARE

- Give both the patient and the caregiver *verbal* and *written* instructions. Provide them with the name and telephone number of a physician or nurse to call if questions arise.
- *General information*
  —Review the procedure, answering any questions about the purpose or the physician's explanation of the findings.
- *Wound/incision care*
  —Provide instruction on care of the puncture site.
- *Warning signs*
  —Review the signs and symptoms that should be reported to a physician or nurse.
    Pain, swelling, or discoloration of puncture site
    Chest pain
    Elevated temperature
- *Activity*
  —Unless otherwise instructed, the patient may resume all normal activities within 1 week. Strenuous activities such as running, biking, or heavy lifting should be avoided for 5-7 days after the procedure.

## FOLLOW-UP CARE

- Stress the importance of regular follow-up visits. Make sure the patient has the necessary names and telephone numbers.

# Carotid Endarterectomy

—**Carotid endarterectomy: surgical removal of atherosclerotic plaque or thrombus from the carotid artery to increase blood flow through the carotid arteries to the brain.**

## INDICATIONS

- Transient ischemic attacks
- Syncope
- Dizziness
- Asymptomatic high-grade carotid lesions

## PREPROCEDURAL TEACHING

- Review the physician's explanation of the procedure and the reason for it; encourage the patient to ask questions and to discuss any fears or anxieties. Review the location of the lesion. Explain the need for written consent.

### Review of Preprocedural Care

- Explain that the operation may be performed under local (cervical block) or general anesthesia. An incision is made on the side of the neck where the diseased artery is located. The incision extends down from the jawline to the base of the neck. Explain that the patient may experience transient numbness in the earlobe after surgery.
- Review diagnostic tests that will be done to confirm the diagnosis: cerebral angiography, carotid ultrasound, and photoangiography.
- Discuss preoperative laboratory tests: blood and urine test, chest x-ray, electrocardiogram.
- Explain the need for the patient to be NPO for 12-24 hours before the operation.
- Explain that the patient may be admitted to the hospital on the day of surgery.
- Tell the patient that the operative site will be cleansed and shaved.

### Review of Postprocedural Care

- Inform the patient that ambulation will be permitted on the day of surgery if there are no complications.
- Explain that the patient may remain in the intensive care unit for 24 hours after surgery for monitoring and then transferred to a regular room.

## SIDE EFFECTS/COMPLICATIONS

- Stroke
- Heart attack

- Transient episodes of postoperative hypertension and hypotension
- Cranial nerve injuries
- Wound hematoma
- Infection
- Shock
- Seizure activity

## HOME CARE

- Give both the patient and the caregiver *verbal* and *written* instructions. Provide them with the name and telephone number of a physician or nurse to call if questions arise.
- *Wound/incision care*
  —Provide instruction regarding daily care of the surgical incision and dressing changes.
- *Warning signs*
  —Review the signs and symptoms that should be reported to a physician or nurse.
      Unusual pain or swelling in the operative area
      Signs of infection: redness, pain, swelling, soreness, feeling of tenderness, drainage
      Sudden changes in vision, gait, or muscle strength
- *Special instructions*
  —Describe the atherosclerotic process and discuss the importance of risk factor modification to reduce the chance of future plaque buildup in the carotid and other arteries (see Coronary Artery Disease, p. 204).
  —For any neurologic deficit or stroke complications, see p. 611.
- *Medications*
  —Explain the purpose, dosage, schedule, and route of administration of any prescribed drugs, as well as side effects to report to a physician or nurse.
- *Activity*
  —Tell the patient to exercise to tolerance but to avoid bending from the waist or lifting and straining.

## FOLLOW-UP CARE

- Stress the importance of regular follow-up visits. Make sure the patient has the necessary names and telephone numbers.

# Carpal Tunnel Syndrome

—Carpal tunnel syndrome: a combination of symptoms affecting the functioning of the wrist, hand, and fingers. Carpal tunnel syndrome occurs when inflammation and fibrosis of the tendon sheaths that pass through the carpal tunnel structures of the hand cause swelling and compression of the median nerve at the wrist, resulting in pain and numbness. Carpal tunnel syndome is one of the most common industrial or work-related conditions. It occurs most frequently in women between 30 and 60 years of age.

## CAUSES/CONTRIBUTING FACTORS

- Trauma, injury: wrist fractures, dislocation, sprains (but may occur with no prior history of trauma)
- Repetitive hand or wrist movement such as wrist twisting, turning, or pounding as occurs in some occupations (e.g., painters, computer users, jackhammer operators)
- Chronic medical disorders: rheumatoid arthritis, renal failure, Raynaud's disease
- Pregnancy: last trimester because of fluid retention and edema
- Menopause

## SIGNS/SYMPTOMS

Signs and symptoms may affect one or both hands. They are worse in the morning or at night and may awaken the patient. They may occur while the patient is holding the hand in one position, such as while driving or typing.
- Pain, numbness, tingling
- Grip strength loss, inability to make a fist
- Muscle weakness
- Wrist swelling
- Burning
- Palmar thenar (base of thumb) atrophy
- Comparative sensations loss over palmar thumb, index, middle, and radial half of ring finger

## COMPLICATIONS

- Prolonged muscle weakness and atrophy
- Rupture of tendon sheath from inadvertent injection of corticosteroid

## DIAGNOSTIC TESTS

- Describe each procedure, its purpose, and the normal feelings or sensations that are likely, as well as any preprocedural and postprocedural care.
  —Compression tests of the median nerve
  > Positive Tinel's sign: tingling over the median nerve with a light tapping over the tendon sheath on the ventral (inner) surface of the wrist
  > Positive Phalen's test: appearance of symptoms with the forearm in vertical position and wrist held in complete flexion for 1 minute
  > Positive compression test: pain, numbness, and tingling provoked when blood pressure cuff is inflated above systolic pressure on the forearm for 1-2 minutes
  —Electroconductive tests
  > Electromyogram: detects denervation of thenar muscles (base of thumb)
  > Nerve conduction velocity study: measures speed of electricity along nerve; may show delayed nerve response
  —X-ray: may show bony pressure on tunnel area; rules out fractures, arthritis

## TREATMENT

*Medical*

- Therapy
  —Conservative treatment usually tried first if symptoms have been present for less than 2 months
  —Wrist immobilization:
  > Splint to relieve pressure and decrease wrist flexion
  > Ice application to volar (ventral) wrist
  > Elevation to decrease edema
  > Restriction of twisting and turning of wrist
- Drugs
  —Local injection of hydrocortisone (into tendon sheath) to relieve inflammation
  —Antiinflammatory agents

*Surgical*
- Carpal tunnel release

**HOME CARE**

- Give both the patient and the caregiver *verbal* and *written* instructions. Provide them with the name and telephone number of a physician or nurse to call if questions arise.
- *General information*
  —Describe the disorder, causes, and contributing factors.
- *Warning signs*
  —Review the signs and symptoms that should be reported to a physician or nurse. Sensory changes are indicative of increased compression of the median nerve.
    Increased burning, tingling of fingers
    Increased pain
    Numbness
    Discoloration of fingers (i.e., red, blue, or white rather than pink)
- *Medications*
  —Explain the purpose, dosage, schedule, and route of administration of any prescribed drugs, as well as side effects to report to a physician or nurse.
- *Activity*
  —Instruct the patient to avoid activities that increase stress on inflamed tissues (grasping and gripping action of hand and wrist); to keep wrist in neutral position; to avoid using wrist in bent (flexed), twisted, turned position; and to minimize repetitive movements, including holding an object for extended periods of time. Advise the patient to wear a wrist splint to help keep the wrist in neutral position.
  —Discuss the role prevention plays in controlling carpal tunnel syndrome; review preventive measures.
    Limit wrist movement as flexion increases compression and tension of the inflamed nerve.
    Instruct patient how and when to apply night or occupational wrist splint, explaining that its purpose is to decrease wrist flexion and movement, especially at night or when engaging in repetitive wrist movement. Advise patient where to obtain splints.
  —Elevate hand above heart level to decrease swelling.
  —Apply ice to the wrist to decrease swelling.

—Teach patient range-of-motion exercises and explain their importance for maintaining strength of muscles. If patient is wearing splint, tell patient to remove it to perform daily exercises.

**FOLLOW-UP CARE**
- Stress the importance of regular follow-up visits. Make sure the patient has the necessary names and telephone numbers.

# Carpal Tunnel Release

—**Carpal tunnel release: surgical decompression of the nerve by releasing the carpal ligament to restore sensation and mobility to the hand.**

**INDICATIONS**
- Persistent or progressive signs and symptoms of carpal tunnel syndrome, unrelieved by conservative treatment

**PREPROCEDURAL TEACHING**
- Review the physician's explanation of the procedure and the reason for it; encourage the patient to ask questions and to discuss any fears or anxieties. Discuss the need for written consent for the surgery and local anesthesia.

### Review of Preprocedural Care
- Explain the need to be NPO from midnight of the night before surgery.
- Discuss the properative blood and urine tests.
- Inform the patient about the skin preparation: arm, wrist, and hand shaved and cleansed with bactericidal soap.
- Explain that hospital admission may be on the day of surgery.
- Explain that the procedure takes about 45 minutes and is done under local anesthesia.

### Review of Postprocedural Care
- Explain that the hand will be bandaged and the arm will be elevated in a cast or splint.

- Inform the patient that vital signs and neurovascular status will be checked every 15 minutes for the first hour and then at increasing intervals.
- Discuss the need to move all fingers of the affected hand frequently to improve circulation.

## SIDE EFFECTS/COMPLICATIONS

- Infection
- Neurovascular injury
- Keloid formation

## HOME CARE

- Give both the patient and the caregiver *verbal* and *written* instructions. Provide them with the name and telephone number of a physician or nurse to call if questions arise.
- *General information*
  —Review any explanation about the procedure and specific follow-up care.
- *Wound/incision care*
  —Instruct the patient on care of the hand and dressing: to keep arm and hand elevated above heart level to reduce swelling and promote healing.
  —Tell the patient to check the dressing daily for signs of increased bleeding or drainage. Discuss the need to keep the dressing clean, dry, and intact. Explain that when bathing is permitted (usually as soon as the patient feels strong), the patient should shower with the dressing covered by a plastic bag.
- *Warning signs*
  —Review the signs and symptoms that should be reported to a physician or nurse.
      Neurovascular impairment: burning, tingling sensation of fingers; increased pain or throbbing in fingers unrelieved by prescribed analgesics; inability to move fingers; discoloration of fingers; fingers that are cool and do not warm up after being covered
      Infection: fever >101° F, malaise, increased pain, foul odor from dressing
- *Medications*
  —Explain the purpose, dosage, schedule, and route of administration of any prescribed drugs, as well as side effects to report to a physician or nurse.

- *Activity*
    —Review activity allowances and limitation. Encourage discussion regarding return to work, recreational sports, and activities.
    —Discuss any prescribed exercises to maintain circulation and improve range of motion, such as sponge squeezing.

**FOLLOW-UP CARE**

- Stress the importance of regular follow-up visits. Make sure the patient has the necessary names and telephone numbers.

# Cast Care

—**Cast care: maintenance of a cast, a plaster- or synthetic-coated bandage that comes in strips or rolls. Casts are applied to immobilize musculoskeletal tissues following trauma or surgery. They are made of plaster, synthetic materials such as fiberglass or plastic, or cast tape. Fiberglass, plastic, and cast tape have some advantages over plaster because they may get wet without being seriously damaged, are lightweight, and last longer. In addition, x-rays can be taken with the cast on to evaluate the healing process, whereas the x-rays do not penetrate plaster well. The cast bandage, which comes in strips or rolls, is dipped in water and applied to the injured body part. It molds to the shape and then hardens as it dries.Types of casts include extremity casts (short arm, short leg, long leg), body casts (chest and abdomen), hip spica or spica casts (cover hips and one or both legs), cervical casts, and Minerva casts (cover chest, neck, and hand).**

**PREPROCEDURAL TEACHING**

- Review the physician's explanation of the procedure and the reason for it; encourage the patient to ask questions and to discuss any fears or anxieties.

**Review of Preprocedural Care**

- Explain the need for x-rays to ascertain the extent of trauma and assess bone alignment (before and after reduction).

- Describe how casts are applied.
  —A sedative, narcotic, or anesthetic may be given before application. The skin surface is checked for open lesions and blisters, then the skin is cleansed and rubbing alcohol is applied to dry the skin surface to be casted.
  —Soft padding is applied to the skin to protect it and underlying bones from direct contact with or pressure from the cast.
  —The cast is applied to fit snugly so that the injured bones are held immobilized and in the correct position. Explain that the cast will be looser after swelling of the injury subsides.

## SIDE EFFECTS/COMPLICATIONS

- Neurovascular impairment
- Fever
- Infection
- Skin impairment
- Compartment syndrome
- Cast syndrome

## HOME CARE

- Give both the patient and the caregiver *verbal* and *written* instructions. Provide them with the name and telephone number of a physician or nurse to call if questions arise.
- *Cast care*
  —Instruct the patient on the importance of protecting the cast until it dries: 2-3 days for plaster; usually less than a day for synthetic material.
    While the cast is still damp, elevate it on firm pillows without plastic covers to prevent it from becoming deformed.
    Explain that the skin underneath the cast will feel warm until it dries. However, warm areas after the cast has dried may indicate infection, which should be reported to the physician.
    While the cast is drying, it should be handled as little as possible. When necessary the cast is lifted by supporting it under two joints using the palms of the hands. Avoid pressing fingers into the cast, which would put pressure on the skin inside.
    The cast should be left uncovered to facilitate drying. Fans placed 18-24 inches from the cast may be used to speed drying except after open reduction. Heat lamps should not be used because they could burn the skin under the cast.

—Review daily care once the cast is completely dried.

Plaster casts must be kept dry; use plastic bags when bathing, using the toilet (for spica cast), or going out in rain or snow.

A damp cloth and scouring powder can be used to clean soiled spots.

For a synthetic cast such as fiberglass, immersion in water may be permitted if there are no wounds under the cast. The cast should be rinsed inside and out to flush out dirt and chemicals. The cast and stockinette should be dried thoroughly to avoid excess moisture on skin. A hair dryer set on the cool setting can be used.

—Instruct the patient on the importance of maintaining good skin care under and around the cast.

Do not insert objects such as coat hangers under the cast, since this could scrape the skin and cause infection.

Powders and lotions should be used only outside the cast so that the skin stays clean and soft.

Explain the importance of keeping dirt, sand, and powder away from the inside of the cast, since they can cause sore areas.

Instruct the patient to massage the skin distal to the cast.

Instruct the patient to notify the physician if skin irritation develops: redness, swelling, breaks in skin.

—Explain how to reduce swelling.

Elevate the injured part above the heart by propping it up on pillows or some other support (tell the patient to recline if the cast is on the leg).

Apply ice to the cast over the fractured area; ice should be put into a dry plastic bag or ice pack and should go half-way around the cast.

Advise the patient that swelling or edema around the site of injury is common at first and creates pressure against the inside of the cast. Advise the patient that for the first 48 hours or so after the cast is applied, it will feel tight.

As swelling subsides and the cast becomes loose, it may be necessary for the physician to replace the cast to ensure that broken bones do not move out of place.

• *Warning signs*

—Review the signs and symptoms that should be reported to a physician or nurse.

If soft spots or cracks develop in the cast or if it feels too loose

Pain or soreness under the cast, especially around bony prominences, such as the wrist or ankle, that is not relieved by repositioning of the body

Red, blue, or white color of the skin; when a finger or toe protruding from the cast is squeezed until it is white, the pink color should return within 4-6 seconds

Fingers or toes that are cool and do not warm up after 20 minutes of being covered

Increased swelling

Tingling or burning sensation

Inability to move the muscles around the cast

Foul odor around the cast edges

Any breaks or cracks in the case

For spica or body casts: shortness of breath, nausea, vomiting, abdominal distention (cast syndrome) caused by air swallowing

- *Activity*
  —Advise the patient not to walk on a leg cast for the first 48 hours unless otherwise instructed by the physician. Once allowed to walk on the cast, the patient should be sure to use a walking heel if weight bearing is permitted.
  —Describe and demonstrate proper use of ambulatory aids, such as crutches, cane, or walker. Refer the patient to a physical therapist as needed.
  —Discuss the need for active range-of-motion exercises to unaffected extremities and show the patient how to perform them.
- *Diet*
  —Encourage at least 3000 ml of fluids per day to maintain skin turgor.

# Cataract and Cataract Surgery

—**Cataract: growing opacity of the lens and lens capsule usually associated with aging, although it can be congenital or caused by trauma, heat, toxins, intraocular inflammation, or chronic disease.**

## RISK FACTORS

- Women over 65 years of age
- Residence in warm, sunny climate
- High-dose radiation
- Long-term use of drugs such as corticosteroids, phenothiazine, chemotherapy agents
- Diabetes
- High blood pressure
- Blunt trauma
- Maternal rubella in first trimester
- Down's syndrome

## SIGNS/SYMPTOMS

- Painless, gradual blurring
- Decreased peripheral vision
- Photophobia, glare, especially at night
- Milky white appearance of pupil
- Poor reading vision

## DIAGNOSTIC TESTS

- Ophthalmoscopy with dilatation
- Slit lamp examination

## TREATMENT

*Surgical*

- Cataract surgery if patient has diminished visual acuity or cataracts that may cause eye damage
- Cataract extraction: surgical extraction of the defective lens
  —Intracapsular: most common procedure; removal of the entire lens, including surrounding capsule
  —Extracapsular: removal of the anterior portion of the capsule and lens, leaving the posterior capsule intact; done on children and adults
  —Phacoemulsion: breaking the lens into fragments and particles using ultrasonic vibrations and removing them by suction; performed on patients under 30 years
  —Lens implantation: insertion of an intraocular lens implant following cataract excision; done to avoid the need to wear cataract glasses or contact lenses postoperatively; used for the following indications:

    Patients who are unable to manage self-care and insertion or removal of contact lenses (e.g., mentally impaired or with limited manual dexterity)

Other eye conditions that contraindicate contact lens wear (dry eyes, severe allergies, severe astigmatism)

Adverse work environment (presence of dust or fumes)

Only one eye affected

## PREPROCEDURAL TEACHING

- Review the physician's explanation of the procedure and the reason for it; encourage the patient to ask questions and to discuss any fears or anxieties.

### Review of Preprocedural Care

- Explain that the procedure is done as same-day surgery.
- Explain the need for the patient to be NPO from midnight of the night before surgery.
- Discuss routine preoperative laboratory tests: blood and urine.
- Discuss preoperative medications.
  - —Topical antiinfective agents, usually prescribed 1 week before surgery
  - —Mydriatic-cycloplegic agents, usually prescribed 2 hours before surgery
  - —Hyperosmotic agents
  - —Sedatives/hypnotics

### Review of Postprocedural Care

- Discuss the necessity of wearing an eye patch postoperatively for 24-72 hours.
- Discuss the need to wear a protective eye shield at night.
- Discuss postoperative medications.
  - —Mydriatic-cycloplegic agents (not used in patients with lens implants)
  - —Antiinfective eyedrops and ointments
  - —Corticosteroids
  - —Antiemetics
  - —Analgesics
- Explain that medication will be administered to prevent nausea, vomiting, and straining with elimination to avoid increasing ocular pressure.

## SIDE EFFECTS/COMPLICATIONS

- Cataract
  —Glaucoma
  —Blindness
- Cataract surgery
  —Wound rupture (from sutures loosening)
  —Hyphema
  —Hemorrhage
  —Prolapse of the iris into the anterior chamber
  —Loss of vitreous
  —Adhesions
  —Infection
  —Retinal detachment
  —Corneal edema
  —Lens displacement (if lens implant performed)

## HOME CARE

- Give both the patient and the caregiver *verbal* and *written* instructions. Provide them with the name and telephone number of a physician or nurse to call if questions arise.
- Advise the patient to avoid squeezing the eyelids shut or touching the eyes postoperatively; encourage elderly patients to wear glasses during the day to avoid rubbing eyes.
- *Warning signs*
  —Review the signs and symptoms that should be reported to a physician or nurse.
    Increased intraocular pressure: sudden onset of eye pain, photophobia, sudden decrease in vision
    Infection: redness and watering of eyes, swelling, blurred vision, pain
- *Special instructions*
  —Discuss the need to wear an eye shield at night for 2-6 weeks to avoid eye injury.
  —Warn that depth perception may be lost and that 50% of peripheral vision will be lost because of eye patch; review safety precautions:
    Instruct the patient to avoid falls by turning the head fully to the affected side to view objects.
    Advise the patient to use up and down head movements to judge stairs and oncoming objects and to move slowly.
    Discuss the need to wear dark glasses during the day

to avoid pupil constriction and glare, since the eye is sensitive to light after surgery.

—If the patient had cataract surgery without a lens implant, warn that vision will be diminished in one or both eyes until prescription eyeglasses or contact lenses are obtained (in about 4-8 weeks).

—If the patient is receiving eyeglasses, explain that images will be magnified 30%, peripheral vision will be impaired and distorted, and lenses will be bifocal or trifocal. Review safety precautions.

Turn head side to side to see peripherally.

Judge distances when descending stairs or viewing oncoming objects.

—If the patient is receiving contact lenses, explain that images will be magnified 7%-10%, peripheral vision will be intact, and reading glasses may also be prescribed.

—Review the care, insertion, and removal of lenses. Advise the patient of the importance of routine appointments with the physician for removal, cleansing, and reinsertion of extended wear lenses.

—If the patient is receiving an intraocular lens implant, explain that the lens implant aids in focusing but that glasses will be prescribed for close vision in 8-12 weeks; there will be no loss in depth perception.

• *Medications*

—Explain the purpose, dosage, schedule, and route of administration of any prescribed drugs, as well as side effects to report to a physician or nurse.

—Review the correct procedure for instilling eyedrops and ointments and applying eye shield (without touching or applying pressure on the eyeball) to avoid self-inflicted injury.

—Advise the patient to avoid over-the-counter medications, eyedrops, or ointments without checking with the physician.

• *Activity*

—Explain the need to avoid activities that can increase intraocular pressure: heavy lifting, straining with elimination, bending over at the waist, coughing, vomiting.

—Instruct the patient to take medications for nausea and constipation as ordered.

—Instruct the patient to avoid sleeping on the operative side.

—Explain the need to avoid any strenuous exercise for 6 weeks;

tell the patient to check with the physician before resuming occupational or recreational activities.
—Explain that it will be necessary to adjust to mild magnification when performing daily activities.

**FOLLOW-UP CARE**
• Stress the importance of regular follow-up visits. Make sure the patient has the necessary names and telephone numbers.

# Catheter Care
## (External Venous Catheter: Central Line, Hickman-Broviac)

—Catheter: convenient way to deliver medications and withdraw blood samples without having to insert a needle in the patient's vein. The catheter is a soft plastic tube. One end of the tube is placed in a large vein, the other stays outside the body. The catheter has a cap that can be removed when blood samples are needed or drugs must be given. The venous catheter is inserted percutaneously into the superior vena cava through the subclavian or external jugular vein.

**INDICATIONS**
• Administration of cancer drugs
• Frequent blood drawing

**SIDE EFFECTS/COMPLICATIONS**
• Infection at the site of insertion of the catheter
• Venous thrombosis
• Catheter migration
• Occlusion of catheter

**HOME CARE**
• Give both the patient and the caregiver *verbal* and *written* instructions. Provide them with the name and telephone number

of a physician or nurse to call if questions arise. Use visual aids and permit time for return demonstration of procedures before discharge.

• *Warning signs*
  —Review the signs and symptoms that should be reported to a physician or nurse.

    Pain, redness, and puffiness around the catheter site
    Drainage from catheter site
    Temperature above 100° F
    Catheter slippage
    Blood in catheter
    Inability to flush catheter
    Difficulty breathing
    Sudden chest pain at insertion site

• *Special instructions*
  —Review purpose of catheter insertion. If for infusion of medication:

    Discuss type and amount of solution to be infused.
    Discuss proper storage of medication; if refrigerated bring to room temperature before administration.
    Advise and assist patient to obtain medications and supplies for infusion.

  —Review dressing change and catheter care procedures (see below).

    Instruct patient to inspect insertion site daily.
    Teach proper handwashing techniques; instruct patient to wash hands before changing dressings.
    Dressing on catheter must be changed frequently, at least every other day, until the wound site has healed.
    After the site has healed, the patient may be allowed to clean around the wound site with soap and water while showering, then dry the area and apply a small gauze pad or adhesive bandage to the exit site.
    Before changing the dressing, assemble the following equipment: hydrogen peroxide, small container in which to pour hydrogen peroxide, alcohol wipes, antibiotic ointment, dressing, tape, cotton-tipped ear swabs.
    Wash hands.
    Remove old dressing and wash hands again.
    Pour hydrogen peroxide into container, dip cotton swab into hydrogen peroxide. Starting at wound site and using circular motion, clean skin around wound site, work-

ing outward. Use new cotton swab whenever more hydrogen peroxide is needed.

Clean length of catheter with alcohol wipe.

Apply antibiotic ointment to wound site with cotton swab.

Tape new dressing over wound site.

—Review procedure for changing catheter cap.

Cap should be changed every 7 days.

Assemble the following equipment: catheter cap, catheter clamp, alcohol wipes.

Wash hands.

Clamp catheter.

Unscrew old cap; wipe around end of catheter with alcohol wipes.

Screw on new cap. Unclamp catheter.

—Review the procedure for flushing catheter.

Catheter is flushed based on policy (as often as once a day) to prevent blood clots from forming inside it.

Assemble the following equipment: vial of heparin-saline solution, disposable syringe and needle, alcohol wipes.

Wash hands.

Open bottle of heparin-saline solution; wipe vial opening with alcohol wipe.

Remove needle guard from syringe and pull back plunger; insert needle into vial, turn vial upside down, and pull back on syringe to fill it. Tap on side of syringe to remove air bubbles.

Clean catheter cap with alcohol wipe, insert needle into cap, and push down on plunger to inject solution into catheter.

Remove needle; carefully discard it and syringe.

—Review procedure for catheter maintenance.

Have a catheter repair kit to use when a leak occurs.

Call the physician or nurse if the catheter continues to leak even after repair.

• *Medications*

—Explain the purpose, dosage, schedule, and route of administration of any prescribed drugs, as well as side effects to report to a physician or nurse.

## FOLLOW-UP CARE

• Stress the importance of regular follow-up visits. Make sure the patient has the necessary names and telephone numbers.

# Catheter Care
## (Implanted Port)

—Infusion port: catheter and port placed under the skin to provide vascular access for patients requiring repeated infusions of drugs, solutions, and blood products and to take blood samples needed without damaging veins. The port consists of a soft plastic catheter and port with a metal base and rubber top through which medications are given and blood is drawn. There are no external parts. The port is surgically placed in the chest or abdomen. The catheter is threaded into the superior vena cava or right atrium via the subclavian or internal jugular vein.

### INDICATIONS

- Administration of:
  - —Cancer drugs
  - —Total parenteral nutrition
  - —Blood, blood products
- Repeated blood drawing

### HOME CARE

- Give both the patient and the caregiver *verbal* and *written* instructions. Provide them with the name and telephone number of a physician or nurse to call if questions arise. Use visual aids and permit time for a return demonstration of the procedure before discharge.
- *Warning signs*
  - —Review the signs and symptoms that should be reported to a physician or nurse.
      Redness, pain, or puffiness around port
      Drainage from incision site
      Temperature above 100° F
      Shortness of breath
      Chest pain
- *Special instructions*
  - —Review the purpose of the port insertion, how long it will stay in, and how frequently it will be changed.

—Discuss protection of the skin over the port.

> Instruct the patient not to wear bra straps or clothing that may rub the port site and to adjust the car seat belt if it rubs the port site.
>
> Unless receiving infusion the patient may shower, bathe, and swim without worry.
>
> When receiving an infusion the patient should keep the site dry and protected.

—Review the procedure for changing the drug reservoir bag.

> Directions for changing the bag vary with the type of pump.
>
> Provide the patient with a diagram and complete instructions.
>
> Advise and assist the patient to obtain the necessary medical supplies. Explain how to order the medicine and total parenteral nutrition solution. Remind the patient to renew the prescription before medicine or supplies run out.

—Review procedures for administration of drugs or solutions.

> If treatment is needed for an extended period, a bent needle (Huber needle) is inserted into the port and connected to an ambulatory infusion pump. The needle is left in the port until treatment is finished.
>
> The pump is attached to the body by a belt or pouch and worn for the duration of treatment.
>
> The dressing is taped over the needle and must be checked to ensure that the tape is holding the dressing and the needle has not slipped. The dressing may need to be changed periodically.

—Review the infusion of medications.

> Discuss the type, amount, and preparation of solution to be infused.
>
> Teach the patient how to use the infusion pump if ordered.
>
> Discuss the proper storage of medication.
>
> Review any side effects of medication that should be reported.

—Review the administration of total parenteral nutrition solution.

> Review the preparation, schedule of infusion, and use of infusion pump as indicated.
>
> Instruct the patient on storing total parenteral nutrition solution and the need to inspect the solution for contamination.

Instruct the patient on measuring and recording intake and output and testing urine for sugar and acetone as ordered. Review the signs and symptoms to report: rapid weight loss or gain, glucose in urine.

**FOLLOW-UP CARE**

- Stress the importance of regular follow-up visits. Make sure the patient has the necessary names and telephone numbers.

# Cellulitis

—Cellulitis: a suppurative inflammation of the dermis and subcutaneous tissue, usually from bacterial invasion through a broken area of the skin. Cellulitis may occur without an evident site of entry and spreads throughout the tissue spaces. Lymphangitis may occur. *Streptococcus pyogenes* and *Staphylococcus aureus* are the most common infecting organisms.

**CAUSES/CONTRIBUTING FACTORS**

- Skin trauma
- Ulceration of skin
- Lymphedema

**SIGNS/SYMPTOMS**

- Localized pain, redness, swelling, skin tenderness
- "Peau d'orange": skin resembling that of an orange
- Lymphangitic streaks: red streaks on skin
- Pitting of skin with pressure
- Fever, chills, malaise
- Headache
- Characteristic lesion or open wound
- Purulent discharge from wound

**COMPLICATIONS**

- Abscesses
- Sepsis
- Gangrene

## DIAGNOSTIC TESTS

- Describe each procedure, its purpose, and the normal feelings or sensations that are likely, as well as any preprocedural and postprocedural care.
    - Tests to identify causative organism: group A beta-hemolytic *Streptococcus* or *Staphylococcus aureus*
    - Culture of skin lesion
    - Blood culture
    - Blood tests

        Complete blood count and white blood cell count: to detect inflammatory process

        Erythrocyte sedimentation rate: will be elevated

## TREATMENT

*Medical*

- Therapy
    - Intraveous antibiotic therapy for severe infection requiring hospitalization, usually about 2 days
    - Immobilization and elevation of the affected limb to reduce edema
    - Cool compresses for discomfort alternating with warm compresses or soaks to increase circulation to promote wound healing
- Drugs
    - Analgesics and antipyretics (acetylsalicylic acid or Tylenol)

*Surgical*

- Incision and drainage for formation that is unresponsive to treatment or in which tissue damage has occurred
- Debridement of devitalized structures: to remove damaged tissues

## HOME CARE

- Give both the patient and the caregiver *verbal* and *written* instructions. Provide them with the name and telephone number of a physician or nurse to call if questions arise.
- *General information*
    - Explain the disorder and contributing causes.
- *Warning signs*
    - Review the signs and symptoms that should be reported to a physician or nurse.

        Headache, fever, chills

        Pain, redness, swelling, heat

Purulent discharge

Odor from dressing

- *Special instructions*

    —Explain the importance of elevation and immobilization of the affected limb for at least 2-3 days or until redness and swelling have subsided.

    —Instruct the patient in wound care and dressing changes.

    Explain how to wash an open wound or draining wound gently with a clean washcloth and soap and water and how to apply dressings using aseptic technique.

    Instruct the patient to wash hands before and after changing dressings and explain how to dispose of dirty dressings.

    Advise the patient on handling soiled linens and clothing; washing them separately in hot water prevents spread of infection.

    —Demonstrate how to apply cool compresses for discomfort, alternating with a warm compress or warm soak to increase circulation to the affected area.

- *Medications*

    —Explain the purpose, dosage, schedule, and route of administration of any prescribed drugs, as well as side effects to report to a physician or nurse.

    —Explain the need to take oral antibiotics for 1 week after infection has cleared. Tell the patient that it may be necessary to prolong the treatment for several weeks, depending on the severity of infection.

- *Activity*

    —Inform the patient that activity to tolerance using supportive devices (e.g., sling, crutches) is permitted. Instruct in the use of ambulatory aids as needed.

## FOLLOW-UP CARE

- Stress the importance of regular follow-up visits. Make sure the patient has the necessary names and telephone numbers.

# Cervical Cancer

—Cervical cancer: cancer of the cervix, the second most common cancer in women. The incidence is greater among women of lower socioeconomic status. Cervical cancers are classified as preinvasive and invasive. Preinvasive cancers are limited to the cervix and are curable in 75%-90% of cases. Invasive cancers involve the cervix and other pelvic structures. The incidence of invasive cervical cancer is decreasing, but premalignant changes, referred to as "carcinoma in situ," are increasing, especially in young women. Cervical cancers are predominantly of the squamous cell type. Some are adenocarcinomas; the clear cell type is seen most commonly in younger women and is increasing in incidence. The term "cervical intraepithelial neoplasia" is used to describe the malignant changes in the squamocolumnar junction that progress to involve full thickness. Cervical cancer spreads by direct extension and via the lymphatics and blood. Seventy-five percent of recurrence is local; 25% is distant metastases to the liver, bones, and mediastinal and supraclavicular nodes.

## RISK FACTORS

- Initial intercourse at an early age, especially between 15 and 17 years of age
- Multiple sex partners
- Sexually transmitted diseases (particularly human papillomavirus, possibly herpes simplex virus)
- Pregnancies in the teen years
- Smoking history
- Long-term use of hormones such as progestin

## SIGNS/SYMPTOMS

- Abnormal vaginal bleeding: painless, thin, watery, blood-tinged vaginal discharge that progresses to spotting and frank bleeding
- Prolonged menstrual period or intermittent periods
- "Contact" bleeding after intercourse
- Anemia caused by chronic blood loss
- Advanced disease: vaginal discharge becomes dark and foul

smelling; pain in lower back, legs, and groin (pelvis); leg edema; difficulty voiding, urgency, and hematuria; rectal tenesmus and bleeding

## DIAGNOSTIC TESTS

• Describe each procedure, its purpose, and the normal feelings or sensations that are likely, as well as any preprocedural and postprocedural care.

   —Cervical examination and biopsy via colposcopy: to detect mass or malignant cells or both

   —Computed tomography of abdomen: to determine retroperitoneal lymph node involvement

   —Magnetic resonance imaging: to estimate tumor volume

   —Lymphangiography: to determine lymph system involvement

   —Chest x-ray, excretory urography, cystoscopy, proctosigmoidoscopy: to detect evidence of tumor spread

## TREATMENT

*Medical*

• Therapy

   —Cryotherapy (freezing of malignant lesion with portable cautery) or laser ablation

      Complications: immediate: hemorrhage, uterine perforation; delayed: cervical stenosis, infertility, cervical incompetence, increased incidence of preterm (low-birth-weight) delivery

   —Radiation therapy: external beam, intracavity

   —Chemotherapy

      Cisplatin

      Carboplatin

      Cyclophosphamide

      Melphalan

      5-Fluorouracil

      Vincristine

      Methotrexate

      Hydroxyurea

*Surgical*

• Conization: to treat carcinoma in situ in women of childbearing age

• Abdominal or vaginal radical hysterectomy and pelvic node dissection

   —Complications: ureteral fistulas, bladder dysfunction, pulmonary embolus, pelvic infection, bowel obstruction, rectovaginal fistulas, hemorrhage

- Pelvic exenteration: nodal dissection and removal of bladder, urethra, uterus, cervix, vagina, rectum, and all lateral supporting tissues; patient will have permanent fecal stoma and urinary diversion
  —Complications: pulmonary embolus or edema, cerebrovascular accident, hemorrhage, myocardial infarction, sepsis, small bowel obstruction

## PREPROCEDURAL TEACHING

- Review the physician's explanation of the procedure, the reason for it, and any specific preprocedural or postprocedural care; encourage the patient to ask questions and to discuss any fears or anxieties, especially about changes in body image and function, fertility, and sexual function.
- For radiation therapy, explain that therapy induces menopause.
- For conization, tell the patient to expect spotting and bleeding for as long as a week after the procedure. Explain that cramping may occur.
- For hysterectomy and pelvic exenteration, see general preprocedural teaching in Abdominal Surgery, p. 3.
- For pelvic exenteration, encourage a preoperative visit by a rehabilitated person who has undergone similar surgery, including vaginal reconstruction when appropriate. The visitor may be from the United Ostomy Association. Offer to make referral to a sexual counselor.

### Review of Postprocedural Care

- Encourage the patient to turn, cough, and deep breathe at regular intervals.
- Prepare the patient for the presence of bulky dressings on the surgical site, urethral catheters, and colostomy or ileostomy depending on the type of surgical procedure.
- Explain that the dressing will be inspected frequently and changed as needed.
- Encourage early ambulation.

## HOME CARE

- Give both the patient and the caregiver *verbal* and *written* instructions. Provide them with the name and telephone number of a physician or nurse to call if questions arise.

- Review the explanation of the type of cancer and the therapeutic or surgical procedures to be performed. For radiation treatment see p. 559; for chemotherapy see p. 178.

## Patient Undergoing Surgery

- *General information*
  —See Abdominal Surgery, p. 3.
- *Warning signs*
  —Review the signs and symptoms that should be reported to a physician or nurse.
  
    Infection: redness, edema, drainage, warmth, fever, pain at incision site
- *Activity*
  —Explain that the patient should avoid coitus and douching for 2-6 weeks after surgery as indicated by physician.
  —Stress the importance of walking at regular intervals and not sitting for long periods.
  —Avoid heavy lifting and vigorous activity for 6-8 weeks after surgery.

## Patient Undergoing Cryosurgery/Laser Therapy

- *Special instructions*
  —Explain that perineal drainage is clear and watery initially, progressing to a foul-smelling discharge that contains dead cells. Report drainage that lasts longer than 8 weeks.
  —Review perineal care and hygiene. Advise the patient that showers and sponge baths are permitted but that tub baths and sitz baths should be avoided.
  —Discuss the need for regular Papanicolaou smears and pelvic examinations because of the high percentage of recurrence.

## Patient Undergoing Pelvic Exenteration

- *Special instructions*
  —Assist patient to obtain appropriate supplies for ostomy care (see Fecal Ostomy, p. 299).
  —Provide instruction on perineal care. Explain that drainage may continue for several months and that the patient should take sitz baths as directed. Demonstrate wound irrigation procedures and application of sanitary pads as needed.
  —Tell the patient to avoid prolonged sitting.
  —Encourage the patient to express feelings of loss of sexuality and body image.

**FOLLOW-UP CARE**

- Stress the importance of regular follow-up visits. Make sure the patient has the necessary names and telephone numbers.

**REFERRALS**

- Assist the patient to obtain services as needed for support groups and sexual and fertility counseling.

# Charcot's Syndrome
## (Neurogenic Arthropathy)

—Charcot's syndrome: a progressive degenerative disease of the stress-bearing portion of joints caused by impaired sensory nerve innervation. The resulting loss of sensation to the joints permits further destruction from trauma or from the underlying disease, which leads to laxity of supporting ligaments and disintegration of the affected joints. The weight-bearing joints are most commonly affected: knees, hips, ankles, and lower spine. The condition is most common in men over 40 years of age.

**CAUSES/CONTRIBUTING FACTORS**

- Diabetes mellitus: affects joints of feet
- Tabes dorsalis: degeneration of dorsal vertebrae affecting the large weight-bearing joints (knee, hip, ankle, lower spine)
- Syringomyelia: affects shoulder and upper extremity joints
- Charcot-Marie-Tooth disease: progressive atrophy of the peroneal nerve
- Intraarticular injection of corticosteroids: affects hip or knee joint
- Spinal cord trauma
- Paraplegia
- Peripheral nerve injury
- Myelomeningocele in children
- Leprosy
- Pernicious anemia

**SIGNS/SYMPTOMS**

- Neuropathy: loss of sensation in affected area
- In affected joint
  —Swelling
  —Warmth
  —Increased mobility
  —Instability
  —Deformity
  —Backache (if vertebral joints are affected)

**COMPLICATIONS**

- Joint subluxation or dislocation
- Articular (joint) fractures
- Pathologic fractures
- Amputation

**DIAGNOSTIC TESTS**

- Describe each procedure, its purpose, and the normal feelings or sensations that are likely, as well as any preprocedural and postprocedural care.
  —X-rays: to confirm the diagnosis and assess the severity of joint damage
  —Vertebral examination: to document narrowing of the disk spaces and vertebral deterioration
  —Synovial biopsy: to detect bony fragments and bits of calcified cartilage
  —Neuromuscular test: to look for sensory or motor defects

**TREATMENT**

*Medical*

- Therapy
  —Immobilization: to protect the joint from stress and injury
      Crutches, braces, splints
      Restriction from weight bearing
      Wheelchair
  —Protective footwear
- Drugs
  —Analgesics

*Surgical*

- Arthrodesis (joint fusion) for immobilization
- Amputation

**HOME CARE**

- Give both the patient and the caregiver *verbal* and *written* instructions. Provide them with the name and telephone number of a physician or nurse to call if questions arise.
- *General information*
  —Explain the causes or contributory factors of the disorder and identify affected joints.
  —Assist the patient to become familiar with his or her own pain pattern and sensory perceptions so that a baseline can be established against which to measure changes and responses to medication and treatment.
  —Caution the patient that because of loss of sensation (neuropathy), injury can occur without causing pain or discomfort.
- *Warning signs*
  —Review the signs and symptoms that should be reported to a physician or nurse.
     Increasing joint pain, swelling, or instability
- *Special instructions*
  —Explain how to apply warm compresses to relieve local joint pain and tenderness.
  —Instruct the patient to inspect the skin of affected joints daily, checking for abrasions, cuts, or ulcers, and to report any lesions that do not heal. Alert the patient to the need to check water temperature to avoid burns.
  —Provide instruction in the proper technique for crutches or other immobilization devices. Refer the patient to the physical therapy department for proper fitting and the readjustment of devices.
  —Advise the patient to wear prescribed protective footwear and to avoid tight-fitting shoes and heels higher than 1 inch.
- *Medications*
  —Explain the purpose, dosage, schedule, and route of administration of any prescribed drugs, as well as side effects to report to a physician or nurse.
- *Activity*
  —Explain the importance of developing life-style techniques to protect the joints.
     Avoid fatigue.
     Pace daily activities and plan regular rest periods even when not feeling tired.

Avoid physical activities that may cause pathologic fractures, such as walking and running.

Take safety precautions at home to avoid falls or other injuries: remove throw rugs and keep passageways clear of clutter.

—Encourage the discussion of allowances and limitations with regard to exercise, occupation, and recreation.

## FOLLOW-UP CARE

• Stress the importance of regular follow-up visits. Make sure the patient has the necessary names and telephone numbers.

## REFERRALS

• Provide referral for home health care as indicated.

# Chemotherapy

—**Chemotherapy: systemic cancer treatment using cytotoxic drugs to destroy malignant cells; used for widespread disease or when there is high risk of recurrence in the body. Chemotherapy may be used alone as a curative measure or can be used as an adjuvant to surgery or radiation therapy. As a palliative treatment, it is used to relieve obstruction or pain.**

## CANCER CHEMOTHERAPEUTIC AGENTS

• Alkylating agents: chlorambucil, cyclophosphamide, ifosfamide, mechlorethamine, melphalan
• Nitrosoureas: carmustine, lomustine, streptozocin, busulfan, carboplatin, cisplatin, thiotepa
• Antimetabolites: cytarabine, floxuridine, fluorouracil, mercaptopurine, methotrexate, thioguanine
• Antibiotics: bleomycin, dactinomycin, daunorubicin, doxorubicin, mitomycin, plicamycin
• Plant alkaloids: etoposide, vincristine, vinblastine
• Miscellaneous drugs: asparaginase, dacarbazine, levamisole, procarbazine

- Hormones and antihormonal drugs: androgens, estrogens, progestins, corticosteroids, antiestrogens
- Biologic response modifiers: interferons, interleukins, erythropoietin, colony-stimulating factors

**C**

## CONTRAINDICATIONS/PRECAUTIONS

- Based on patient's pretreatment condition, stage of disease, response to therapy, and allergies or sensitivities
- Patient's functional status may be used to monitor tolerance to therapy

## ROUTES OF ADMINISTRATION

- Oral
- Intravenous
- Vascular access: central venous catheter (Hickman; see p. 163), implantable port devices (see p. 166), peripheral inserted catheter
- Intraarterial
- Intracavitary: intraperitoneal, intrapleural
- Intrathecal via Ommaya reservoir (reservoir placed in ventricle of the brain)
- Intramuscular and subcutaneous routes used less frequently

## LABORATORY TESTS

- Specific to each type of chemotherapeutic agent used
- General: serum: complete blood count, electrolytes, cultures; liver function test; urinalysis, Hematest
- Bone marrow biopsy
- Pulmonary function studies
- Electrocardiogram

## PREPROCEDURAL TEACHING

- Review the physician's explanation of the type of chemotherapy and the reason for it. Discuss when it will be scheduled, where it will be administered (hospital versus outpatient), route of administration, frequency of treatments, and length of time required to complete the treatment. Encourage the patient to ask questions and to discuss any fears or anxieties.

### Review of Postprocedural Care

- Review the side effects associated with the type of drug to be used and explain that medications will be used to reduce the effects of chemotherapy.

- Inform the patient about possible hair loss and the need to buy a wig or wear a hat, scarf, or turban. Women should have hair cut short before treatment begins, purchase a wig, and have natural hair styled to resemble the wig.

## SIDE EFFECTS/TOXICITY

- Specific toxic side effects and problems depend on the type of medication.
  —Gastrointestinal disturbances: anorexia, nausea, vomiting, diarrhea
  —Bone marrow suppression
  —Hair loss, skin rash, stomatitis
  —Electrolyte and chemical imbalance
  —Hematologic abnormalities
  —Hepatic toxicity
  —Renal dysfunction
  —Cardiac and pulmonary dysfunction

## HOME CARE

- Give both the patient and the caregiver *verbal* and *written* instructions. Use visual aids to assist in instruction. Provide them with the name and telephone number of a physician or nurse to call if questions arise.
- *General information*
  —Explain that fatigue and other side effects begin during the first week and gradually disappear during the 2-4 weeks after therapy ends.
  —Teach the patient the importance of oral hygiene (see Cancer, p. 138).
  —Advise the patient on skin care. Instruct the patient to inspect the skin and report any signs of abrasions or skin breaks. Mild soap and warm water should be used on irritated areas.
- *Warning signs*
  —Review the signs and symptoms that should be reported to a physician or nurse.
     Infection: pain, swelling, redness, drainage
     Excessive nausea, vomiting, diarrhea
     Bleeding
     Excessive fatigue
     Shortness of breath

C

      Palpitations

      Mucositis

      Difficulty with urination

      Paresthesias

      Confusion, memory loss

      Itching, burning

- *Special instructions*
  - —Discuss immunosuppression and the need to monitor the blood count. If the white blood count is low, the patient should avoid persons with infections or colds, large crowds, and recently vaccinated children.
  - —For specific problems see Bone Marrow Suppression (p. 100) and Cancer (p. 138).
- *Medications*
  - —Explain the purpose, dosage, schedule, and route of administration of any prescribed drugs, as well as side effects to report to a physician or nurse.
- *Activity*
  - —Encourage the patient to continue work and other activities of daily living as tolerated, including regular exercise.
  - —Teach the patient how to manage fatigue and maintain mobility, for example, by planning important activities before treatment and after treatment based on energy level.
  - —Stress the need to avoid injury; contact sports should not be played.
- *Diet*
  - —Teach the patient the importance of a high-protein, high-carbohydrate diet. Encourage small, frequent meals if the patient is nauseated. Advise the patient to take an antiemetic ½ hour before meals.
  - —Encourage a fluid intake of 3000 ml per day.

## FOLLOW-UP CARE

- Stress the importance of keeping all scheduled treatment, laboratory, and medical follow-up appointments. Make sure the patient has the necessary names and telephone numbers.

## REFERRALS

- Refer the patient to a support group and other community resources as needed.

# Chest Trauma
## (Flail Chest)

—Chest trauma: chest cage injury causing multiple fractures of ribs. Types of chest injury include penetrating (e.g., bullet and knife wounds, impaled objects) and nonpenetrating (e.g., falls, blunt trauma, deceleration injuries from automobile accident).

### CAUSES/CONTRIBUTING FACTORS

• Automobile accidents
• Assaults
• Explosions
• Other types of accidents

### SIGNS/SYMPTOMS

• Sharp chest pain
• Difficulty in breathing
• Shallow, rapid respirations
• Uneven chest wall movement
• Tachycardia
• Cyanosis
• Copious, blood-tinged sputum

### COMPLICATIONS

• Tension pneumothorax
• Hemothorax
• Pulmonary edema
• Cardiac tamponade
• Respiratory arrest
• Shock

### DIAGNOSTIC TESTS

• Explain that the following diagnostic procedures help confirm the diagnosis. Describe each procedure, its purpose, and the normal feelings or sensations that are likely, as well as any preprocedural and postprocedural care.

   —Chest x-ray: to examine for atelectasis, pneumothorax, evidence of fractured ribs

—Arterial blood gases: to monitor for hypoxemia (decreased $Pao_2$) and hypercapnia (increased $Paco_2$)

—Pulmonary function tests: performed by measuring the volume of air moving in and out of the lungs and then calculating lung capacities

## TREATMENT

*Medical*

• Therapy
  —Oxygen therapy
  —Chest tube insertion
  —Intubation and mechanical ventilation
  —Pain management
• Drugs
  —Antibiotics
  —Neuromuscular blocking agents

## HOME CARE

• Give both the patient and the caregiver *verbal* and *written* instructions. Provide them with the name and telephone number of a physician or nurse to call if questions arise.
• *General information*
  —Explain the underlying cause or contributing factors.
  —Show how to splint the chest when coughing to avoid pain.
• *Warning signs*
  —Review the signs and symptoms that should be reported to a physician or nurse.
     Upper respiratory infection
     Shortness of breath
     Persistent cough
     Persistent chest pain
• *Medications*
  —Explain the purpose, dosage, schedule, and route of administration of any prescribed drugs, as well as side effects to report to a physician or nurse. Explain the need to avoid taking over-the-counter medication without checking with a physician.
• *Activity*
  —Advise the patient of the importance of exercising to tolerance and the need to avoid overexertion and excessive participation in sports and activities.

**FOLLOW-UP CARE**

- Stress the importance of regular follow-up visits. Make sure the patient has the necessary names and telephone numbers.

---

# Cholelithiasis, Cholecystitis

—Cholelithiasis: abnormal formation of stones in the gallbladder.

—Cholecystitis: acute or chronic inflammation of the gallbladder caused by blockage of the cystic duct by gallstones.

**CAUSES/CONTRIBUTING FACTORS**

- Diet: high fat, high caloric
- Obesity
- Diabetes
- Liver disease
- Pancreatitis
- In women: elevated estrogen levels, oral contraceptives, hormone replacement therapy, pregnancy
- Use of clofibrate (anticholesterol drug)

**SIGNS/SYMPTOMS**

- After fatty snacks or meals: indigestion, belching, flatulence, nausea, vomiting
- Pain: acute and colicky; midepigastric area, may spread to back and between shoulder blades or right shoulder
- Fever: low grade or high with chills
- Jaundice
- Dark, concentrated urine
- Clay-colored stools

**COMPLICATIONS**

- Jaundice
- Infection
- Electrolyte imbalance

- Bowel obstruction
- Peritonitis
- Bleeding tendencies (lack of vitamin K)
- Pancreatitis

## DIAGNOSTIC TESTS

- Describe each procedure, its purpose, and the normal feelings or sensations that are likely, as well as any preprocedural and postprocedural care.
  —Radiographic tests: cholecystography, x-rays
  —Ultrasound: to differentiate location and size of stones
  —Blood studies: to show increase in certain enzymes (serum bilirubin, serum amylase)
  —White blood cell count: to check for infection
  —Percutaneous transhepatic cholangiography: to confirm the presence of stones or obstruction

## TREATMENT

*Medical*
- Therapy
  —Hydration (parenteral fluids with electrolytes)
  —Gallstone dissolution therapy (bile acid therapy): to dissolve certain types of stones; indicated for small stones
  —Percutaneous transhepatic biliary catheterization: to remove gallstones; catheter is inserted through small abdominal incision under fluoroscopy; catheter may remain temporarily and drain into small external bag; procedure done on outpatient basis under local anesthesia
  —Endoscopic retrograde sphincterotomy: flexible endoscopic tube inserted through mouth to stomach and through to common bile duct to permit stones to pass; done on an outpatient basis with local anesthesia to throat
  —Endoscopic retrograde cholangiopancreatography: flexible endoscopic tube passed as above but used to remove stones
  —Extracorporeal shock wave lithotripsy: use of high-energy shock waves to break up stones without damaging surrounding tissue (see Extracorporeal Shock Wave Lithotripsy, p. 668).
- Drugs
  —Analgesics
  —Antibiotics
  —Antiemetics

—Anticholinergics

—Vitamin K

*Surgical*

• Cholecystectomy: surgical removal of the gallbladder

## HOME CARE

• Give both the patient and the caregiver *verbal* and *written* instructions. Provide them with the name and telephone number of a physician or nurse to call if questions arise. Explain the disease, causes, and contributing factors.

• *Warning signs*

—Review the signs and symptoms that should be reported to a physician or nurse.

  Biliary colic: severe pain, tachycardia, pallor, diaphoresis

• *Special instructions*

—Review the explanation for prescribed medical therapies (see above).

  Describe the procedure and its purpose, reviewing any specific preprocedural preparation.

  After the procedure, provide instruction on postprocedural care.

  Review catheter care if a catheter is present.

  ○ Explain that the catheter is to remain taped securely in place. Teach the patient how to empty the bag.

  ○ Review the signs and symptoms that should be reported to a physician or nurse: no drainage coming out of the tube, signs of infection (redness, swelling, tenderness around site, fever, chills).

—Review the explanation of surgery if prescribed.

• *Medications*

—Explain the purpose, dosage, schedule, and route of administration of any prescribed drugs, as well as side effects to report to a physician or nurse.

• *Diet*

—Explain that the patient should follow a low-fat diet and take vitamin supplements (A, D, E, and K); refer the patient to the dietary department for specific instructions.

—Discuss the need to decrease dietary fat and cholesterol. Explain the role diet plays in controlling biliary colic.

—Discuss the need to maintain weight control. Advise weight reduction as necessary.

**FOLLOW-UP CARE**

- Stress the importance of regular follow-up visits. Make sure the patient has the necessary names and telephone numbers.

# Cholecystectomy

**—Cholecystectomy: removal of the gallbladder for gallstones or because of inflammation to restore flow of bile from the liver to the small intestine. The procedure may be done as abdominal surgery (open cholecystectomy) or as a laparoscopic procedure.**

## PREPROCEDURAL TEACHING

- Review the physician's explanation of the procedure and the reason for it; encourage the patient to ask questions and to discuss any fears or anxieties.

### Review of Preprocedural Care

- Review the physician's explanation of the procedure. Explain the need for consent forms and signature for surgery, anesthesia, blood transfusions, and photographs, if needed.
- Inform the patient that admission is usually on the day of surgery and that the procedure is performed under general anesthesia.
- Review routine preprocedure tests: complete blood count, urinalysis, chest x-ray, and electrocardiogram.
- Tell the patient that NPO status must be maintained from the night before surgery.
- Review skin preparation; the patient will shower with bactericidal soap (e.g., Safeguard, Dial, Hibiclens).
- Inform the patient that a small cleansing enema (e.g., Fleet) is necessary the night before the procedure.
- For open cholecystectomy:
  - Explain that an incision will be made below the right rib cage.
  - Explain that the procedure may take 2-4 hours if x-rays are done during surgery.

- For laparoscopy:
  —Tell the patient that NPO status must be maintained from the night before surgery.
  —Explain that the procedure usually takes 2-3 hours.
  —Inform the patient that the largest incision will be 2-4 inches below the umbilicus (for removal of the gallbladder) and that three or four punctures will be made in the abdomen to insert other scopes (to inject gas into the abdominal cavity, which makes vision and maneuvering easier), to hold, and to cut.

**Review of Postprocedural Care**

- For open cholecystectomy:
  —See Abdominal Surgery (p. 3).
  —Inform the patient that the hospital stay will be 4 days or more.
  —Explain that drainage tubes will be inserted: nasogastric tube, T-tube for bile drainage, possibly Penrose or Jackson-Pratt drain.
- For laparoscopy:
  —Tell the patient that fluids will be permitted on the evening of surgery if the patient is not nauseated.
  —Explain that the patient will be encouraged to get out of bed and walk.
  —Inform the patient that the abdomen will be distended from gas.
  —Tell the patient what analgesics will be provided for pain.
  —Explain that the patient will be discharged the day after surgery.

**SIDE EFFECTS/COMPLICATIONS**

- Hemorrhage
- Shock
- Paralytic ileus
- Peritonitis
- Electrolyte imbalance
- Wound infection
- Pulmonary problems
- Postcholecystectomy syndrome (fever, jaundice, pain)
- From laparoscopy:
  —Bleeding
  —Wound infection
  —Abdominal cramps and shoulder pain
  —Sepsis
  —Biliary peritonitis

## HOME CARE

- Give both the patient and the caregiver *verbal* and *written* instructions. Provide them with the name and telephone number of a physician or nurse to call if questions arise.
- *Wound/incision care*
  —Explain any specific care of the surgical incision and dressing changes as indicated.
  —Teach the patient how to care for the T-tube and drainage bag.
    Secure the tube by taping it to the body.
    Keep the tube and bag level with the abdomen when lying flat to prevent excessive drainage.
    Do not disconnect the tube and drainage.
    Avoid kinks in the tubing.
    When emptying the bag: wash hands, wipe the connection with alcohol, disconnect and drain into a receptacle, reconnect and wipe connection if drainage is apparent, measure drainage, record the amount, discard drainage into the toilet, rinse receptacle.
    Inspect the insertion side daily for leakage, redness, tenderness, or swelling. Wash with soap and water and replace dressing.
    Clamp the T-tube 1 hour before and after eating (unless instructed otherwise).
- *Warning signs*
  —Review the signs and symptoms that should be reported to a physician or nurse.
    Wound infection: redness, tenderness, swelling
    Biliary obstruction: persistent pain, jaundice, itching (pruritus); lack of bowel movements or clay-colored stools; dark urine
    Fever, chills
    Nausea, vomiting
- *Medications*
  —Explain the purpose, dosage, schedule, and route of administration of any prescribed drugs, as well as side effects to report to a physician or nurse.
- *Activity*
  —For laparoscopy:
    Encourage the patient to increase mobility to reduce abdominal distention.
    Explain that normal activities are usually possible in 2 days.

Explain that the patient should avoid heavy lifting (over 10 pounds) or strenuous work or sports for 1 week or longer as prescribed by the physician.
- *Diet*
  —Tell the patient that a low-fat (for 6 weeks, and then fat may be increased gradually), high-carbohydrate, high-protein diet is needed.
  —Inform the patient that alcohol should be avoided for the first 2 months after surgery to minimize the risk of pancreatic involvement.

## FOLLOW-UP CARE
- Stress the importance of regular follow-up visits. Make sure the patient has the necessary names and telephone numbers.

# Cirrhosis

—**Cirrhosis: chronic, progressive liver disease characterized by diffuse destruction and fibrotic regeneration of hepatic cells, resulting in changes in liver structure and portal blood flow.**

## CAUSES/CONTRIBUTING FACTORS/RISK FACTORS
- Chronic alcoholism
- Viral hepatitis
- Exposure to industrial and chemical toxins, such as arsenic, carbon tetrachloride, phosphorus
- Biliary obstruction or inflammation
- Right-sided congestive heart failure
- Genetic factors

## SIGNS/SYMPTOMS
- Fatigue
- Weakness
- Anorexia

- Weight loss or gain
- Abdominal pain or tenderness
- Diarrhea or constipation
- Nausea and vomiting
- Dyspepsia
- Pruritus
- Petechiae, ecchymosis, bleeding tendencies
- Palmar erythema
- Spider angioma
- Edema of extremities
- Ascites
- Jaundice
- Umbilical hernia
- Distended abdominal veins
- Fetor hepaticus: fruity, musty breath odor
- Asterixis: coarse tremors of the hands
- Changes in reproductive system: amenorrhea, testicular atrophy, gynecomastia, impotence

## COMPLICATIONS

- Portal hypertension
- Bleeding, esophageal varices
- Hepatic encephalopathy
- Hepatorenal syndrome
- Death

## DIAGNOSTIC TESTS

- Describe each procedure, its purpose, and the normal feelings or sensations that are likely, as well as any preprocedural and postprocedural care.
  —Blood studies: liver enzymes, bilirubin levels, total serum albumin, serum protein, prothrombin time, complete blood count, serum electrolytes
  —Urine and stool studies: to measure urobilinogen levels
  —Abdominal x-rays: to detect liver size, cysts, calcification, ascites
  —Liver biopsy: to detect hepatic tissue destruction and fibrosis
  —Computed tomography of liver: to determine liver size, identify masses, and visualize hepatic blood flow
  —Esophagogastroduodenoscopy: to detect esophageal varices, duodenal bleeding, irritation, ulceration

## TREATMENT

Treatment goals are to alleviate the underlying cause for cirrhosis, prevent further hepatic damage, and prevent or treat complications.

*Medical*

- Therapy
  —Gastric intubation: to assess bleeding
  —Esophageal balloon tamponade: to control bleeding esophageal varices
  —Sclerotherapy: to control hemorrhage by inducing sclerosis in the bleeding tissues
  —Low-sodium diet
  —Fluid restriction
  —Vitamin supplements
  —Total parenteral nutrition
- Drugs
  —Antacids
  —Diuretics
  —Vasopressin

*Surgical*

- Peritoneovenous shunt: to drain ascites into the venous circulation, decreasing portal hypertension
- Portal-systemic shunt: to divert portal venous blood flow, decreasing portal hypertension
- Paracentesis: to relieve abdominal pressure
- Liver transplantation

## HOME CARE

- Give both the patient and the caregiver *verbal* and *written* instructions. Provide them with the name and telephone number of a physician or nurse to call if questions arise.
- *General information*
  —Explain cirrhosis, its causes, and contributing factors. Patient education is individualized, depending on the cause of the disease.
- *Warning signs*
  —Review the signs and symptoms that should be reported to a physician or nurse.
     Changes in weight, edema, abdominal girth
     Behavioral or neurologic changes: stupor, lethargy, restlessness, hallucinations, neuromuscular function
     Excessive bleeding, bloody vomitus or stools

C

- *Special instructions*
  —Advise the patient to avoid using soap. Suggest the use of emollients and antipruritic lotions. Emphasize the importance of maintaining skin integrity.
  —Instruct the patient to weigh self daily and to record daily weights and abdominal girth measurements.
  —Instruct the patient to minimize the risk of bleeding by not straining during defecation, blowing the nose forcefully, or using razor blades or hard-bristled toothbrushes.
- *Medications*
  —Explain the purpose, dosage, schedule, and route of administration of any prescribed drugs, as well as side effects to report to a physician or nurse.
  —Stress the importance of avoiding over-the-counter medications.
- *Activity*
  —Encourage the patient to discuss allowances and limitations with respect to occupation, recreation, and activities.
  —Instruct the patient to alternate periods of rest or activity.
  —Instruct the patient in energy conservation methods in activities of daily living.
- *Diet*
  —Stress the importance of abstaining from alcohol.
  —Advise the patient to eat small, frequent meals.
  Assist the patient to plan a diet low in sodium and high in carbohydrates, protein, vitamins, and calories. For advanced-stage disease or encephalopathy, tell the patient to limit protein intake.
  —Instruct the patient and caregiver in total parenteral nutrition, if appropriate.

## FOLLOW-UP CARE

- Stress the importance of regular follow-up visits. Make sure the patient has the necessary names and telephone numbers.
- Encourage the patient to obtain a Medic-Alert bracelet and identification card listing the diagnosis, medications, and treatment.

## REFERRALS

- Assist the patient to obtain referral to home health services.
- Assist the patient and caregiver to participate in Alcoholics Anonymous, if appropriate.

# Colorectal Cancer

—Colorectal cancer: cancer of the colon and rectum. Colorectal cancer occurs more frequently in the elderly; prognosis in the young is very poor. Ninety-five percent of tumors begin with the development of a benign, adenomatous polyp in the large bowel or rectum. Most colon and rectal tumors are adenocarcinomas; others are carcinoid tumors, leiomyosarcomas, and lymphomas.

## RISK FACTORS

- Age over 40 years
- Diet heavy in fats and refined carbohydrates
- Family history of colorectal cancer
- Past history of colorectal adenocarcinoma or cancer; breast cancer, endometrial cancer
- Ulcerative colitis
- Familial polyposis
- Exposure to asbestos
- Member of higher socioeconomic group and urban population

## SIGNS/SYMPTOMS

- Rectal bleeding
- Changes in bowel pattern (constipation or diarrhea)
- Excessive flatus
- Distention
- Cramps
- Unexplained anemia
- Altered bowel habits caused by left-sided colonic lesions: decreased stool caliber (pencil like), urgency to defecate, vague abdominal pain, hemorrhoids
- Unexplained iron deficiency, anemia, and gastrointestinal tract bleeding caused by right-sided lesions
- Obstruction owing to napkin ring growth of tumors of sigmoid colon
- Gross rectal blood and tenesmus with feeling of incomplete evacuation caused by rectal tumors

**COMPLICATIONS**

- Infection
- Paralytic ileus
- Leak of anastomosis with possible fistula formation

**DIAGNOSTIC TESTS**

- Describe each procedure, its purpose, and the normal feelings or sensations that are likely, as well as any preprocedural and postprocedural care.
  - —Hematocrit: to detect blood loss
  - —Occult fecal blood test: to detect blood loss
  - —Digital rectal examination: to determine presence of lesion
  - —Colonic visualization (barium enema, colonoscopy): to determine size, shape, and location of lesion
  - —Biopsy: to determine type of malignant cells
  - —Carcinoembryonic antigen: nonspecific tumor marker elevated in presence of colorectal tumor

**TREATMENT**

*Medical*

- Therapy
  - —Radiation therapy
    - Intraoperative radiation therapy
    - Radiation seeds
    - External beam for inoperable obstructing rectal rumors
    - Transanal irradiation
  - —Postoperative adjuvant therapy with radiation sensitizers for tumors dissecting bowel wall or with positive lymph nodes
  - —Endoscopic laser for inoperable obstructing rectal tumors
  - —Chemotherapy
    - Adjuvant regimen of 5-fluoruracil (5-FU) with levamisole
    - Radiation sensitizers with 5-FU and metronidazole

*Surgical*

- Local excision of well-defined rectal tumors
- Resection of primary colon lesion with mesentery (containing lymph nodes to which tumor is likely to spread) and end-to-end anastomosis
- En bloc resection of colon, small bowel, bladder, uterus, ovaries
- Surgical bypass for inoperable obstructing tumors, with creation of fecal stoma

## PREPROCEDURAL TEACHING FOR SURGERY

- Review the physician's explanation of the procedure and the reason for it; encourage the patient to ask questions and to discuss any fears or anxieties.
- For general preprocedural and postprocedural teaching, see Abdominal Surgery (p. 3).
- Review bowel preparation: liquid diet 2-3 days before surgery, laxatives, enemas, and antibiotics to cleanse and sterilize bowel.
- If a stoma is expected, arrange to meet with the enterostomal therapist before surgery to mark the site of the stoma. The stoma should avoid the waistline and skin folds and should be located where the patient can see and reach the pouch easily.
- Provide emotional support. Encourage questions and discussion to correct any misconception and alleviate fears and concerns regarding changes in body image and life-style.

## HOME CARE

- Give both the patient and the caregiver *verbal* and *written* instructions. Provide them with the name and telephone number of a physician or nurse to call if questions arise. Use visual aids to assist in instruction.
- *General information*
  —Review the disease process and the type of surgical procedure performed or scheduled. Discuss follow-up care.
- *Warning signs*
  —Review the signs and symptoms that should be reported to a physician or nurse.
    - Infection: purulent drainage, pain, incision warm to the touch, fever, redness
    - Paralytic ileus: inability to defecate, distention, abdominal pain and swelling
    - Leak at site of anastomosis: increased drainage around the surgical site
    - Stoma retraction or prolapse
    - Rectal bleeding
- *Special instructions*
  —Review the care of the surgical dressing, explaining how to inspect the incision.
  —For patient with colostomy, explain how to care for the ostomy (see Fecal Ostomy, p. 299).
  —Review prevention and detection procedures to avoid recurrence.

Maintenance of regular bowel movements: eat a high-fiber, low-fat diet; drink up to 8 glasses of fluids per day unless contraindicated; avoid constipation; check with physician or nurse regarding use of laxatives and enemas.

Inspect stools regularly and report any signs of bleeding. Show the patient how to perform a Hemoccult test procedure.

**FOLLOW-UP CARE**

- Stress the importance of regular follow-up visits. Because of the high recurrence rate, discuss the importance of having yearly screening (rectal examination, stool test for occult blood). Make sure the patient has the necessary names and telephone numbers.

# Compartment Syndrome

—**Compartment syndrome: increased pressure within anatomic compartments caused by constriction of edematous tissues, leading to progressive degeneration of muscle, impaired circulation, nerve damage, and tissue necrosis. The elbow, wrist, knee, and ankle are the most commonly affected areas. The cause of constriction is unyielding fascial coverings over muscles. When an injury, such as a fracture, frostbite, or burn, causes swelling, there may be no room for edema within the muscle group or compartment. Thus blood flow is interrupted, causing damage to the blood vessels, nerves, and muscles within this limited space.**

**CAUSES/CONTRIBUTING FACTORS**

- Trauma or surgery
- Bleeding disorders (e.g., hemophilia)
- Major vascular surgery
- Thermal injury: burns, frostbite
- Snakebite
- Intravenous infiltration
- Tight casts or dressings

**SIGNS/SYMPTOMS**

- Pain: in compartment area; increasing, unrelenting, and unrelieved by narcotics
- Paresthesia: of hand or foot; numbness, decreased sensation or burning
- Pallor: caused by decreased circulation in the compartment
- Polar (coolness); from decreased circulation
- Swelling and localized redness
- Progressive loss of motor function
- Paralysis
- Pulselessness: absence of pulse below level of compartment

**COMPLICATIONS**

- Neurovascular dysfunction of extremity
- Muscle weakness
- Tissue necrosis
- Chronic infection, osteomyelitis
- Amputation
- Shock

**DIAGNOSTIC TESTS**

- Describe each procedure, its purpose, and the normal feelings or sensations that are likely, as well as any preprocedural and postprocedural care.
  —Compartment pressure: measured by various methods, such as slit, wick, or large-bore catheter introduced into the compartment and attached to a saline-primed transducer
  —Arteriogram/venogram: to rule out blood vessel blockage or damage
  —Magnetic resonance imaging: to show muscle damage
  —Ankle or brachial index
  —Blood tests: complete blood count, prothrombin time

**TREATMENT**

*Medical*

- Therapy
  —Dressing removed; cast removed, bivalved, or windowed to limit the swelling
  —Immobilization with posterior cast or splint if fracture is involved
  —*Caution:* Extremity should *not* be iced and elevated, since this contributes to decreased blood flow to the affected area

—Continuous fascial pressure monitoring: normal 0-30 mm Hg; sustained pressure >30 mm Hg can damage blood vessels, nerves, and muscles
- Drugs
    —Analgesics: often larger than normal levels of narcotics are needed to control pain
    —Antibiotics

*Surgical*

- Fasciotomy: surgical incision of the fascia for the entire length of the involved compartment to remove restriction or swelling: before procedure, explain that it is necessary to control progressive symptoms of neurovascular compromise and that after several days the surgical incision will be closed or that a skin graft may be necessary
- Surgical repair of lacerated artery: for arterial injury
- Amputation: for severe tissue necrosis or infection

## HOME CARE

- Give both the patient and the caregiver *verbal* and *written* instructions. Provide them with the name and telephone number of a physician or nurse to call if questions arise.
- *General information*
    —Describe the disorder, explaining causes or contributing factors.
- *Warning signs*
    —Review the signs and symptoms of recurrence of the syndrome that should be reported to a physician or nurse.
        Increasing pain
        Numbness, tingling
        Paralysis
        Changes in color: pallor, redness, cyanosis
        Coolness
- *Special instructions*
    —If fasciotomy was performed:
        Explain that there is an increased potential for infection.
        Review the signs of infection to be reported immediately to the physician or nurse: increased temperature, increased pain, foul odor from wound.
        Instruct the patient in the proper technique for care of the surgical incision and aseptic procedures for dressing changes; advise the patient how to dispose of soiled dressings.

Instruct the patient to inspect the wound daily to check for increased drainage.

—If vascular surgery to repair blood vessels was performed:

Review signs of vascular changes requiring attention: pallor, cyanosis, pulselessness, decreased or absent capillary refill (when extremity is pinched, it turns white; pink color returns in 4-6 seconds).

• *Medications*

—Explain the purpose, dosage, schedule, and route of administration of any prescribed drugs, as well as side effects to report to a physician or nurse.

• *Activity*

—Explain the need for rest and elevation of the extremity postoperatively.

—Review the use of assistive devices and ambulatory aids as prescribed by the physician.

**FOLLOW-UP CARE**

• Stress the importance of regular follow-up visits. Make sure the patient has the necessary names and telephone numbers.

# COPD: Chronic Obstructive Pulmonary Disease
## (Chronic Obstructive Lung Disease)

—Chronic obstructive pulmonary disease: a progressive disorder of the lungs and airways. Chronic obstructive pulmonary disease (COPD) affects oxygen and carbon dioxide gas exchange and causes chronic inflammation and narrowing of the small airways, affecting air outflow. COPD includes such diseases as emphysema and chronic bronchitis.

—Emphysema: destruction of lung tissue, causing a reduced expiratory flow rate and overinflated alveoli (air sacs); a progressive disease that is irreversible.

—**Chronic bronchitis: inflammation of the mucous membrane of the bronchus with excessive mucus secretion in the bronchial tree; occurs as a result of irritation to tissue that causes swelling and hypertrophy of the mucus-producing cells.**

### CONTRIBUTING FACTORS

- Cigarette smoking
- Exposure to pollutants: industrial, air
- Chronic respiratory infections

### SIGNS/SYMPTOMS

- Dyspnea on exertion
- Shortness of breath
- Wheezing
- Thick mucus production
- Restlessness
- Fatigue
- Anorexia, weight loss
- Persistent cough: productive, nonproductive
- Malaise
- Somnolence
- Peripheral cyanosis with clubbing

### COMPLICATIONS

- Cor pulmonale
- Acute respiratory failure
- Peptic and esophageal reflux
- Pneumonia
- Polycythemia
- Dysrhythmias
- Hepatomegaly

### DIAGNOSTIC TESTS

- Describe each procedure, its purpose, and the normal feelings or sensations that are likely, as well as any preprocedural and postprocedural care.
  —Chest x-ray
  —Pulmonary function studies: to assess the presence and severity of disease in the large and small airways
  —Sputum specimen analysis

—Laboratory tests: complete blood count, electrolytes, arterial blood gases

—Electrocardiogram

## TREATMENT

*Medical*

- Therapy
  - —Oxygen therapy
  - —Chest physiotherapy: postural drainage and chest percussion
  - —Ultrasonic or mechanical nebulizer treatments
  - —Physical training program
- Drugs
  - —Bronchodilators
  - —Antibiotics
  - —Corticosteroids

## HOME CARE

- Give both the patient and the caregiver *verbal* and *written* instructions. Provide them with the name and telephone number of a physician or nurse to call if questions arise.
- *General information*
  - —Explain the disease process and underlying cause. Assist the patient to identify individual factors that contribute to the disease process.
- *Warning signs*
  - —Review the signs and symptoms that should be reported to a physician or nurse.

    Elevated temperature

    Sore throat

    Increase in sputum production

    Change in color of sputum from clear white to yellow-green

    Upper respiratory infection

    Increased difficulty in breathing

    Decreased activity tolerance

    Decreased appetite
- *Special instructions*
  - —Discuss the importance of avoiding bronchopulmonary irritants.

    Cigarette smoking

    Industrial air pollutants

    Dust

Powders and perfumes

Aerosol sprays

Smoke

—Demonstrate the use of bronchodilator nebulizers. Watch for side effects such as rapid heart rate. Avoid overuse.

—Teach and demonstrate to the patient and caregiver adaptive breathing techniques, such as deep-breathing exercises, coughing techniques, pursed-lip breathing, abdominal breathing, and positions for postural drainage if needed.

—Explain the need to avoid persons with infections, especially upper respiratory tract infections. Urge the patient to seek medical care at the beginning of infections.

—Explain the importance of taking vaccines for influenza and pneumococcal pneumonia.

—Instruct the patient and caregiver on cleaning of all home respiratory equipment (see Oxygen Therapy, p. 492).

—Explain the importance of environmental control: avoid dry air by using a humidifier; provide a warm house (75°-80° F [23.8°-26.6° C]). Explain the need to keep warm and avoid chilling.

—Explain the need to avoid going out in cold temperatures, which may cause bronchospasm.

—Stress the importance of not smoking and of avoiding secondhand smoke. Explain that tobacco smoke is an irritant and can increase the risk of respiratory infection. Provide information about and referral to community-based smoking cessation programs and the local chapter of the American Lung Association.

• *Medications*

—Explain the purpose, dosage, schedule, and route of administration of any prescribed drugs, as well as side effects to report to a physician or nurse.

Bronchodilators: to open the airways and make breathing easier

Antibiotics: to prevent or treat respiratory infections

Corticosteroids: to reduce swelling in bronchi and bronchioles

—Explain the need to avoid taking over-the-counter medications without checking with the physician. Avoid sedatives and narcotics, which can depress respiration.

- *Activity*
  —Advise the patient to exercise to tolerance and to avoid fatigue by planning rest periods during the day.
  —Explain the need to limit activity on days of high air pollution.
  —Instruct the patient to breathe deeply and slowly during periods of activity.
  —Discuss energy conservaton techniques (e.g., perform such activities as bathing and shaving in a seated position).
  —Teach the patient and caregiver to watch for signs of extreme fatigue, chest pain, or diaphoresis during and after activity.
  —Instruct the patient to avoid emotional stress. Teach and demonstrate stress reduction techniques.
  —Explain the need to avoid constipation and straining at stool.
- *Diet*
  —Explain the need to maintain high-calorie diet as indicated.
  —Encourage fluid intake of 2000-3000 ml per day, unless contraindicated, to keep secretions liquid.
  —Suggest that the patient rest before and after meals if shortness of breath increases at mealtime.

**FOLLOW-UP CARE**

- Stress the importance of regular follow-up visits. Make sure the patient has the necessary names and telephone numbers.
- Discuss the need to wear a Medic-Alert band.

# Coronary Artery Disease

—**Coronary artery disease: a progressive disease process characterized by narrowing or blockage of the coronary arteries resulting in decreased blood flow to the heart muscle. Coronary artery disease (CAD) results from atherosclerosis, the buildup of fatty plaques (made up of cholesterol) and lipids on the inside walls of the arteries. Restriction of blood flow deprives the heart muscle of oxygen and nutrients, causing tissue damage. Chest pain occurs when the demand for oxygen by the heart muscle is greater than can be delivered by the blood vessels. CAD can present itself as angina pectoris or as**

**myocardial infarction. Symptomatic CAD is also referred to as ischemic heart disease.**

## CAUSES/CONTRIBUTING FACTORS OF ATHEROSCLEROSIS

- Family history
- Gender and age: males aged 35-55, females >50 or postmenopausal
- Hyperlipidemia
- Hypertension
- Diabetes
- Cigarette smoking
- Physical inactivity; sedentary life-syle
- Personality traits:
  —Hostility
  —Competitiveness
  —Aggression
  —Anger
- In premenopausal females:
  —Severe hypertension
  —Use of estrogen oral contraceptives
  —Smoking history

## ANGINA

Angina is chest pain that typically occurs during periods of exertion or emotion but is relieved by rest or nitroglycerin. It is caused by an imbalance in the supply and demand of oxygen-rich blood to the heart muscle resulting from a narrowed coronary artery, which is usually more than 70% blocked. Types of angina include stable, which comes on with effort and is relieved by rest and nitroglycerin; unstable, which can increase in frequency, duration, and severity even when little effort is expended; Prinzmetal's (variant angina), which is unrelated to exercise and is usually caused by coronary artery spasm; and intractable, which is frequent or continuous pain unrelieved by therapy. Complications of angina include myocardial infarction (heart attack), arrhythmias, sudden death, and heart failure.

## MYOCARDIAL INFARCTION

Myocardial infarction, or heart attack, is the death of myocardial tissue from lack of oxygen, caused by severe or complete occlusion of a coronary artery. The area of dead tissue is eventually replaced by scar tissue. Types of myocardial infarction and the associated blocked arteries are anterior wall (left anterior descending artery), anteroseptal (left anterior descending artery septal perforator), anterolateral (left anterior descending artery diagonal branch), inferior wall (right coronary artery in 90% of cases, circumflex artery in 10%), and lateral wall (circumflex artery).

## SIGNS/SYMPTOMS

- Chest pain and discomfort, such as tightness, squeezing, aching
- Indigestion above the waist
- Aching in the neck, jaw, throat, shoulder, or back (between the shoulder blades)
- Breathlessness, weakness, sweating, dizziness
- Diaphoresis or nausea associated with the above symptoms

## COMPLICATIONS

- Arrhythmias
- Heart failure
- Cardiogenic shock
- Arterial embolism
- Phlebothrombosis and pulmonary embolism
- Pericarditis
- Left ventricular aneurysm
- Cardiac rupture
- Ventricular septal defect
- Dressler's syndrome
- Valvular dysfunction

## DIAGNOSTIC TESTS

- Describe each procedure, its purpose, and the normal feelings or sensations that are likely, as well as any preprocedural and postprocedural care.
  - —Electrocardiogram: to identify ischemic or infarcted area
  - —Chest x-ray: to visualize enlarged heart and signs of left ventricular failure
  - —Echocardiography: to detect abnormalities of left ventricular wall motion and mechanical defects
  - —Coronary arteriography
  - —Blood tests
    - Serum lipids: lactate dehydrogenase, high-density lipoprotein, cholesterol

Cardiac enzymes: to determine amount of heart muscle damage

Complete blood count, erythrocyte sedimentation rate, and white blood cell count: to detect an inflammatory process

—Indium-111 antimycin antibody imaging: to detect infarcted cells and tissue

—Graded exercise test: to determine amount of exercise that causes angina, detect lack of blood supply to the tissues during exercise, and assess the risk to heart muscle

—Radionuclide studies

Thallium treadmill: to determine if areas of the heart muscle are receiving inadequate circulation during exercise

Technetium scan: to determine the amount of damage to the heart muscle

—Multigated acquisition scan: to evaluate ventricular function and detect aneurysms and wall motion abnormalities

## TREATMENT
### General

*Medical*
- Therapy
  - —Control of hypertension and diabetes
  - —Stress management
  - —Reduction of cholesterol and lipid levels
  - —Weight reduction
  - —Exercise
  - —Smoking cessation

### Angina

*Medical*
- Drugs
  - —Nitrates: to improve circulation to the heart muscle
  - —Beta blockers: to decrease heart rate, blood pressure, and force of contraction of the heart muscle and prevent cardiac arrhythmias
  - —Calcium entry blocking agents, such as nifedipine, verapamil, diltiazem
  - —Antiplatelets (aspirin): to reduct the risk of clot formation

*Surgical*
- Percutaneous balloon coronary angioplasty
- Coronary atherectomy

**Myocardial Infarction**

*Medical*
- Drugs
  - —Nitrates: to increase circulation to the muscles
  - —Beta blockers: to decrease heart rate, blood pressure, and force of contraction of the heart muscle and prevent cardiac arrhythmias
  - —Antiplatelets (aspirin): to reduce clot formation
  - —ACE inhibitors: to improve the healing of heart muscle by reducing its work
  - —Thrombolytic therapy: to restore circulation and prevent further damage that begins within 4-6 hours of the onset of chest pain

*Surgical*
- Coronary artery bypass surgery

## HOME CARE

- Give both the patient and the caregiver *verbal* and *written* instructions. Provide them with the name and telephone number of a physician or nurse to call if questions arise.
- Use a heart model or other visual aids to help the patient understand coronary anatomy. Discuss the atherosclerosis process, plaque formation, the role of lipids (high-density versus low-density lipoprotein) and cholesterol in plaque formation, and the various manifestations of coronary artery disease.

### Coronary Artery Disease

- *General information*
  - —Review ischemic heart disease, discussing the differences between angina and myocardial infarction. Angina is a temporary lack of blood supply, whereas myocardial infarction is a complete blockage that results in heart muscle damage. Damaged tissue heals into a scar in 6-8 weeks.
  - —Review the physician's explanation of the patient's form of coronary artery disease and the recommended treatment. Point out the location of the patient's coronary lesion.
  - —Discuss the importance of controlling any coexisting disease such as hypertension, diabetes, or hyperlipidemia.
  - —Discuss risk factors, assist the patient to identify his or her risk factors, and outline a plan for risk factor modification.
- *Medications*
  - —Explain the purpose, dosage, schedule, and route of adminis-

tration of any prescribed drugs, as well as side effects to report to a physician or nurse.

- *Special instructions*
  —Stress the importance on not smoking or using tobacco products. Explain the effect nicotine has on the cardiac system: causing the heart to work faster, constricting blood vessels, decreasing the amount of oxygen delivered to the heart, and in the presence of coronary artery disease, increasing the likelihood of chest pain. Refer the patient to a community-based smoking cessation program.
  —Discuss the role that stress plays in aggravating coronary artery disease. Help the patient to identify stress-producing factors and discuss methods of stress management. Discuss the need to recognize and deal with feelings of denial, anger, and depression. Provide the patient with a referral to psychologic and support groups to contact as needed.
- *Activity*
  —Discuss the benefits of exercise: decrease in high-density lipoproteins, which lowers blood pressure; weight loss; improved cardiovascular status.
  —Encourage a regular home exercise program that includes aerobic activities: walking, jogging, swimming, bicycling. Refer the patient to community-based cardiac fitness programs.
- *Diet*
  —Explain how the diet can modify cholesterol and lipid levels.
  —Discuss dietary modifications: limit intake of eggs, saturated fats (e.g., butter and cream), foods high in animal fat (e.g., bacon, red meat, luncheon meat); use polyunsaturated fats (e.g., vegetable oils) for cooking; restrict table salt and sodium intake.
  —Explain the importance of controlling weight and avoiding obesity. Inform the patient of the appropriate weight range for age, gender, and body frame.

### Angina Pectoris

- *Activity*
  —Assist the patient to identify and avoid physical and emotional factors that precipitate pain.
  —Tell the patient to avoid exercise in extremes of weather (hot or cold days), after heavy meals, when emotionally upset, and on smoggy days.

—Caution the patient to reduce the intensity and effort of activities such as shoveling snow; work slower and in as easy a manner as possible.

—Inform the patient that sexual activity should be avoided when fatigued. If chest pain occurs during sexual activity, the patient should stop and take nitrate if ordered. If pain persists or extreme fatigue occurs, the patient should notify the physician or nurse.

—Discuss self-management during episodes of chest pain: stop activity and rest; take nitrates as ordered (e.g., place a nitroglycerin tablet under the tongue and wait; pain will subside within 20 seconds); seek medical attention if pain persists longer than 20 minutes or diaphoresis and shortness of breath appear.

- *Diet*
  —Tell the patient to avoid eating heavy meals and exercising after eating.

  —Explain that caffeine and heavy alcohol intake should be avoided.

## Myocardial Infarction

- *General information*
  —Review the physician's explanation of infarction and associated complications.
- *Warning signs*
  —Review the signs and symptoms of escalation of angina to myocardial infarction that should be reported to a physician. Angina is chest pain or pressure that is associated with physical or emotional strain and is usually relieved by rest or vasodilators. Myocardial infarction is chest pain or discomfort that is not necessarily associated with physical exertion and is unrelieved by medication or rest. Stress the importance of seeking medical attention if chest pain lasts longer than 20 minutes or is associated with other symptoms.
- *Activity*
  —Discuss activity limitations during recovery.

    The patient should have 1-2 weeks of relative rest with short periods of activity, followed by 2-3 weeks of slowly increasing activity, such as walking and stair climbing, then several weeks of progressive activity be-

fore returning to work. Refer the patient to a cardiac rehabilitation program as indicated.

The physician should be consulted for specific exercise
limitations. Encourage questions about resumption of
work and recreational or sports activities.

The patient should avoid or modify activities after heavy
meals or alcohol intake and during periods of emotional
stress and temperature extremes.

—Discuss long-term modification of activity.

The patient should begin a lifelong aerobic exercise program.

Sexual activity can be resumed when the patient can climb
two flights of stairs without shortness of breath.

If symptoms occur, the patient should take nitroglycerin.
If no relief occurs within 15 minutes, the patient should
contact a physician or go to the nearest emergency room.

Explain the importance of maintaining independence in
self-care activities.

## PSYCHOSOCIAL CARE

• Encourage discussion about the need to deal with feelings about
possible role changes. Discuss the importance of communication between the patient and the caregiver or significant others.

# Coronary Artery Bypass Graft Surgery

—**Coronary artery bypass graft surgery: a surgical procedure
that increases blood flow to the heart muscle. Increasing the
supply of oxygen and nutrient to the myocardium prevents
myocardial infarction. Coronary artery bypass grafting
(CABG) is an open heart procedure that requires cardiopulmonary bypass, is performed under general anesthesia, and
generally involves two incisions. A leg (calf or thigh) incision
is made to remove a segment of the saphenous vein and a second incision is made in the chest (sternum) to allow one end
of the vein to be connected to the aorta and the other to be**

connected to the affected coronary artery below the level of
blockage. Multiple vein grafts can be done. Alternatively, a segment of the internal mammary artery may be used.

## INDICATIONS

• Acute or chronic ischemic heart disease

## PREPROCEDURAL TEACHING

• Review the physician's explanation of the procedure and the reason for it; encourage the patient to ask questions and to discuss
any fears or anxieties. Discuss the need to obtain written consent.

### Review of Preprocedural Care

• Review preparation of the skin of the chest and leg: the patient
is shaved from chin to toes and takes an antiseptic shower or
bath.
• Explain that a sedative will be given the night before and the
morning of surgery.
• Inform the patient that an anesthesiologist and respiratory therapist will visit the patient before surgery.

### Review of Postprocedural Care

• Explain that the patient will be taken to the surgical intensive
care unit right after the procedure; the usual stay in the unit is
1-2 days.
• Describe the unit, the noises the patient may hear, visiting privi-
leges, the pain the patient will feel, and the medications that
will be provided.
• Discuss the number of tubes (nasogastric tube, endotracheal
tube, chest tube, Foley catheter) and the intravenous and arterial lines. Explain that they will be removed as the patient's condition is stabilized.
• Explain the method of communication that will be used after
the operation while the patient is intubated.
• Inform the patient about routine care: frequent turning, coughing, deep breathing, and monitoring of vital signs.
• Emphasize the importance of coughing, deep breathing, and using the incentive spirometer; permit time for practice.
• Tell the patient that dangling and sitting in a chair may be permitted as early as the evening of surgery.

- Explain that the patient may be disoriented because of medications or lack of sleep and that sedation is used to keep the patient comfortable.

## SIDE EFFECTS/COMPLICATIONS

- Arrhythmias
- Bleeding or hemorrhage
- Hypotension/hypertension
- Cardiac tamponade
- Intraoperative myocardial infarction (2.5%-5% of patients)
- Pericarditis
- Postpericardiectomy syndrome
- Shock
- Postpump psychosis

## HOME CARE

- Give both the patient and the caregiver *verbal* and *written* instructions. Provide them with the name and telephone number of a physician or nurse to call if questions arise.
- *General information*
  —Review the operative procedure, discussing any specific precautions and complications associated with the surgery and what to expect with recovery.
  —Explain that complete healing and recovery take 8-12 weeks.
  —Inform the patient that the sternum was wired together and that a feeling of movement or a clicking sound is normal during the healing period.
  —Tell the patient that mild itching, redness, numbness, soreness, swelling, or a drawing feeling is normal during the healing period.
- *Wound/incision care*
  —Inform the patient that showers are allowed within a few days after surgery. The patient should use warm water and wash the incision gently.
  —Explain that most sutures dissolve slowly and do not require removal by a medical team.
  —Suggest that the patient wear loose, comfortable clothing. Women who have a submammary incision should not wear a bra for the first few days. When a bra can be worn again, it should not be an underwire bra, which could cause irritation.

- *Warning signs*
  —Review the signs and symptoms that should be reported to a physician or nurse.
    Wound infection: swelling, drainage, redness, pain
    Swelling of hands, legs; weight gain; shortness of breath
    Fever, rapid pulse
    Chest pain with inspiration or exertion
- *Medications*
  —Explain the purpose, dosage, schedule, and route of administration of any prescribed drugs, as well as side effects to report to a physician or nurse.
- *Activity*
  —Discuss activity limitations and allowances.
    Instruct the patient to increase activities gradually and to begin a daily exercise program such as walking. Refer the patient to a hospital- or community-based cardiac exercise program.
    Advise the patient to avoid fatigue by alternating activity with rest.
    Tell the patient to avoid prolonged standing or sitting. When sitting, the patient should not cross the legs or elevate the leg with the incision.
    Caution the patient to avoid lifting or carrying heavy objects or performing isometric activities. Driving should be restricted for the first few weeks or as ordered.
  —Encourage questions about when specific activities can be resumed, for example:
    Sexual activity when the patient and partner feel comfortable
    Sports such as swimming, golf, and tennis at 6 weeks
    Vacuuming, snow blowing, and moving at 6 weeks
    Return to work usually at 4-6 weeks; depends on occupation
  —Explain that CABG does not cure coronary artery disease. Emphasize the importance of life-style changes to prevent the recurrence of obstructions (see Coronary Artery Disease, p. 203).
- *Diet*
  —Explain that the diet should be low fat or as ordered and that salt intake should be restricted.

**FOLLOW-UP CARE**

• Stress the importance of regular follow-up visits. Make sure the patient has the necessary names and telephone numbers.

**PSYCHOSOCIAL CARE**

• Explain that emotions, irritability, and depression are commonly associated with recovery. Reassure the patient that they are temporary.

**REFERRALS**

• Refer the patient to local and national support groups, such as the Mended Heart Club.

# Craniotomy and Craniectomy

—**Craniotomy: a surgical opening into the skull to provide access to intracranial structures for surgical revision, resection, or removal of abnormalities.**

—**Craniectomy: surgical removal of a portion of the skull.**

**INDICATIONS**

• Removal of tumor or hematoma
• Repair of aneurysms
• Intracranial bleeding
• Relief of intracranial pressure

**PREPROCEDURAL TEACHING**

• Review the physician's explanation of the procedure and the reason for it; encourage the patient to ask questions and to discuss any fears or anxieties. Discuss the need to obtain written consent.

**Review of Preprocedural Care**

• Discuss the use of antiseptic shampoo, the administration of corticosteroids and anticonvulsants, and the need for a baseline neurologic assessment.

**Review of Postprocedural Care**

- Discuss the intensive care unit environment, intracranial pressure monitoring, ventilatory support, cardiac monitoring, intravenous lines, postoperative neurologic checks, fluid balance management, surgical drains, proper positioning, bed rest, and potential for cervical collar.
- Reassure the patient that precautions for seizures will be taken.
- Discuss anticipated body changes: loss of hair at the surgical site, head dressing, and potential for and duration of periorbital and facial edema.
- Warn the patient against pulling or tugging at the head dressing and drains.
- Stress the importance of deep breathing and avoiding coughing and sneezing. Maintain NPO until otherwise indicated, then provide fluids and diet within restrictions as ordered. Assess for swallowing and chewing ability.

**SIDE EFFECTS/COMPLICATIONS**

- Increased intracranial pressure
- Seizures
- Meningitis
- Respiratory distress
- Cardiac dysrhythmias
- Wound infection
- Diabetes insipidus
- Hemorrhage
- Thrombophlebitis
- Visual disturbances
- Personality changes
- Motor and sensory disturbances

**HOME CARE**

- Give both the patient and the caregiver *verbal* and *written* instructions. Provide them with the name and telephone number of a physician or nurse to call if questions arise.
- *General information*
  —Review the physician's explanation of the surgery and specific follow-up care.
  —Encourage the caregiver to verbalize anxieties related to the procedure, underlying conditions, and rehabilitative process.

- *Wound/incision care*
  —Demonstrate proper wound management and dressing changes: procedure, frequency of dressing change, and inspection of incision with each dressing change.
  —Instruct the patient to avoid scratching sutures and to keep the incision dry.
  —Advise the patient that hair may be shampooed when the sutures are removed but to avoid scrubbing around the suture line.
  —Advise the patient to avoid using a hair dryer until the hair grows back.
- *Warning signs*
  —Review the signs and symptoms that should be reported to a physician or nurse.
    Infection: fever, erythema, tenderness, pain, warmth, purulent drainage from the incision
    Meningitis: fever, chills, malaise, back stiffness and pain, nuchal rigidity
    Neurologic changes: behavioral, personality, motor, or sensory changes
    Increased intracranial pressure: altered level of consciousness, nausea, vomiting, seizures, headache
    Leakage of cerebrospinal fluid: clear or bloody drainage from ear, nose, or throat; complaints of salty taste or frequent swallowing; presence of "halo ring" on pillowcase
- *Special instructions*
  —Teach the caregiver seizure precautions as indicated.
    Try to prevent or break the fall.
    Ease the patient onto the floor.
    Support and protect the patient's head.
    Turn the patient to one side.
    Remove surrounding furniture and any hard or sharp objects.
    Loosen constrictive clothing around the neck.
    Stay with the patient and call the physician immediately.
  —Stress the importance of maintaining proper positioning and body mechanics as indicated by the surgical procedure.
    Teach the patient to avoid bending from the waist: keep back straight, bend knees, and lower body to pick up objects.

Use straight, flat chairs; avoid soft-cushioned chairs.

Avoid crossing knees.

Avoid lifting while back is flexed or twisted.

Keep head and neck in proper alignment with the cervical collar.

Avoid hyperextension of the spine: avoid sleeping in a prone or supine position; sleep on one side with knees and hips in flexion.

—Teach the patient to avoid extreme hot and cold temperatures of the lower extremities because of possible sensory nerve loss.

—Instruct the patient to avoid straining during defecation and to avoid constipation through the use of prescribed stool softeners and laxatives.

—Instruct the patient to avoid coughing, sneezing, and nose blowing. If unavoidable, they must be done with an open mouth to control intracranial pressure.

• *Medications*

—Explain the purpose, dosage, schedule, and route of administration of any prescribed drugs, as well as side effects to report to a physician or nurse.

—Advise the patient against taking over-the-counter medications without consulting the physician.

• *Activity*

—Encourage the patient to discuss allowances and limitations with respect to occupation, recreation, and activities.

—Encourage independent activities as the patient is able. Assist the patient and caregiver to identify and implement measures that assist with reorientation and communication, if indicated.

—Discuss safety measures specific for postoperative residual motor deficits, sensory deficits, cognitive deficits, and seizure activity. Assist the patient and caregiver to identify and correct hazards in the home.

## FOLLOW-UP CARE

• Stress the importance of regular follow-up visits with the physician, physical therapist, occupational therapist, speech therapist, and rehabilitation therapist as indicated. Make sure the patient has the necessary names and telephone numbers.

• Assist the patient in obtaining a Medic-Alert bracelet and identification card listing diagnosis and medications.

## REFERRALS

- Refer the patient to local support groups available through the American Cancer Society, American Brain Tumor Association, Acoustic Neuroma Association, or home health support services.

# Crutch Walking

—Crutch walking: use of ambulatory aids to limit or eliminate the amount of weight on the lower extremities. Use of crutches permits the patient to be mobile while the extremity is healing from traumatic injury or surgery.

## PREPROCEDURAL TEACHING

- Discuss the selection of proper crutches.
    - Underarm crutches with double uprights and hand bars are the most commonly used. Crutches may be made of wood or aluminum.
    - Shoulder pieces must have a rubber cover to prevent axillary pressure from hard wood or aluminum.
    - Rubber suction tips over each crutch base prevent slipping.
- Measure the patient for crutches.
    - Crutch length is measured from the anterior fold of the axilla to the lateral side of the heel, and 2 inches are added.
    - The level of the hand piece is in a positon that allows a slight bend at the elbow (25-30 degrees).

## SIDE EFFECTS/COMPLICATIONS

- Reinjury caused by falls
- Axillary nerve damage

## HOME CARE

- Give both the patient and the caregiver *verbal* and *written* instructions. Provide them with the name and telephone number of a physician or nurse to call if questions arise.

- *General information*
  —Review the physician's explanation of the use of crutches.
- *Warning signs*
  —Review the signs and symptoms that should be reported to a physician or nurse.

    Numbness and tingling down the arms to the thumb that does not go away quickly when leaning on the crutch tops is stopped

    Explain that leaning too long or putting too much pressure in the axillary (armpit) area can injure nerves and cut off circulation down the arms.

- *Special instructions*
  —Review the specific walking procedures, permitting time to practice before discharge.

    For crutch walking with some weight bearing on both legs: move one foot and leg and the crutch in the opposite hand forward at the same time, then move the other crutch and opposite foot and leg forward.

    For crutch walking with no weight bearing on one leg (i.e., one leg in cast with no weight bearing allowed): move both crutches and the affected leg forward about 8-10 inches. Shift weight to wrists and hands and step forward with the unaffected leg. Always move crutches, foot, and leg forward at the same time.

  —Review safety measures.

    Keep the crutches even as they are advanced ahead a comfortable and stable distance, approximately 10-12 inches.

    Pressure (weight) goes on the hands and not the armpits.

    Keep elbows into sides of body to help stabilize the crutches under the arms.

    Do not walk with crutches too close to feet, since this may result in tripping on them. Crutches should be placed 2-3 inches out to the side of the feet.

    Remove loose throw rugs, electrical cords, toys, and other objects on the floor at home to prevent falls.

    Avoid walking on slick or wet floors to prevent falls.

    Keep crutch tips clean, since dirt and dust can build up on them and make them slippery. Advise the patient of the importance of replacing worn tips.

  —Discuss and demonstrate sitting and rising with crutches.

Sitting down in a chair with crutches: walk up close to the chair. Turn, then back up until the chair touches the back of the legs. Hold the handgrips of both crutches with one hand, and with the other hand reach for the arm or seat of the chair. Bearing weight on the handgrips of the crutches and the arm or seat of the chair, lower into the chair. Slide the affected leg forward.

Getting up from a chair with crutches: slide forward in the chair as far as possible. Position the unaffected foot slightly farther back than the affected foot. Both crutches should be on the affected side. Holding on to the handgrips of the crutches, use the other hand to push from the edge or armrest of the chair when leaning forward to stand.

Stress the importance of not sitting down with crutches under the arms, since this can cause damage to the axillary nerve from undue pressure.

—Discuss and demonstrate walking up and down stairs.

Walking up stairs with one crutch in each hand: walk close to the bottom of the steps. Put all weight on the handgrips and step up to the next step with the unaffected leg and foot. Bring the body, affected leg, and crutches up to the same step, making sure the crutches are centered on the step.

Walking down stairs with one crutch in each hand: walk to the edge of the top step. Bend the hips and place both crutches and the affected leg on the next lower step. Put weight on crutches and bring the unaffected leg down to the same step.

Walking up stairs with railing: place both crutches under the arm opposite the banister and grasp both handgrips. Grasp the railing with the free hand. Put all weight on hands and lift the unaffected foot and leg up to the next step. Bring crutches, body, and affected leg up to the same step.

Walking down stairs with railing: put both crutches in one hand, holding them together at handgrips and under the arm. Put the other hand on the railing. Move the affected leg and crutches down to the next step. (Do not put any weight on the affected leg if it should not bear weight.) Put all weight on hands and wrists of the crutches and the railing, and step down with the unaffected leg.

# Cushing's Disease and Cushing's Syndrome

—Cushing's disease and Cushing's syndrome: a condition resulting from the overproduction of adrenal steroid, particularly cortisol. The high levels of circulating glucocorticoids affect protein, carbohydrate, and lipid metabolism. The disease may occur as a primary disease or secondary to a pituitary tumor. It more commonly affects females.

## CAUSES/CONTRIBUTING FACTORS
### Cushing's Disease
- Hypersecretion of the pituitary gland, which secretes an excess of adrenocorticotropic hormone (ACTH) in the face of high levels of plasma cortisol

### Cushing's Syndrome
- ACTH-secreting tumors of the adrenals
- Iatrogenic causes, such as excessive doses of cortisol or ACTH

## SIGNS/SYMPTOMS
- Physical changes
  - Central obesity (large trunk, thin legs and arms)
  - Buffalo hump
  - Round face ("moonface")
  - Supraclavicular fat pads
- Other changes
  - Weight gain
  - Muscle weakness
  - Thin, transparent skin
  - Bruising
  - Impaired wound healing
  - Susceptibility to infections
  - Hypertension, fluid retention with pitting edema
  - Emotional and mental disturbances
- Orthopedic changes
  - Kyphosis and back pain
  - Osteoporosis

- In women
  —Masculinization
  —Menstrual changes
- In men
  —Feminization
  —Impotence
  —Decreased libido

## COMPLICATIONS

- Pathologic fractures
- Congestive heart failure
- Peptic ulcers
- Diabetes insipidus: with adrenalectomy
- Diabetes mellitus

## DIAGNOSTIC TESTS

- Describe each procedure, its purpose, and the normal feelings or sensations that are likely, as well as any preprocedural and postprocedural care.
  —Computed tomography or magnetic resonance imaging: to identify causative tumor of the pituitary gland
  —Serum tests
    Blood glucose: increased (tested after meals)
    Potassium: decreased
    Overnight dexamethasone suppression test: plasma cortisol levels decreased to 50% of baseline
  —Urine tests
    24-Hour for free cortisol (17-ketosteroid and 17-hydroxycorticosteroid) levels: elevated

## TREATMENT

*Medical*
- Therapy
  —Irradiation of the pituitary gland: used for mild disease or poor surgical risk
- Drugs
  —Adrenocortical inhibitors
    Metopirone
    Mitotane
    Aminoglutethimide
    Cyproheptadine

*Surgical*
- Transsphenoidal pituitary surgery
- Adrenalectomy: unilateral or bilateral

## HOME CARE

- Give both the patient and the caregiver *verbal* and *written* instructions. Provide them with the name and telephone number of a physician or nurse to call if questions arise.
- *General information*
  —Review the physician's explanation of Cushing's disease and Cushing's syndrome, the causes, and contributing factors.
  —Review skin care, explaining the need to avoid bruising and cuts.
    Advise the patient to inspect the skin for reddened areas, signs of excoriation, and breakdown.
    Keep the skin clean and dry. Use moisturizing skin lotions.
    Advise the patient against using razor blades for shaving.
- *Warning signs*
  —Review the signs and symptoms that should be reported to a physician or nurse.
    Excessive adrenal hormone: weight gain, polydipsia, polyuria, easy bruising, and muscle weakness
    Insufficient adrenal hormone: easy fatigability, weight loss, abdominal pain
    Infection of upper respiratory tract, urinary tract, oral cavity: fever, cough, malodorous sputum; burning, frequency, urgency with urination, malodorous urine; red, swollen, bleeding, painful oral mucosa, painful mucosal lesions, painful teeth
- *Special instructions*
  —For patients with bilateral adrenalectomy: provide the patient with an emergency kit incuding alcohol, prefilled syringes (hydrocortisone) for episodes of severe adrenal insufficiency (see p. 10).
  —Instruct the patient to self-monitor laboratory values and assist the patient to identify personal baseline levels.
  —Discuss the need to prevent injury associated with osteoporosis.
    Keep rooms free of throw rugs and hazardous furniture to prevent falls.
    Use ambulatory aids (e.g., walker, cane) as necessary.

- *Medications*
  —Explain the purpose, dosage, schedule, and route of adminis-
  tration of any prescribed drugs, as well as side effects to re-
  port to a physician or nurse.
  —Teach the patients with bilateral adrenalectomy about the need
  for lifelong hormonal therapy.
  —Discuss hormonal replacement (see Steroid Therapy, p. 608).
  —Discuss the need to avoid over-the-counter medications with-
  out first consulting the physician or nurse.
- *Activity*
  —Encourage the patient to discuss allowances and limitations
  with respect to occupation, recreation, and activities.
  —Encourage the patient to pace activites, allow for frequent rest
  periods, and avoid overexertion.
  —Teach the importance of using protective devices (decubitus
  matrices, well-fitting shoes) and practices (changing position
  frequently, range-of-motion exercises) to avoid injury.
  —Discuss the relationship between stress and cortisol levels.
  Teach stress reduction methods: imagery, progressive relaxation, breathing exercises, and meditation.
- *Diet*
  —Discuss the importance of a well-balanced diet that is high in
  potassium and low in sodium, calories, and carbohydrates.
  High-potassium foods include avocadoes, apricots, bananas,
  meat, poultry, potatoes, and milk.

**FOLLOW-UP CARE**

- Stress the importance of regular follow-up visits for medical and
  laboratory evaluation. Make sure the patient has the necessary
  names and telephone numbers.
- Emphasize the need to wear a Medic-Alert bracelet and carry
  an identification card at all times.

**PSYCHOSOCIAL CARE**

- Explain the effects of hormones on emotional status.
- Discuss methods for managing labile emotional states.
- Encourage open communication between the patient and care-
  givers.

# Cystic Fibrosis

—Cystic fibrosis: an autosomal recessive disorder of the exocrine (mucus-secreting) glands: respiratory, pancreatic, and sweat. Cystic fibrosis (CF) causes respiratory glands to produce and accumulate abnormally thick, tenacious secretions. Pancreatic function is affected by a deficiency of trypsin and lipase, which prevents the absorption of fat and protein in the intestinal tract and interferes with the digestion of food. A chronic, progressive, and incurable genetic disease, CF may manifest itself soon after birth or may take years to develop. Survival rates have been improving, with patients living into their thirties and forties.

## SIGNS/SYMPTOMS

- Gastrointestinal system
  - —Poor weight gain
  - —Thin extremities with abdominal distention
  - —Stool (steatorrhea): frequency: large, bulky, frothy, greasy; float in toilet; foul smelling
  - —Anorexia
- Pulmonary system
  - —Dry, chronic cough followed by loose, productive cough
  - —Thick, tenacious mucus
  - —Shortness of breath with activity
  - —Wheezing
  - —Cyanosis, clubbed fingers

## COMPLICATIONS

- Respiratory
  - —Severe atelectasis
  - —Emphysema
  - —Pneumonia
  - —Pneumothorax
  - —Cor pulmonale
  - —Pulmonary hypertension
- Gastrointestinal
  - —Intestinal obstruction
  - —Esophageal varices

—Portal hypertension
—Cirrhosis
• Other
   —Dehydration
   —Arthralgia of distal long bones and associated joints (e.g., knees, ankles, wrists)
   —Sterility: secondary amenorrhea in women, azoospermia (lack of sperm) in men

## DIAGNOSTIC TESTS

• Describe each procedure, its purpose, and the normal feelings or sensations that are likely, as well as any preprocedural and postprocedural care.
   —Sweat electrolytes: elevated sweat chloride level (>60 mEq/L)
   —Pancreatic enzymes: decreased or absent trypsin, lipase, and amylase
   —Stool examination: minimal or absent trypsin in stool, elevated fat in stool, and increased albumin (azotorrhea, >20 mg/dl)
   —Chest x-ray: identifies pulmonary complications
   —Pulmonary function tests

## TREATMENT

*Medical*
• Therapy
   —Respiratory management: pulmonary hygiene, oxygen therapy, postural drainage
• Drugs
   —Bronchodilators, mucolytics, expectorants
   —Antibiotics; to treat pulmonary infections
   —Pancreatic enzyme replacement with meals and snacks
   —Fat-soluble vitamins
   —Daily iron supplements
   —Salt tablet supplements during hot weather
*Surgical*
• Pulmonary lavage or bronchial washings
• Resection of blebs and pleural scars

## HOME CARE

• Give both the patient and the caregiver *verbal* and *written* instructions. Provide them with the name and telephone number of a physician or nurse to call if questions arise.

- *General information*
  - —Explain the disease process, causes, and prescribed treatments.
- *Warning signs*
  - —Review the signs and symptoms that should be reported to a physician or nurse.
      Excessive number of large, bulky, foul-smelling stools
      Change in sputum characteristics or color (e.g., thickened and contains blood)
      Decreased activity tolerance
      Poor appetite
      Fatigue
      Weight loss
      Fever
      Stress symptoms
- *Special instructions*
  - —Stress the importance of breathing exercises and postural drainage techniques. Demonstrate and permit time to practice.
  - —Teach the patient and family the use of the home nebulizer and other respiratory equipment necessary to loosen secretions and dilate bronchi. Assist the patient to obtain equipment from a pharmacy or medical supply company.
  - —Explain the need to avoid persons with upper respiratory infections and known respiratory irritants such as smoke and air pollutants.
- *Medications*
  - —Explain the purpose, dosage, schedule, and route of administration of digestive agents, bronchodilators, and antibiotics, as well as side effects to report to a physician or nurse.
  - —Advise the patient against taking over-the-counter medications without consulting the physician.
- *Activity*
  - —Encourage the patient to participate in a program of aerobic exercise. Swimming helps strengthen the muscles of respiration and promotes good breathing habits.
  - —Tell the patient to perform respiratory treatment before participating in physical activity.
  - —Discuss modifications needed during warm day to prevent dehydration: avoid activities on hot and polluted days, drink plenty of fluid, and take salt supplements.

- *Diet*
  —Review the prescribed diet, which is high in calories and protein and low in fat.
  —Discuss the need to include vitamin supplements (A, D, E, K).
  —Encourage the patient to eat salty foods and add salt at the table.
  —Explain the need to mix supplemental pancreatic enzymes with carbohydrate foods such as applesauce. Protein foods cause enzymes to break down immediately. Instruct the patient to take supplements with snacks as well as meals and to adjust pancreatic enzyme replacement as necessary in accordance with food intake and stool patterns.
  —Tell the patient to avoid known dietary irritants.
  —Assist the patient and caregiver to consult a dietitian for special diet instructions and counseling, alternative ways to prepare foods, and modification of family recipes.

## FOLLOW-UP CARE

- Stress the importance of regular follow-up visits. Make sure the patient has the necessary names and telephone numbers.
- Obtain influenza and pneumonia vaccines as recommended.

## PSYCHOSOCIAL CARE

- Encourage the patient and caregiver to communicate feelings and concerns to health care professionals and each other. Encourage the caregiver and patient to talk with another family living with cystic fibrosis and its prognosis.
- Discuss with the caregiver the need for everyone to participate in the care of a family member with cystic fibrosis.

## REFERRALS

- Refer the patient to the Cystic Fibrosis Foundation.
- Provide referral for counseling and financial assistance if necessary.

# Decubitus Ulcers
## (Pressure Sores, Bedsores)

—Decubitus ulcers: an area of tissue necrosis, usually over a bony prominence, that results from tissue hypoxia caused by pressure. Patients at risk include the elderly, spinal cord injury patients, and debilitated patients who are increasingly immobile.

### STAGES OF DECUBITUS ULCER

I. Erythema only; no break in skin
II. Partial thickness; loss of skin involving epidermis, often into dermis
III. Full thickness; involves epidermis extending into dermis and involves subcutaneous tissue
IV. Deep tissue destruction extending to subcutaneous tissue and into fascia, muscle, bone

### RISK FACTORS

- Old age
- Immobility
- Impaired sensation
- Incontinence
- Malnutrition
- Skin shearing

### SIGNS/SYMPTOMS

- Redness
- Warmth at pressure area
- Disruption of skin integrity with pain, swelling, heat, induration, drainage, tissue necrosis

### COMPLICATIONS

- Infection: bacteremia, septicemia
- Further tissue necrosis

## DIAGNOSTIC TESTS

- Describe each procedure, its purpose, and the normal feelings or sensations that are likely, as well as any preprocedural and postprocedural care.
  —Wound cultures
  —Serum albumin

## TREATMENT

*Medical*
- Therapy
  —Diet, vitamins, mineral supplements
  —Pressure relief devices: pads, mattresses, bed
- Drugs
  —Systemic and topical antibiotics

*Surgical*
- Debridement (surgical or chemical [mechanical]): to remove necrotic tissue
- Surgical repair and grafting

## HOME CARE

- Give both the patient and the caregiver *verbal* and *written* instructions. Provide them with the name and telephone number of a physician or nurse to call if questions arise.
- *General information*
  —Explain the underlying cause or contributing factors. Identify and review the patient's stage of ulcer development, discussing specific procedures to prevent further progression.
  —Explain that treatment depends on the stage of healing. Instruct the caregiver to recognize and record the signs of healing.
- *Warning signs*
  —Review the signs and symptoms that should be reported to a physician or nurse.
  　Weight loss
  　Elevated temperature
  　Increased drainage from the ulcer
  　Foul odor from the dressing
  　Further necrosis around the ulcer and reddened areas at other pressure points
- *Special instructions*
  —Ulcer care, stages I and II
  　Eliminate causative factors.
  　Cleanse the skin every 8 hours with mild soap. Pat dry.

Massage the skin gently to increase circulation. Avoid vigorous rubbing. Do not massage reddened areas.

Protect the skin surface of the affected area with protective skin gels, ointment, and porous dressings as ordered. Avoid using tape directly on the skin. Demonstrate proper application techniques. If necessary, tape lightly. Use special protective pads and mattresses.

If the patient is on bed rest, turn every 1-2 hours. Show the patient how to use a turn sheet; instruct not to slide on sheets. Keep bedsheets wrinkle free; change linens frequently if the patient is diaphoretic or incontinent.

Encourage the patient to position self on unaffected areas.

If the patient is incontinent, encourage frequent use of the commode. Tell the patient to avoid use of heavy or excessive incontinent pads, which can increase perspiration and irritate skin.

—Ulcer care, stages III and IV

After debridement, inspect the wound for size, color, odor, and drainage and record information. Cleanse the wound using prescribed procedure. Provide the caregiver with written instruction. Review the signs and symptoms to report: elevated temperature, increased drainage, foul odor.

Explain debridement or skin grafting procedures as indicated.

Discuss with the caretaker the importance of daily hygiene to prevent infection and skin breakdown. Stress the importance of regular (three times a day or more) inspections of bony prominences and maintaining skin integrity by keeping skin clean and dry. Use mild soap and water. Provide perineal care after voiding or bowel movement.

Avoid use of skin-damaging products: harsh soaps, alcohol-based lotions, tincture of benzoin, hexachlorophene.

Instruct the patient and caregiver not to use a heat lamp because it increases the metabolic rate of the tissues, resulting in increased demand for blood flow in an area with impaired perfusion. As a result, ulcer diameter and depth can be increased.

Instruct the patient and caregiver to gently massage the area around the bony prominence (not on it) and administer gentle back rubs with bland emollient; remove any excess and avoid use of alcohol.

Instruct the patient and caregiver in protecting the heels, elbows, back of head, iliac crests, sacrum, and coccyx against skin breakdown by using foam rubber pads.

Demonstrate wound care, including cleansing procedure and application of medication and dressing changes.

Arrange to obtain equipment, such as pressure-reducing mattress, footboard, bed cradle, and wound care supplies, that will be used at home. Explain the function of pressure relief devices and demonstrate how to use the equipment properly. Advise the patient and caregiver on where to buy equipment, such as drugstores and medical supply stores.

Consult with an enterostomal therapist for specific wound care instruction if necessary.

- *Medications*
  —Explain the purpose, dosage, schedule, and route of administration of any prescribed drugs, as well as side effects to report to a physician or nurse.
- *Activity*
  —Explain the importance of increasing activity as tolerated, changing positions every 2-3 hours while in bed or in chair, and avoiding pressure on affected area.
  — Instruct the caregiver in assisting the patient out of bed and into a chair.
  —Teach active and passive range-of-motion exercises to all extremities and explain that they should be performed every 4 hours.
- *Diet*
  —Encourage a high-calorie, high-protein diet with adequate fluid intake (2 liters per day), unless contraindicated, to maintain body weight and promote healing.
  —For debilitated patient, instruct the patient to eat small, frequent meals that include protein- and caloric-rich supplements.

## FOLLOW-UP CARE

- Stress the importance of regular follow-up visits for medical and laboratory evaluation. Make sure the patient has the necessary names and telephone numbers.

# Diabetes Insipidus

—**Diabetes insipidus: a transient or permanent disturbance of water metabolism that results in the excretion of a large volume of dilute urine. The disease may be pituitary, nephrogenic, or psychogenic in nature.**

## CAUSES/CONTRIBUTING FACTORS

- Central (pituitary)
- Nephrogenic
- Psychogenic (polydipsia)

## SIGNS/SYMPTOMS

- Excretion of large volumes of dilute urine (polyuria; 4 liters per day)
- Polydipsia, unquenchable thirst, preference for cold or iced water
- Low specific gravity (1.001-1.005)
- Poor skin turgor, dry skin, weight loss
- Constipation

## DIAGNOSTIC TESTS

- Describe each procedure, its purpose, and the normal feelings or sensations that are likely, as well as any preprocedural and postprocedural care.
    —Dehydration test
        Central and nephrogenic: no change in urine concentration
        Psychogenic: urine will become concentrated
    —Administration of vasopressin following dehydration
        Central: urine becomes concentrated
        Nephrogenic and psychogenic: no change
    —Visual field testing: defects suggest hypothalamic pituitary lesions
    —Computed tomography scan: useful for detection of hypothalamic pituitary lesions

## TREATMENT

*Medical*
- Drugs
    —Pituitary hormones

Vasopressin (Aqueous Pitressin): short acting, emergency and diagnostic use

Vsopressin (Pitressin Tannate in oil): longer acting, chronic and diagnostic use

Lypressin nasal solution (Diapid Nasal Spray; synthetic lysine): may be used alone or with Pitressin Tannate

Desmopressin (DDAVP; synthetic arginine, vasopressin): drug of choice for chronic treatment

## HOME CARE

- Give both the patient and the caregiver *verbal* and *written* instructions. Provide them with the name and telephone number of a physician or nurse to call if questions arise.
- *General information*
  —Explain and discuss with the patient diabetes insipidus, its specific causes, and contributing factors.
- *Warning signs*
  —Review the signs and symptoms that should be reported to a physician or nurse.

    Polydipsia
    Polyuria
    Dilute urine
    Weight loss or gain

- *Special instructions*
  —Show the patient how to measure and record intake and output, stressing that intake should equal output.
  —Demonstrate how to check the urine's specific gravity. Advise the patient where to obtain supplies.
  —Instruct the patient to weigh self daily at the same time with the same clothing and to record weight.
  —Advise the patient to avoid fluids that may have diuretic effect: coffee, tea, alcohol.
- *Medications*
  —Explain the purpose, dosage, schedule, and route of administration of any prescribed drugs, as well as side effects to report to a physician or nurse.
  —Demonstrate how to administer vasopressin. Discuss with the patient side effects or toxic effects to report to the physician and how to use urine volume and characteristics as parameters for the need for administration.

- *Activity*
  —Encourage the patient to discuss allowances and limitations with respect to occupation, recreation, or activities.
  —Discuss the need to plan rest periods and avoid overexertion.

**FOLLOW-UP CARE**

- Stress the importance of regular follow-up visits for medical and laboratory evaluation. Make sure the patient has the necessary names and telephone numbers.
- Discuss the importance of wearing a Medic-Alert bracelet and having a disease identification card.

---

# Diabetes Mellitus
## (Ketoacidosis)

---

**—Diabetes mellitus: a metabolic disorder characterized by glucose intolerance. It is a systemic disease caused by a relative or absolute lack of insulin, affecting carbohydrate, protein, and fat metabolism.**

## CAUSES/CONTRIBUTING FACTORS

- Primary
  —Insulin-dependent diabetes mellitus (IDDM) (type I, juvenile, brittle, labile)
  —Non-insulin-dependent diabetes mellitus (NIDDM) (type II, adult)
- Secondary
  —Impaired glucose tolerance
  —Gestational diabetes mellitus

## RISK FACTORS

- Familial tendency (heredity)

## SIGNS/SYMPTOMS

- Polyphagia
- Polydipsia
- Polyuria

- Weight loss or gain
- Blurred vision, headaches
- Lethargy
- Impotence, vaginal discharge, increased vaginal infections
- Increased wound healing time
- Orthostatic hypotension, decreased pedal pulses
- Paresthesias, decreased sensations (extremities)

**COMPLICATIONS**

- Diabetic neuropathies (loss of sensation in extremities)
- Charcot's syndrome
- Retinopathy, kidney failure
- Atherosclerosis of the heart and large vessels
- Amputation

**DIAGNOSTIC TESTS**

- Describe each procedure, its purpose, and the normal feelings or sensations that are likely, as well as any preprocedural and postprocedural care.
  —Serum
   Fasting blood sugar
   Glucose tolerance test
   Blood insulin levels
   Plasma proinsulin
   Plasma C-peptide
   Glycosylated hemoglobin
  —Urine
   Urinalysis (ketone, glucose, protein)

**TREATMENT**

*Medical*

- Therapy
  —American Diabetes Association (ADA) diet
  —Insulin infuser pens, open-loop infusion pumps
  —Photocoagulation
- Drugs
  —Insulin preparations: human, pork, beef-pork
   Short acting: regular, semilente
   Intermediate acting: NPH, lente
   Long acting: ultralente, protamine zinc
   Premixed insulins

—Oral hypoglycemic agents: sulfonylureas

—First generation: tolbutamide (Orinase), chlorpropamide (Diabinese), acetohexamide (Dymelor), tolazamide (Tolinase)

—Second generation: glipizide (Glucotrol), glyburide (Diabeta, Micronase)

## HOME CARE

- Give both the patient and the caregiver *verbal* and *written* instructions. Provide them with the name and telephone number of a physician or nurse to call if questions arise. Include visual aids and permit time before discharge for return demonstration.

- *General information*

  —Explain and discuss with the patient the specific type of diabetic disorder, the causes, and contributing factors.

- *Warning signs*

  —Review the signs and symptoms of hyperglycemia and hypoglycemia that should be reported to a physician or nurse.

    Polydipsia

    Polyuria

    Lethargy

    Shakiness

    Nausea

    Blood glucose >200

  —Discuss complications associated with diabetes, their signs and symptoms, and measures to prevent them.

- *Special instructions*

  —Discuss blood glucose monitoring and urine ketone testing.

    Discuss when the test will take place, the technique, the desirable blood sugar range, how to read test results, what to do for abnormal results, the cleaning of equipment, and quality control measures (expiration of strips, calibration of equipment).

    Discuss the importance of washing the hands before using equipment.

  —Discuss self-care when the patient is sick.

    Monitoring is increased to every 4 hours when the patient is sick because illness or injury increases glucose demand. A change in food and medication also is usually required.

    Test results and symptoms should be reported to a physician: blood glucose level >300, urine results 1% for two successive tests, inability to take oral fluid and food, signs and symptoms of hyperglycemia.

The patient should keep a log of blood and urine results near the phone as a reference when talking to the physician.

Hydration should be maintained with broth, tea, nondietetic soda, gelatin, or fluid with electrolytes.

Insulin administration should be based on test results and discussions with the physician.

—Discuss issues of safety and personal hygiene, stressing specifics related to dental, foot, and skin care.

Maintain meticulous dental hygiene to prevent infection.

Wear shoes or slippers at all time to prevent foot injury.

Inspect the feet daily with a handheld mirror to detect cuts, abrasion, and sores.

Visit a podiatrist to have nails, calluses, and corns trimmed.

Keep skin surfaces clean and dry to prevent injury and infection. Report any nonhealing lesions to the physician or nurse for follow-up.

Wear gloves while gardening.

—Advise a female patient to monitor for vaginal infections (fungal) and report them to a physician or nurse for follow-up.

—Discuss with the patient the need to carry fast-acting sugar (Life-Savers, sugar packets) for treatment of hypoglycemia.

—Advise the patient to obtain appropriate items, equipment, and assistive devices for various diabetic needs (glucose monitor, urine chemstrips, Medic-Alert bracelet and identification card, protective shoes).

—Discuss the need to prepare for travel.

Inform the physician.

Obtain immunizations. Have duplicate prescriptions (medications, syringes, needles). Have a letter describing the condition. Obtain a Medic-Alert bracelet.

Arrange for special meals en route.

Carry insulin and supplies in hand luggage to prevent loss or exposure to extreme temperature changes. Carry emergency medications to treat travel complications. Carry food.

Be aware of the need to adjust meal and medication schedules as time zones change.

Find out where to obtain emergency assistance if needed.

Travel with a companion if possible.

—For women of childbearing age:

Stress the importance of planning all pregnancies. Explain that pregnancy presents serious risks to the mother and infant.

Encourage the patient to discuss her particular risks with the physician or nurse.

- *Medications*

—Explain the purpose, dosage, schedule, and route of administration of any prescribed drugs, as well as side effects to report to a physician or nurse.

—Demonstrate insulin administration (see discussion of subcutaneous injection below). Review the following:

Peak action times

Insulin storage

Preparation and injection

Site selection and rotation

Techniques for self-injection

—Discuss the use and side effects of oral hypoglycemic agents.

—Tell the patient that new supplies and medication prescriptions should be refilled 1-2 weeks before stocks run out.

—Instruct the patient to keep a daily log of blood glucose and urine ketone levels and doses of insulin and oral hypoglycemics.

—Review subcutaneous insulin injection. Demonstrate and explain the following steps of the procedure, and permit sufficient time for the patient or caregiver to practice.

Rotate the injection sites weekly to prevent hypertrophy or lipoatrophy of the subcutaneous tissues.

Wash hands and use aseptic technique when holding the syringe and needle.

Mix insulin correctly (rolling, not shaking).

Withdraw the correct amount of insulin.

Select the injection site: use subcutaneous fatty tissue and avoid the area within 2 inches of the umbilicus.

Cleanse the skin with alcohol and allow to dry.

Hold the syringe filled with correct insulin dosage like a dart.

Pinch up the skin, forming a fat roll between the fingers.

Using a dartlike motion, quickly insert the needle up to the hub or syringe at a 45-degree angle into the subcutaneous tissue.

Inject the insulin. After completing the injection, pull the needle out quickly and cover the site with cotton. Apply slight pressure for 5-8 seconds. *Do not rub.* Rubbing can cause too rapid absorption.

Record the date, time, site, and dosage of each infection on the home record.

Dispose of needles/sharps in a stiff plastic container (gallon bleach container, sharps container). Tape lid or lock closed when two thirds full.

—Arrange to have the necessary equipment available at home.

- *Activity*
  —Stress the importance of regular exercise and activity to control blood sugar level and weight.
  —Tell the patient to carry simple carbohydrates (raisins, Life-Savers) while exercising in case of emergency.
  —Encourage the patient to discuss allowances and limitations with respect to occupation, recreation, or activities.
  —Explain that aerobic exercise such as walking, swimming, running, and cycling is preferable because it decreases glucose and benefits cardiovascular status.
  —Refer the patient to a community-based exercise program such as those offered by the YMCA or YWCA.
- *Diet*
  —Obtain a dietary consult and review the prescribed diet.
  —Discuss with the patient the need to spread meals throughout the day and to eat meals and snacks at regular times and in prescribed amounts. ADA guidelines suggest 55%-60% carbohydrates, 30% fat, 12%-20% protein.
  —Instruct the patient in methods for adjusting the diet to meet a change in activity (greater caloric intake is required for prolonged or strenuous activity to prevent hypoglycemia).

## FOLLOW-UP CARE

- Stress the importance of regular medical and laboratory follow-up visits. Make sure the patient has the necessary names and telephone numbers.

## PSYCHOSOCIAL CARE

- Discuss with the patient and significant others the need for support for required life-style changes Make sure the patient has the necessary names and telephone numbers.

**REFERRALS**

• Encourage participation in and provide information about local diabetes support groups, the ADA, and the Juvenile Diabetes Foundation.

# Dialysis
## (Hemodialysis, Peritoneal Dialysis)

—Dialysis: a temporary or permanent process that artificially replaces the excretory function of the kidney. Dialysis is used to remove excessive amounts of drugs, fluids, or toxic waste products from the body and to correct serious electrolye and fluid imbalances.

—Hemodialysis: removal of toxins from the body by shunting the patient's blood from the body through a machine for filtration and diffusion and then returning the blood to the patient's circulation. Hemodialysis requires access to the patient's bloodstream by special vascular catheters called shunts. An external shunt involves two cannulas from an artery and vein connected outside the body, usually on the arm. An internal arteriovenous fistula is a connection made between an artery and vein or an artificial graft implanted between the artery and vein. This is done on the arm or thigh. Hemodialysis may be a temporary measure, as for acute renal failure or hepatic coma, or a permanent measure, as for chronic renal failure or end-stage renal disease. The sessions last 3-5 hours and take place three or four times a week.

—Peritoneal dialysis: instillation of dialyzing solution directly into the abdominal cavity through a silicone catheter (Tenckhoff). The body tissue acts as a filter to remove the toxins. The fluid is left in for a specified time and then drained. Peritoneal dialysis can be performed by machine or manually by gravity. There are three types: intermittent, continuous ambulatory, and continuous cycling. Intermittent peritoneal dialysis is performed in 8- to 10-hour sessions four or five times a week. It can be done manually or by a cycling machine. The patient is restricted to the bed or chair during the procedure. In continuous ambulatory peritoneal dialysis, exchanges take place every 4 hours during the day and every 8 hours at night. The patient can be up and about, continuing daily activities. After fluid instillation, the bag remains connected and is placed under the clothing until time to drain and change it. Continuous cycling peritoneal dialysis is a combination of the other types. Three exchanges are done at night by a cycling machine and one cycle is done during the day. The patient is ambulatory during the day and confined to bed at night.

## INDICATIONS

- Acute poisoning (aspirin, methanol, phenobarbital)
- Acute renal failure
- Chronic renal failure
- End-stage renal failure
- Hepatic coma
- Hyperkalemia
- Metabolic acidosis

## PREPROCEDURAL TEACHING

- Review the physician's explanation of the type of procedure, the reason for it, and whether it is permanent or temporary. Encourage the patient to ask questions and to discuss any fears or anxieties.

### Review of Preprocedural Care

- Discuss preprocedural tests.
  - —Blood studies: to determine drug and electrolyte levels and kidney function
      Blood urea nitrogen
      Creatinine
      Protein
      Clotting levels
      Platelets
  - —Urine studies
      Urinalysis
      Culture and sensitivity
- Discuss the specific type of *hemodialysis*.
  - —For temporary hemodialysis: written consent for insertion of

the catheter into a large vein in the shoulder or groin area; procedure performed under local anesthetic

—For permanent hemodialysis: written consent for insertion of the shunt; procedure done as same-day surgery under general anesthetic; patient may stay in hospital overnight or longer; NPO status from midnight of the night before

- *Peritoneal dialysis:* written consent needed for surgery and local anesthesia; same-day surgery with overnight or longer stay; small incision made on the abdomen below the umbilicus to insert a Silastic catheter; procedure may be performed at the bedside under certain conditions

### Review of Postprocedural Care

- Stress the need to protect the operative site from compression.
- For hemodialysis, explain that the extremity will be elevated and monitored for pulses, excessive bleeding, and temperature.
- For peritoneal dialysis, see Abdominal Surgery, p. 3.

### SIDE EFFECTS/COMPLICATIONS

- After insertion of shunt
  —Clot formation
  —Bleeding
  —Anemia
  —Infection of operative site: redness, warm to touch, tenderness, purulent drainage
- During or after hemodialysis
  —Hypotension
  —Hypertension
  —Dysrhythmias
  —Muscle cramps (potassium imbalance)
  —Air embolus
  —Hemorrhage from heparinization
  —Hepatitis B
  —Dialysis disequilibrium syndrome
  —Restless leg syndrome
  —Mechanical problems
- During or after peritoneal dialysis
  —Peritonitis
  —Catheter displacement
  —Catheter plugging
  —Shortness of breath
  —Hyperglycemia

—Hypoglycemia
—Bowel adhesions
—Leakage and extravasation of dialysate
—Mechanical cycling problems

**HOME CARE**

- Give both the patient and the caregiver *verbal* and *written* instructions. Provide them with the name and telephone number of a physician or nurse and the dialysis center to call if questions arise. Use visual aids to assist in instruction.
- *General information*
  —Explain the disease, the underlying cause for dialysis, and the type of dialysis treatment to the patient and family.

**Hemodialysis**

- *Warning signs*
  —Review the signs and symptoms that should be reported to a physician or nurse or the dialysis center.
  > Swelling and pain over the access site
  > Numbness or tingling in the extremity
  > Coolness in the extremity distal to the access site
  > Loss of thrill or bruit
  > Blood that is cool to touch in the external shunt
  > Disconnection of the external shunt
  > Infection at the site: redness, tenderness, swelling, warm to touch, possible drainage
- *Special instructions*
  —Discuss shunt care: clean with hydrogen peroxide solution (or other solution as prescribed) daily until completely healed and sutures removed (10-14 days); keep site clean and dry; wash site with mild soap and water between dialysis treatments; keep sterile dressing over site.
  —Tell the patient to avoid infection by not showering, bathing, or swimming for several hours after dialysis.
  —Instruct the patient to watch the access area for bleeding or bruising under the skin after dialysis starts; demonstrate how to monitor vascular access, including palpating thrill (vibration) and auscultating for bruit daily or as ordered.
  —Review precautions to take with the shunt: avoid lying, tugging, or pulling on the affected extremity; avoid wearing tight clothing or jewelry over the access site; do not lift heavy ob-

jects or strain with the affected extremity; never permit blood drawing, blood pressure monitoring, or injection on the affected extremity.

—For an external shunt:

Explain the need to have a bandage wrapped loosely around the area to prevent accidental removal or disconnection.

Emphasize the importance of having clamps attached to the bandage at all times. Discuss what to do if the shunt connection comes loose or is disconnected.

—For internal shunt:

Show the patient how to check pulsations.

## Peritoneal Dialysis

• *Warning signs*

—Review the signs and symptoms that should be reported to a physician or nurse.

Infection of cannula insertion site: redness, swelling, warmth to touch, tenderness, possible drainage

Increase in abdominal girth, abdominal distention or pain

Absence of bowel movements or inability to pass gas

• *Special instructions*

—Discuss the need for and teach the peritoneal dialysis procedure. Permit time for practice. Refer the patient to a dialysis nurse for specific instructions.

—Review and teach skin and peritoneal catheter care.

Change dressing daily or whenever wet or soiled.

Inspect site carefully.

Cleanse area with hydrogen peroxide or prescribed solution, using sterile applicators; pat area dry.

Apply a sterile dressing over the site, taping all sides securely.

Protect the catheter from damage. Keep sterile cap in place.

Stress the importance of maintaining sterile technique when opening and closing catheter connections.

—Discuss the procedure for peritoneal dialysis infusion.

Review the signs and symptoms that should be reported to a physician or nurse.

○ Shortness of breath or trouble breathing

○ Slow outflow even after repositioning or no outflow

○ Abdominal pain

○ Leakage around catheter

○ Outflow solution foul smelling, cloudy, fecal colored, or bloody (new site will have blood-tinged outflow for the first or second day after catheter insertion)

○ Presence of fibrin (clear or white strands) in outflow

Review self-administration technique. Refer the patient to the dialysis nurse for a specific demonstration.

Discuss the need for the following:

○ Urinate before the procedure.

○ Wash hands.

○ Check solution for intact bag and clarity.

○ Warm solution slightly if desired (with warming pad at lowest setting, never in microwave).

○ Put on a surgical mask and use sterile gloves.

○ Prepare all materials necessary for exchange.

○ Clean the connections per protocol and connect the solution bags.

Review the amount of dialysis solution to be infused.

Review common symptoms with infusion: fullness of abdomen or rectum; cramping; shoulder aching; aching in penis, scrotum, or vagina, especially at the beginning (should decrease during the dwell).

## General Care

• *Special instructions*

—Instruct the patient to monitor and maintain the following:

Dialysis record

Daily log of weights, using same scale, clothing, and time of day when weighing

Blood pressure, pulse, temperature

Intake and output

—Refer the patient to the dialysis nurse for assistance in obtaining appropriate equipment and supplies.

• *Medications*

—Explain the purpose, dosage, schedule, and route of administration of any prescribed drugs, as well as side effects to report to a physician or nurse.

—Instruct the patient to omit hypertensive medications before hemodialysis as instructed.

—Instruct the patient to avoid using over-the-counter medications without checking with the physician or nurse.

- *Activity*
  - —Encourage the patient to discuss allowances and limitations with respect to occupation, recreation, and activities.
  - —Tell the patient to avoid lifting heavy objects or straining of the extremity with access. Inform the patient of the need to avoid contact sports (football, soccer, basketball) or unusually strenuous exercise.
  - —Explain the need for frequent rest periods, especially after dialysis.
- *Diet*
  - —Discuss the diet prescribed by the physician for the underlying condition.
  - —Refer the patient to a dietitian as indicated.
  - —Explain the need to restrict liquids and define the limits.

**FOLLOW-UP CARE**

- Stress the importance of keeping regular follow-up medical and laboratory appointments. Remind the patient to bring the daily log to appointments. Make sure the patient has the necessary names and telephone numbers.
- Encourage or assist the patient to obtain a Medic-Alert bracelet and identification card listing the diagnosis and medication.

**PSYCHOSOCIAL CARE**

- Assist the patient, family, and significant others to obtain counseling if needed.

**REFERRALS**

- Assist the patient to obtain referral services through the social worker and discharge planner.

# Diarrhea

—**Diarrhea: frequent passage of loose stools (>200 grams a day) containing 70%-90% water. Stools may contain mucus,** pus, or blood. **Diarrhea is usually a symptom of some under-lying disorder or a side effect of treatment, such as chemotherapy or radiation therapy.**

## CAUSES/CONTRIBUTING FACTORS

- Acute diarrhea
  —Diet alteration
  —Improper cooking
  —Spoiled food
  —Drug reaction
  —Infection
  —Ingestion of toxins
- Chronic diarrhea
  —Lactase insufficiency
  —Laxative abuse
  —Stress and anxiety
  —Inflammatory bowel syndrome
  —Irritable bowel syndrome
  —Cancer of the colon
  —Chemotherapeutic agents
  —Radiation
  —Gastrointestinal surgery
  —Malabsorption disease

## SIGNS/SYMPTOMS

- Abdominal pain
- Cramping
- Increased stool frequency
- Loose, liquid stools
- Urgency
- Change in color of stool

## COMPLICATIONS

- Dehydration
- Electrolyte imbalance

## HOME CARE

- Give both the patient and the caregiver *verbal* and *written* instructions. Provide them with the name and telephone number of a physician or nurse to call if questions arise.

- *General information*
  —Explain the disease and the underlying cause.
- *Warning signs*
  —Review the signs and symptoms that should be reported to a physician or nurse.
    Uncontrolled diarrhea lasting longer than 24 hours
    Stools with blood, pus, or mucus
    Increasing fatigue or weakness
    Abdominal pain or severe discomfort that accompanies diarrhea and is not relieved by passage of stools or gas
    Fever of 101° F or greater
    Chills, vomiting, or fainting
    Excessive thirst
- *Special instructions*
  —Instruct the patient to maintain a record of stools, including the number per day, time, color, amount, consistency, odor, and presence of mucus, blood, or pus.
  —Teach the patient to perform perianal and perineal skin care after every bowel movement, including washing gently with mild soap and warm water, applying protective ointment and gels, and drying area by gently patting with a soft towel. Sitz baths may be used as necessary.
  —Discuss the need for good hygiene: wash hands after each stool, clean bathroom after each stool if bathroom is shared with others.
- *Medications*
  —Explain the purpose, dosage, schedule, and route of administration of any prescribed drugs, as well as side effects to report to a physician or nurse.
  —Explain the need to avoid use of antidiarrheal agents if the diarrhea is due to gastrointestinal infection (e.g., *Shigella*) without checking with a physician.
  —Tell the patient to avoid use of antacids that contain magnesium, which aggravates diarrhea.
- *Diet*
  —Discuss the need to rest the stomach and increase fluid intake up to 3000 ml per day. Encourage clear fluids: water, diluted broth, decaffeinated tea, carbonated liquids served flat, gelatin, or sports drinks a sip at a time until the stomach can handle a larger amount. Tell the patient to avoid fluids that are too hot or cold, since these increase peristalsis.

—Tell the patient to avoid irritating foods until all symptoms have disappeared: spicy, fatty, or fried foods; milk; caffeine; raw fruits and vegetables; and alcohol.

—Encourage a low-fat, low-fiber diet: bananas, toast, applesauce, soda crackers. Once stools begin to firm, food as tolerated can be increased: chicken, mashed potatoes, cottage cheese.

**D**

# Dilated Cardiomyopathy

—**Dilated cardiomyopathy: cardiomyopathy is a heart muscle disorder resulting in impaired function of the heart's pumping action. Dilated cardiomyopathy, the most common form, results from damaged myocardial fibers. The heart takes on a globular shape and contracts poorly during systole.**

## CAUSES/CONTRIBUTING FACTORS
- Primary: idiopathic
- Secondary
  —Infection: e.g., viral, streptococcal
  —Immunologic disorders: e.g., rheumatic heart disease, systemic lupus erythematosus, scleroderma
  —Metabolic disorders: e.g., thyrotoxicosis, myxedema
  —Toxic processes: alcohol, immunosuppressive drugs
  —Miscellaneous: pregnancy, post partum, radiation

## COMPLICATIONS
- Congestive heart failure
- Arrhythmias
- Emboli

## DIAGNOSTIC TESTS
- Describe each procedure, its purpose, and the normal feelings or sensations that are likely, as well as any preprocedural and postprocedural care.
  —Chest x-ray: to detect enlarged heart
  —Echocardiogram: to assess heart chamber size and function and valve function

—Radionuclide studies: to assess ineffective wall motion and decreased cardiac output

—Cardiac catheterization: to detect impaired heart function, such as coronary artery disease and valve abnormalities; findings may include impaired cardiac motion, decreased cardiac output, and increased ventricular pressures

—Electrocardiogram: to detect enlarged heart muscle, rhythm disturbances, conduction disturbances, and evidence of previous heart muscle damage

## TREATMENT

*Medical*
- Therapy
  —Bed rest: to reduce the work of the heart
  —Oxygen: to improve the oxygen content of tissues
- Drugs
  —Digitalis: to strengthen the force of contraction by the heart muscle and regulate abnormal rhythms
  —Diuretics: to help the kidney eliminate extra salt and fluid
  —Vasodilators: to reduce the amount of blood coming into the heart and thus reduce the work of the heart
  —Anticoagulants (with prolonged bed rest): to prevent clots from forming

*Surgical*
- Heart transplant

## HOME CARE

- Give both the patient and the caregiver *verbal* and *written* instructions. Provide them with the name and telephone number of a physician or nurse to call if questions arise.
- *General information*
  —Describe the type of cardiomyopathy and contributing causes.
  —Review the prognosis: that in certain cases the prognosis is excellent if the cause is corrected (e.g., if the patient stops using alcohol or delivers a baby, or if toxic agents are removed).
  —For specific home care, see Heart Failure, p. 352.
- *Activity*
  —Explain any limitations imposed on the patient's life-style.

# Diverticulosis and Diverticulitis

**D**

—**Diverticulosis: the development of small pockets along the mucosa of the colon, formed by herniation of mucosal and submucosal linings through the muscular layers of the large intestine. They can occur anywhere throughout the intestine but are most common in the sigmoid colon.**

—**Diverticulitis: the inflammatory process in which a diverticulum ruptures or feces becomes impacted in the diverticulum.**

## CAUSES/CONTRIBUTING FACTORS
- Low-fiber diet
- Increased intracolonic pressures
- Weakened intestinal wall

## SIGNS/SYMPTOMS
- Cramplike pain and tenderness in the left lower quadrant
- Anorexia
- Nausea and vomiting
- Fever
- Changes in bowel function: constipation or diarrhea
- Mucus or blood in stools
- Increased flatulence
- Abdominal distention

## COMPLICATIONS
- Peritonitis
- Fistulas to the bladder, vagina, or abdominal wall
- Hemorrhage
- Intraabdominal abscesses
- Intestinal obstruction or perforation

## DIAGNOSTIC TESTS
- Describe each procedure, its purpose, and the normal feelings or sensations that are likely, as well as any preprocedural and postprocedural care.
  —Water-soluble contrast enema: to locate abscess cavities, fistulas, sinus tracts

- Abdominal x-rays: to detect presence of free air and fluid, obstruction, or ileus
- Complete blood count with differential: to determine the presence of infection as reflected by a shift to the left
- Urinalysis: to rule out bladder involvement
- Computed tomography: to locate diverticula, abscesses, or fistulas
- Stool examination: to assess for occult blood
- Sigmoidoscopy, colonoscopy, or ultrasonography: to reveal the presence of diverticula

## TREATMENT

*Medical*
- Therapy
  —Intravenous fluid replacement with electrolytes
  —Diet NPO for acute diverticulitis; when inflammation is resolved, progression to high-fiber diet
  —Nasogastric tube aspiration: to relieve nausea, vomiting, and abdominal distention
- Drugs
  —Antibiotics
  —Analgesics: meperidine (Demerol) the agent of choice, since it also decreases gastrointestinal motility and spasms
  —Hydrophilic colloid laxatives

*Surgical*
- Bowel resection with anastomosis
- Bowel resection with temporary colostomy

## HOME CARE

- Give both the patient and the caregiver *verbal* and *written* instructions. Provide them with the name and telephone number of a physician or nurse to call if questions arise. Use visual aids to assist in instruction.
- If a temporary colostomy is present, see also Fecal Ostomy, p. 299.
- *General information*
  —Explain and discuss the development of diverticulitis and diverticulosis, the causes or contributing factors, care, and treatment.
- *Warning signs*
  —Review the signs and symptoms that should be reported to a physician or nurse.
  Fever

Nausea or vomiting

Cloudy or malodorous urine

Changes in bowel function: constipation or diarrhea

Wound infection: fever, incisional pain, redness, drainage, or swelling

For temporary colostomy: change in stoma color from the normal bright red or peristomal skin irritation

- *Special instructions*
  —Assist the patient in obtaining appropriate supplies, such as sterile dressings or ostomy devices, if indicated.
  —Demonstrate proper wound care or stoma management and dressing changes: procedure, frequency, and wound or stoma inspection.
  —Advise the patient to avoid straining at stool during defecation, constipation, enemas, and harsh laxatives.
  —Stress the importance of establishing regular bowel habits.
  —Discuss pain management techniques for dealing with chronic pain: visualization, guided imagery, meditation, relaxation, biofeedback, or back rubs.

- *Medications*
  —Explain the purpose, dosage, schedule, and route of administration of any prescribed drugs, as well as side effects to report to the physician or nurse.
  —Instruct the patient to take hydrophilic colloid laxatives as prescribed; advise against taking other laxatives without consulting a physician.

- *Activity*
  —Encourage the patient to discuss allowances and limitations with respect to occupation, recreation, or activities.
  —Instruct the patient to resume activities of daily living gradually but to avoid heavy lifting (>10 pounds), pushing, or pulling for 6 weeks to prevent herniation.
  —Advise that baths or showers may be taken when drains or sutures are removed.

- *Diet*
  —Explain the relationship between diet and diverticular disease.
  —Assist the patient to plan a high-fiber diet, including fruits, vegetables, and bran. Provide a list of high-fiber foods and ways to make bran more palatable.
  —Instruct the patient to increase bran gradually because bran may cause abdominal distention and increased flatus.

—Advise the patient to avoid large meals, alcohol, or extremely cold foods.

—Advise the patient to drink plenty of fluids, up to 2-3 liters per day, unless contraindicated.

**FOLLOW-UP CARE**

• Stress the importance of regular follow-up visits with the physician and enterostomal therapy (ET) nurse (if indicated). Make sure the patient has the necessary names and telephone numbers.

**REFERRALS**

• Assist the patient to obtain referral to the ET nurse, home health support services, and dietitian.

---

# Dysrhythmia
## (Arrhythmia)

---

—Dysrhythmia: disturbance of the normal heart rhythm. Normal heart rhythm begins at the sinus node and follows a normal sequence through the heart's electrical system. Normal resting heart rate is 60-100 times a minute. A heartbeat that is too slow (bradycardia) or too fast (tachycardia) can interfere with normal heart function and produce symptoms that can be minor or life threatening. Interruption of the electrical impulse is termed heart block. The heart rate is governed by emotions (nervous system), activities, exercise or rest, drugs, and other stimulants, such as caffeine, tobacco, and electrolytes (body chemicals). Dysrhythmias can be classified by the area where they originate:

—Atrial dysrhythmias: above the atrioventricular node originating in the upper heart chambers (right and left atrium)

—Supraventricular dysrhythmias: involving the upper chamber and atrioventricular node

—Ventricular dysrhythmias: involving primarily the lower heart chambers (right and left ventricles)

## SINUS BRADYCARDIA

Sinus bradycardia is a sinus rhythm of <60 beats per minute. The rhythm is normal. Sinus bradycardia can be normal in well-conditioned athletes; it may occur in response to drugs or increased vagal tone. Slowing heart rates are often found in the elderly.

### Causes/Contributing Factors

- Increased intracranial pressure
- Increased vagal tone (bowel straining or vomiting)
- Hypothyroidism
- Sick sinus syndrome
- Medications (beta blockers and calcium channel blockers: digoxin, quinidine, propranolol, procainamide)
- Diminished blood flow to the sinoatrial node

### Signs/Symptoms

- Usually asymptomatic
- Dizziness
- Weakness
- Altered level of consciousness
- Low blood pressure
- Chest pain
- Fatigue
- Shortness of breath

### Complications

- Syncope

### Treatment

*Medical* (necessary only if symptomatic)
- Therapy
  —Correction of underlying cause
  —Pacemaker: temporary or permanent
- Drugs
  —Atropine: as emergency measure to increase heart rate

## HEART BLOCK

Heart block (first-, second-, or third-degree) is a conduction disturbance that results in a slow heart rate with partial or complete electrical dissociation between the atria and ventricles. In complete, or third-degree, heart block the ventricles function independently, resulting in decreased efficiency of the heart.

**Causes/Contributing Factors**

- Lack of blood supply to the electrical system of the heart
- Ischemic heart disease
- Myocardial infarction
- Hypothyroidism
- Congenital heart disease
- Digitalis toxicity

**Signs/Symptoms**

- Dizziness
- Lightheadedness
- Loss of consciousness
- Low blood pressure
- Weakness
- Difficulty breathing (signs of congestive heart failure)

**Complications**

- Syncope (loss of consciousness)
- Heart failure
- Asystole (heart stops beating)

**Treatment**

*Medical*
- Therapy
  —Observation: heart block associated with myocardial infarction usually corrects itself with time
  —Pacemaker: temporary or permanent
- Drugs
  —Discontinuation of causative drug
  —Atropine
  —Isoproterenol

## JUNCTIONAL RHYTHM

Junctional rhythm originates in the atrioventricular node or junction. The rate is usually 40-60 beats per minute. Atrial activity (corresponding to the P-wave on the electrocardiogram) either is absent or occurs simultaneously with or after the ventricular activity (corresponding to the QRS on the electrocardiogram).

**Causes/Contributing Factors**

- Digitalis toxicity
- Inferior wall myocardial infarction or ischemia (inadequate blood supply to the sinus node)
- Hypoxia
- Vagal stimulation
- Acute rheumatic fever
- Valve surgery

**Signs/Symptoms**

- Asymptomatic
- Dizziness
- Weakness
- Altered level of consciousness

**Treatment**

*Medical*

- Therapy
  —Observation: junctional rhythm is not usually permanent
  —Treatment of underlying cause
  —Permanent pacemaker
- Drugs
  —Atropine: to block effects of vagal stimulation
  —Isoproterenol

**SINUS TACHYCARDIA**

Sinus tachycardia is sinus rhythm that is >100 beats per minute. The origin of the beat and the transmission of the electrical impulse are normal. Rhythm is regular.

**Causes/Contributing Factors**

- Fever
- Exercise
- Anxiety
- Pain
- Dehydration
- Heart disease
- Hyperthyroidism
- Hypovolemia

**Signs/Symptoms**

- Shortness of breath (depending on underlying cause)
- Palpitation
- Fatigue

**Complications**

- Hypotension
- Dizziness
- Syncope

**Treatment**

*Medical*
- Therapy
  —Treatment of underlying cause

## ATRIAL FLUTTER

Atrial flutter is a rapid, regular rhythm disturbance that starts in the right atrium. The atrial rate is 200-300 beats per minute. The electrical impulses are transmitted to the atrioventricular node. Usually the node is blocked so that not all electrical impulses get through to the ventricles. The ventricular rate is 100-150 beats per minute.

**Causes/Contributing Factors**

- Heart failure
- Valvular heart disease
- Congenital heart disease
- Pulmonary embolism
- Digitalis toxicity
- Coronary artery bypass surgery

**Complications**

- Heart failure (shortness of breath)
- Low cardiac output
- Coronary insufficiency
- Embolization

**Treatment**

*Medical*
- Therapy
  —Treatment of the underlying cause

—Synchronized cardioversion: to restore normal sinus rhythm
—Atrial pacemaker: to restore heart rhythm
—Vagal stimulation: to slow heart rate
• Drugs
—Digitalis (unless dysrhythmia is due to digitalis toxicity)
—Propranolol: to decrease heart rate (blocks catecholamine stimulation)
—Quinidine: to decrease heart rate by blocking conduction through the atrioventricular node
—Procainamide: to block abnormal excitation from abnormal focuses in the heart muscle
—Verapamil: to slow conduction through the atrioventricular node and decrease heart tone as a vasodilator
—Antiarrhythmic agents
Amiodarone: to prolong cardiac action
Beta Pace: has beta-blocking and antiarrhythmic properties
Rhythmol: to stabilize heart muscle and has local anesthetic effects

## ATRIAL FIBRILLATION

Atrial fibrillation is rapid irregular rhythm disturbances that originate in the atrium. The atrial rate is greater than 400 beats per minute and is irregular and chaotic. The atrial impulses (electrical) are transmitted to the atrioventricular node. The node is blocked so that not all electrical impulses get through to the ventricle. Ventricular rate varies (90-100 beats per minute), and P-waves are not visible on the electrocardiogram. The condition is common in the elderly.

### Causes/Contributing Factors

• Heart failure
• Chronic obstructive pulmonary disease
• Hyperthyroidism
• Sepsis
• Pulmonary embolism
• Mitral stenosis
• Atrial irritation
• Coronary bypass surgery
• Valve surgery

**Complications**
- Embolization
- Heart failure
- Low cardiac output

**Treatment**

*Medical*
- Therapy
  —Treatment of underlying condition
  —Cardioversion
- Drugs
  —Antarrhythmics
  —Anticoagulants
  —Beta blockers, calcium channel blockers, digitalis: to control
  rate

## VENTRICULAR TACHYCARDIA

Ventricular tachycardia is an abnormally rapid (usually regular) rhythm that originates in the ventricles. Atrial activity is usually unrelated to ventricular activity (dissociated) during ventricular tachycardia. The rate can vary from 120-250 beats per minute. Ventricular tachycardia usually occurs in patients who have had underlying heart disease but rarely may occur in individuals without heart disease, in which case it is usually drug related. Because ventricular tachycardia is usually a precursor to ventricular fibrillation, it is treated as a serious dysrhythmia.

**Causes/Contributing Factors**
- Heart disease
  —Myocardial ischemia
  —Myocardial infarction
  —Congenital heart disease
  —Ventricular aneurysm
  —Left ventricular dysfunction
- Digitalis or quinidine toxicity
- Low potassium levels
- High calcium levels

**Signs/Symptoms**
- Chest pain
- Anxiety

- Palpitations
- Dyspnea
- Low blood pressure
- Loss of consciousness

**Complications/Contributing Factors**

- Ventricular fibrillation/cardiac arrest
- Shock

**Treatment**

*Medical*

- Therapy
  —Treatment of underlying condition
  —Catheter ablation
  —DC cardioversion
  —Implantable defibrillator
- Drugs
  —Antiarrhythmics

## VENTRICULAR FIBRILLATION

Ventricular fibrillation is an abnormally rapid, irregular rhythm that originates in the ventricles. Atrial activity is unrelated to ventricular activity. The heart rhythm becomes so rapid and chaotic that the heart becomes totally ineffective as a pump. Blood no longer flows forward, there is no blood pressure, and the patient loses consciousness. If the fibrillation is untreated, the patient will die within minutes.

**Causes/Contributing Factors**

- Acute or chronic heart disease
- Untreated ventricular tachycardia
- Electrolyte imbalances, such as sodium, potassium, calcium
- Digitalis or quinidine toxicity
- Electric shock (electrocution)
- Hypothermia

**Signs/Symptoms**

- Loss of consciousness
- Possible seizures
- Sudden death

**Treatment**

*Medical*

- Therapy
  —Emergency measures
      Cardiopulmonary resuscitation (CPR): to maintain circulation
      Electrical defibrillation
  —Ongoing treatment to prevent recurrence
      Catheter ablation
      Implantable defibrillator
- Drugs
  —Emergency measures
      Epinephrine
      Isoproterenol

**DIAGNOSTIC TESTS**

- Describe each procedure, its purpose, and the normal feelings or sensations that are likely, as well as any preprocedural and postprocedural care.
- Inform the patient that several diagnostic procedures may be performed to aid in the diagnosis of the dysrhythmia.
  —12-Lead electrocardiogram: to detect dysrhythmias and identify possible cause
  —Serum electrolyte levels: to assess sodium, potassium, calcium, and magnesium levels that might be abnormally high or low
  —Drug levels: to identify toxicities that can precipitate dysrhythmias
  —Ambulatory monitoring (24-hour Holter monitor or cardiac event recorder): to identify dysrhythmias and associate abnormal rhythms to the patient's symptoms
  —Signal averaging electrocardiogram: computerized electrocardiogram used to detect areas of slow electrical conduction that are associated with certain rhythm disturbances
  —Event recorder: 30-day recording device activated during symptoms to correlate symptoms with electrocardiographic rhythm changes
  —Electrophysiologic study: to determine origin of dysrhythmia and inducibility and effectiveness of drug therapy in dysrhythmia suppression
  —Exercise stress testing: to assess cardiac response to an in-

crease in workload that can precipitate rhythm abnormalities, such as premature ventricular contractions caused by lack of blood supply to the heart muscle, and to guide therapy

—Arterial blood gases: to identify lack of oxygen in the blood, caused by a compromise in the heart function and circulation in the presence of dysrhythmias

**D**

## HOME CARE

- Give both the patient and the caregiver *verbal* and *written* instructions. Provide them with the name and telephone number of a physician or nurse to call if questions arise. Use heart models, diagrams of the conduction system, and other visual aids to assist in instruction.
- *General information*
  —Explain what the particular rhythm disturbance is and the identified or suspected cause.
  —Emphasize the importance of not smoking or using tobacco products. Discuss how nicotine can cause dysrhythmias.
  —For a patient receiving an implantable defibrillator, see p. 402.
- *Warning signs*
  —Review the signs and symptoms that should be reported to a physician or nurse.
  
  Palpitations
  Chest pain
  Shortness of breath
  Rapid pulse
  Dizziness
  Syncope
- *Special instructions*
  —Teach the patient how to take the pulse for a full minute (see Pulse Taking, p. 555).
  —Explain the importance of leading a normal, productive life in the patient's present condition.
  —Help the patient understand what precautions to take at work and at home and how to prepare for vacations.
  —For patients with chronic or serious dysrhythmias, explain the need to identify a health care facility near home and work and to have emergency numbers at hand.
  —Advise the patient to use relaxation techniques to reduce stress and prevent dysrhythmias by preventing the release of hormones, such as adrenaline, that stimulate the heart rate.

- *Medications*
  - —Explain the purpose, dosage, schedule, and route of administration of any prescribed drugs, as well as side effects to report to the physician or nurse.
  - —Instruct the patient not to stop taking medications abruptly, because of side effects, but to notify the physician so a plan for changing medications can be developed.
  - —Explain the need for continued follow-up to assess the effectiveness of the medications and to alter treatment if necessary.
  - —Stress the importance of reordering medications before they run out and ordering enough medication when planning a vacation or travel.
  - —Discuss the need to avoid taking over-the-counter drugs.
- *Activity*
  - —Advise the patient to avoid strenuous activity and overexertion. Warn the patient to stop exercise or activity immediately if experiencing dizziness, lightheadedness, or chest pain.
  - —Encourage questions about allowances and limitations with respect to occupation, recreation, and activities.
- *Diet*
  - —Advise the patient to eliminate or reduce intake of products containing caffeine, such as coffee, chocolate, tea, and colas, and alcohol.

## FOLLOW-UP CARE

- Stress the importance of regular follow-up visits. Make sure the patient has the necessary names and telephone numbers.
- Discuss importance of carrying a Medic-Alert bracelet and a card listing all medications.

## PSYCHOSOCIAL CARE

- Explain the psychologic implications of the presence of cardiac disease and life-threatening arrhythmias: loss of control over life-style, anxiety and fear associated with death, possible nightmares or other sleep disturbances, denial, depression, and anger.

# Electrophysiology Study
## (Cardiac Mapping)

—Electrophysiologic study: an invasive procedure used to detect, induce, and treat dysrhythmias. By use of an electrode catheter that is placed through a peripheral vein into the right atrium or ventricle, the heart can be stimulated to recreate and locate the origins of the abnormal heart rhythm, as well as determine the effectiveness of antiarrhythmia therapy.

### CONTRAINDICATIONS

• Acute myocardial infarction

### PREPROCEDURAL TEACHING

• Review the physician's explanation of the procedure and the reason for it; encourage the patient to ask questions and to discuss any fears or anxieties. Explain that the procedure can be done on an outpatient basis and requires informed consent.

### Review of Preprocedural Care

• Instruct the patient not to eat for 6-12 hours before the procedure. Fluids may be permitted until 3 hours before the test.
• Explain what will happen during the procedure.
  —Medications are given before the procedure.
  —A peripheral intravenous infusion is started, and oxygen may be administered.
  —The site of the catheter insertion is shaved and cleansed.
  —Dentures and eyewear are removed.
  —The patient is taken to a special laboratory room and placed on a padded surgical table. The procedure takes about 2-4 hours.
• Review the sensations to be expected during the procedure.
  —Pressure or discomfort in the groin during the catheter insertion; local anesthesia is used to decrease pain and discomfort
  —Discomfort associated with electrical cardioversion; patient is sedated and usually does not remember the discomfort
• Explain that the patient is sleepy and unaware of surroundings, but is arousable and able to communicate with the physician if necessary.

- Instruct the patient to report any feelings of pain, nausea, dizziness, or palpitations felt during or after the procedure.
- Review the procedure.
  —Electrocardiographic leads are attached for continuous cardiac monitoring.
  —Special patches are applied to the chest to be used for defibrillation, if needed.
  —The groin is cleansed and draped.
  —Several catheters are inserted under fluoroscopy, threaded through the vein or artery in the groin, and positioned in the heart.
  —The patient is heavily sedated.
  —Various parts of the heart's electroconduction system are stimulated by atrial or ventricular pacing. The electroconduction system and its defects are mapped, and dysrhythmias are identified.
  —Antiarrhythmic medications are given to see if they are effective in controlling the dysrhythmia. If the medication is effective, the abnormal rhythm can no longer be induced.
  —Dysrhythmias that do not stop spontaneously may be terminated by rapid overdrive pacing or electrical cardioversion.
  —When all necessary information has been obtained, catheters are removed. Pressure is applied to the sites for 10 minutes and the patient is returned to his or her room.

**Review of Postprocedural Care**

- Explain that the patient remains on bed rest and is closely monitored for bleeding or rhythm disturbances. The leg is kept straight for 3-6 hours.

**COMPLICATIONS**

- Ventricular tachycardia or fibrillation
- Perforation of the myocardium
- Catheter-induced embolic events (cerebrovascular accident, myocardial infarction)
- Phlebitis, thrombosis at venipuncture site
- Hemorrhage

**HOME CARE**

- Give both the patient and the caregiver *verbal* and *written* instructions. Provide them with the name and telephone number of a physician or nurse to call if questions arise.

- For specific home management, see Cardiac Catheterization (p. 144) and Dysrhythmia (p. 256).
- *General information*
  —Review the physician's explanation of electrophysiology study findings and explain recommended treatment.
- *Medications*
  —Explain the purpose, dosage, schedule, and route of administration of any prescribed drugs, as well as side effects to report to the physician or nurse.

## PSYCHOSOCIAL CARE

- Encourage expression of fears and concerns regarding any identified dysrhythmias and prescribed treatment.

## REFERRALS

- Provide the patient and caregiver with telephone numbers and names of people to contact with questions and concerns.

# Encephalitis and Meningitis

—Encephalitis and meningitis: inflammation of the tissues of the brain and spinal cord, resulting in altered function of various portions of these tissues. Encephalitis is frequently accompanied by signs of systemic infection. Encephalitis usually follows a systemic viral infection, mosquito exposure, or swimming or diving in fresh water (amebic). Meningitis may result from a direct invasion of the meninges by bacterial, viral, fungal, or parasitic agents or from the iatrogenic introduction of irritating substances. Meningitis usually follows a recent upper respiratory infection or ear infection or contact with infected persons.

## CAUSES/CONTRIBUTING FACTORS

- Encephalitis
  —Toxemia accompanying an infectious disease
  —Allergic response

—Primary infection
  Mosquito-borne viral encephalitides
  Amebic meningoencephalitis
—Secondary infection
  Herpes virus
- Meningitis
  —Meningococcal *(Neisseria meningitidis):* acute communicable
  —Haemophilus *(Haemophilus influenzae):* acute communicable
  —Pneumococcal *(Streptococcus pneumoniae):* high risk of fatality
  —Viral (aseptic or serous): self-limiting and benign

## SIGNS/SYMPTOMS

- Encephalitis
  —Frontal headache, nausea, vomiting, dizziness, fever and chills
  —Tachypnea, tachycardia
  —Level of consciousness/behavioral changes
    Mild listlessness progressing to eventual coma
    Irritability, bizarre behavior, seizures
  —Neurologic: aphasia, olfactory hallucinations, nuchal rigidity, weakness, accentuated deep tendon reflexes, extensory plantar response, ataxia, spasticity, tremors
  —Excess or deficient antidiuretic hormone secretion
- Meningitis
  —Throbbing headache
  —Muscle pains
  —Stiff neck
  —Backache
  —Chills
  —Irritability
  —Fever (38°-41° C)
  —Flushed, hot, dry skin
  —Increased blood pressure with increasing intracranial pressure
  —Delirium progressing to deep coma
  —Positive Brudzinski's sign (flexion of neck elicits flexion of knees and hips)
  —Positive Kernig's sign (pain elicited in hamstring following straight leg lift in supine position)

## COMPLICATIONS

- Encephalitis
  —Mental deterioration

—Paralysis
—Convulsive disorders
• Meningitis
—Bacterial: hydrocephalus, cranial nerve involvement (blindness and deafness), arthritis, myocarditis, pericarditis
—Aseptic: clinical encephalitis

## DIAGNOSTIC TESTS

• Describe each procedure, its purpose, and the normal feelings or sensations that are likely, as well as any preprocedural and postprocedural care.
—Neurologic assessment and eye examination
—Culture and Gram's stain of blood, cerebrospinal fluid, and respiratory secretions: to identify causative organism
—Serologic tests of blood: to identify viral antibodies
—Lumbar puncture: to obtain spinal fluid for culture and micrsopic examination
—Immunofluorescence staining of biopsy specimen of brain
—Petechial skin scrapings for Gram's stain

## TREATMENT

*Medical*

• Therapy
—Fluid and electrolytc therapy
—Nasogastric tube feedings
—Ventilatory and oxygenation support
• Drugs
—Amebic meningoencephalitis
Antiinfective agents (amphotericin B [Fungizone], sulfadiazine, miconazole [Monistat], rifampin [Rifamycin])
—Mosquito-borne encephalitis
No specific treatment
—Infectious viral encephalitides
No specific treatment except for herpes infections: adenine arabinoside (vidarabine, ara-A) intravenously; acyclovir
—Meningitis
Antiinfective agents: ampicillin, chloramphenicol
Immunologic agents: meningococcal polysaccharide, pneumococcal polysaccharide, *H. influenzae* type B
—Encephalitis and meningitis
Sedatives
Antiepilepsy agents

Glucorticorticoids
Osmotic diuretics
Analgesics
Stool softeners and laxatives
Antipyretics

## HOME CARE

- Give both the patient and the caregiver *verbal* and *written* instructions. Provide them with the name and telephone number of a physician or nurse to call if questions arise.
- *General information*
  —Review the physician's explanation of the specific type of disorder, its causes, and contributing factors.
- *Warning signs*
  —Review the signs and symptoms of meningeal irritation that should be reported to a physician or nurse. Emphasize the importance of immediately reporting any exacerbation of symptoms.
    Throbbing frontal headache
    Stiff neck
    Any change in mental status
    Fever
    Nausea and vomiting
- *Special instructions*
  —Encourage the patient with encephalitis to swim only in chlorinated water to avoid amebic infection.
  —For bacterial meningitis:
    Encourage the patient to notify all contacts to be evaluated for detection and treatment.
    Discuss prophylactic measures to prevent bacterial transmission; immunization may be indicated for close contacts.
- *Medications*
  —Explain the purpose, dosage, schedule, and route of administration of any prescribed drugs, as well as side effects to report to the physician or nurse.
    Acyclovir: teach the patient to monitor for side effects involving the kidney: weight gain, respiratory difficulty, imbalance between fluid intake and output, edema
- *Activity*
  —Encourage the patient to discuss allowances and limitations with respect to occupation, recreation, and activities.

—Explain to the patient and significant others that convalescence is of variable duration, depending on the severity of the disease.
—Tell the patient to allow adequate time for recovery before resuming full activities.
—Explain that rest is needed to decrease stimulation of the irritated meninges.

### FOLLOW-UP CARE

- Stress the importance of regular follow-up visits. Make sure the patient has the necessary names and telephone numbers.

# Endocarditis

—Endocarditis: an inflammatory process involving the lining of the heart that may involve the heart valves. Endocarditis results from an infectious process that leads to bacteremia. A number of organisms may cause bacteremia, the most common of which are staphylococci, streptococci, and *Escherichia coli*. Common portals of entry for bacteremias are the mouth, urinary tract, and gastrointestinal tract. While infective endocarditis generally occurs in patients with preexisting heart disease, it can occur in patients with normal heart valves.

### RISK FACTORS

- Preexisting heart disease
  —Valvular heart disesase
  —Congenital heart disease
- Invasive diagnostic and therapeutic procedures
- Intravenous drug use
- Immunosuppression
- Old age

### SIGNS/SYMPTOMS

- Fatigue
- Elevated temperature
- Chills, night sweating

- Joint aches and pains
- Weight loss
- Loss of appetite
- Just not feeling well

## COMPLICATIONS

- Cardiac
  —Abscesses
  —Valvular heart disease
  —Heart failure
  —Myocarditis
- Systemic embolization: cerebral, renal, splenic, coronary
- Other
  —Pulmonary embolism
  —Stroke

## DIAGNOSTIC TESTS

- Describe each procedure, its purpose, and the normal feelings or sensations that are likely, as well as any preprocedural and postprocedural care.
  —Blood tests: to identify the causative organism and look for damage to other organs, including the heart and kidneys
      Blood cultures: to detect causative organism
      Complete blood count: to detect inflammatory process and anemia
      Rheumatoid factor
      Erythrocyte sedimentation rate
  —Echocardiography: to identify any vegetations or abscesses on the heart valves; to evaluate ventricular function
  —Electrocardiogram: to identify any irregular heart rhythms that may result from damage to the heart
  —Radionuclide studies: to identify damage to heart structures and function
  —Other: blood chemistries, special blood studies (e.g., serum assays), chest x-ray

## TREATMENT

*Medical*

- Drugs
  —Intravenous antibiotics: therapy may last 4-6 weeks depending on the infecting organism and heart involvement

—Antipyretics (aspirin)

—Anticoagulants if patient has vegetations on valves and develops atrial fibrillation

*Surgical*

- Generally not indicated, but may be considered in the presence of acute infection with abscess that is unresponsive to intravenous therapy

**HOME CARE**

- Give both the patient and the caregiver *verbal* and *written* instructions. Provide them with the name and telephone number of a physician or nurse to call if questions arise.
- *General information*
    —Review the physician's explanation of the disease, its causes, and contributing factors.
- *Warning signs*
    —Review the signs and symptoms that should be reported to a physician or nurse.
        Persistent temperature
        Chills alternating with diaphoresis
        Fatigue
- *Special instructions*
    —Review factors that can lead to bacteremia and reinfection: poor oral hygiene, dental work (cleaning, gum treatment, extractions), gastrointestinal or genitourinary procedures, vaginal deliveries, furuncles, staphylococcal infections, surgical procedures.
    —Explain the importance of notifying all physicians and dentists of endocarditis risk before having any procedures performed.
    —Explain the need for good oral hygiene and regular dental care. Stress the importance of notifying the dentist at the first sign of oral infection or gum disease.
- *Medications*
    —Explain the purpose, dosage, schedule, and route of administration of any prescribed drugs, as well as side effects to report to the physician or nurse.
    —Explain the need for antibiotic prophylaxis before a procedure that may cause bacteremia.
- *Activity*
    —Explain the need to avoid fatigue and schedule regular rest periods.

**FOLLOW-UP CARE**

- Stress the importance of regular follow-up visits. Make sure the patient has the necessary names and telephone numbers.

# Endometrial Cancer
(Uterine Cancer)

—**Endometrial cancer: cancer of the uterus, the most common gynecologic malignancy. A slow-growing tumor, endometrial cancer is found primarily in postmenopausal women. Most endometrial cancers are adenocarcinomas. Others are adenoacanthomas, clear cell tumors, and squamous cell tumors (these are rare but aggressive and affect younger women). Metastatic spread is most commonly to the pelvic and paraaortic lymph nodes. Bloodborne metastases are most commonly to the lungs, liver, bone, and brain.**

**RISK FACTORS**

- Obesity (>15% over normal weight)
- Nulliparity (never having had a child)
- Endometrial hyperplasia
- Polycystic ovarian disease
- Late menopause (after age 52)
- History of irregular menses
- Failure of ovulation
- History of breast, colon, or ovarian cancer
- Diabetes
- Hypertension
- Prolonged use of exogenous estrogen therapy (unopposed)
- Incidence higher among urban, white, and Jewish women

**SIGNS/SYMPTOMS**

- Postmenopausal bleeding
- Pain in lumbosacral, hypogastric, and pelvic areas
- Advanced disease: bowel obstruction, jaundice, ascites, respiratory difficulty

**DIAGNOSTIC TESTS**

- Describe each procedure, its purpose, and the normal feelings or sensations that are likely, as well as any preprocedural and postprocedural care.
    —Papanicolaou (Pap) smear: to detect malignant cells
    —Endometrial biopsy or fractional dilation and curettage: to detect malignant cells
    —Laparotomy with sampling of peritoneal fluid or washings: to detect malignant cells

**TREATMENT**

*Medical*

- Therapy
    —Radiation therapy
       Preoperative: intracavity radiation therapy
       Postoperative: external beam
    —Chemotherapy
       Progesterone (Megace), hydroxyprogesterone, or medroxyprogesterone acetate
       Single-agent chemotherapy: cisplatin, doxorubicin, hexamethylmelamine, cyclophosphamide

*Surgical*

- Stage I tumors
    —Total abdominal hysterectomy with bilateral salpingo-oophorectomy and pelvic and paraaortic lymph node biopsies
- Stage II tumors
    —Radical hysterectomy

**HOME CARE**

- Give both the patient and the caregiver *verbal* and *written* instructions. Provide them with the name and telephone number of a physician or nurse to call if questions arise. Use visual aids to assist in instruction.
- *General information*
    —Review the physician's explanation of the disease, its causes, and contributing factors.
    —Provide pain management (see Pain Management, p. 501).
    —Prepare the patient for intracavity radiation therapy (see Radiation Therapy, p. 559).
    —Prepare the patient for hysterectomy (see Hysterectomy, p. 400).

- *Warning signs*
  - —Review the signs and symptoms that should be reported to a physician or nurse.
    - Infection: redness, drainage, pain, warmth, fever
    - Bleeding: evidence of vaginal or incisional bleeding
    - Fluid volume deficit: decreased unrinary output, concentrated urine, weakness, change in mental status

## FOLLOW-UP CARE

- Stress the importance of regular follow-up visits. Make sure the patient has the necessary names and telephone numbers.

## REFERRALS

- Assist the patient to obtain referral services for sexual counseling and support groups.

# Endometriosis

—**Endometriosis: abnormal growth of endometrial tissue outside the uterus, commonly on the ovaries, peritoneal cul-de-sac (pouch of Douglas), uterosacral ligaments, and peritoneal surface of the uterus. The ectopic tissue is also responsive to the hormonal changes of the menstrual cycle. A benign disease of unknown cause, endometriosis possesses the ability to infiltrate and spread. It commonly occurs in nulliparous women 30-40 years of age and in older women who delay childbearing.**

## CAUSES/CONTRIBUTING FACTORS/RISK FACTORS

- Congenital obstruction of the vagina or cervix associated with reflux menstruation
- Hormonal or inflammatory factors

## SIGNS/SYMPTOMS

- Changes in menstrual pattern: excessive, prolonged, frequent
- Dysmenorrhea: pain with menstruation
- Pain with defecation during menses
- Vague aching or cramping in pelvic or sacral regions
- Dyspareunia: pain with sexual intercourse

**COMPLICATIONS**

- Infertility
- Decreased fertility
- Spontaneous abortion

**DIAGNOSTIC TESTS**

- Describe each procedure, its purpose, and the normal feelings or sensations that are likely, as well as any preprocedural and postprocedural care.
  —Laparoscopy: to visualize lesions or adhesions; to perform biopsy of lesions

**TREATMENT**

*Medical*

- Therapy
  —Pregnancy for women wishing to have children
- Drugs
  —Gonadotropin-releasing hormone agonists
  —Antigonadotropic agents

*Surgical*

  —Laparoscopic removal, laser therapy, or cauterization of endometrial implants and lysis of adhesions
  —Hysterectomy: maintains normal hormonal patterns
  Total abdominal hysterectomy with bilateral salpingo-oophorectomy: to remove the organs producing hormones that influence disease

**HOME CARE**

- Give both the patient and the caregiver *verbal* and *written* instructions. Provide them with the name and telephone number of a physician or nurse to call if questions arise.
- *General information*
  —Review the physician's explanation of the disease, its causes and contributing factors, care, and treatment.
  —Prepare the patient for hysterectomy (see Hysterectomy, p. 400).
- *Warning signs*
  —Review the signs and symptoms that should be reported to a physician or nurse.
    Fever
    Vaginal bleeding and discharge
    Abdominal pain and distention

- *Special instructions*
  —Provide pain management, offering alternative methods to deal with chronic pain: visualization, guided imagery, meditation, relaxation, biofeedback.

## FOLLOW-UP CARE

- Stress the importance of regular follow-up visits, including pelvic examinations. Make sure the patient has the necessary names and telephone numbers.

## PSYCHOSOCIAL CARE

- Encourage the patient and partner to explore and share feelings, fears, and anxiety about potential infertility, changes in body image, and changes in sexual function.
- Advise the patient and partner not to postpone childbearing, since infertility is a complication.

## REFERRALS

- Assist the patient to obtain referral to community groups, such as RESOLVE, or to a counselor for further support.
- Assist the patient and partner to obtain referral to infertility specialists, if desired.

# Endoscopy

—Endoscopy: visualization of the lining of the digestive tract, used to detect sources of bleeding; to identify abnormalities such as ulcers, tumors, polyps, or inflammation; and to obtain tissue samples (biopsy) for laboratory analysis. Types and organs imaged include gastroscopy (stomach), duodenoscopy (duodenum), gastroduodenoscopy (stomach and duodenum), and esophagogastroduodenoscopy (esophagus, stomach, and duodenum).

## INDICATIONS

- Achalasia
- Cancer of the oral cavity or esophagus

- Esophagitis and esophageal varices
- Mallory-Weiss syndrome
- Acute or chronic gastritis
- Gastric and duodenal ulcers
- Gastric cancer

## PREPROCEDURAL TEACHING

- Review the physician's explanation of the procedure and the reason for it; encourage the patient to ask questions and to discuss any fears or anxieties. Explain that the procedure takes 15-30 minutes, is usually done on an outpatient basis, and involves passage of a long, flexible, lighted tube with an optical head for direct visualization. Explain the need to obtain informed consent.

### Review of Preprocedural Care

- Allow the patient to verbalize fears and concerns about the procedure.
- Explain that the patient will be NPO for 6-12 hours before the procedure.
- Review the procedure.
    —If the procedure is done on an emergency basis, a nasogastric tube is inserted to aspirate gastric contents.
    —An intravenous line or heparin lock is inserted.
    —Dentures and partial plates are removed.
    — Sedatives and analgesics are given.
    —Atropine is given to decrease gastrointestinal motility and prevent aspiration.
    —A local anesthetic is sprayed into the mouth and throat to ease the passage of the endoscope. Explain that the mouth and throat will feel swollen and it will be difficult to swallow. Instruct the patient to allow saliva to drain from the side of the mouth into an emesis basin.

### Review of Postprocedural Care

- Explain what will happen after the procedure.
    —The patient is NPO until the gag reflex returns, about 2-4 hours.
    —Throat lozenges and analgesics are prescribed for throat soreness.
    —The patient is monitored for signs and symptoms of complications.

- Advise the patient to have someone available to drive him or her home because of the effects of sedation.

## COMPLICATIONS
- Hemorrhage
- Esophageal or gastric perforation
- Difficult or painful swallowing
- Fever
- Hematemesis
- Respiratory and hemodynamic instability

## HOME CARE
- Give both the patient and the caregiver *verbal* and *written* instructions. Provide them with the name and telephone number of a physician or nurse to call if questions arise.
- *General information*
  —Review the physician's explanation of the procedure, findings, and specific follow-up care.
- *Warning signs*
  —Review the signs and symptoms that should be reported to a physician or nurse.
      Persistent difficulty in swallowing
      Increased pain
      Bleeding: bloody emesis, black stools
      Respiratory distress
- *Special instructions*
  —Advise the patient that a sore throat or burping may continue for 3 days after the procedure.
  —Suggest throat lozenges or warm saline gargles to ease throat discomfort.
- *Diet*
  —Instruct the patient to resume a regular diet or a diet prescribed for the underlying condition when gag and swallowing reflexes return, in 2-4 hours.
  —Suggest beginning with soft, bland foods until soreness subsides.

## FOLLOW-UP CARE
- Stress the importance of regular follow-up visits. Make sure the patient has the necessary names and telephone numbers.

# Enucleation

—**Enucleation: surgical removal of the eyeball, performed when other treatment of the eyeball is insufficient to prevent pain, disfigurement, or spread of malignant disease.**

**E**

## INDICATIONS

* Severe infections
* Malignancies (melanoma, retinoblastoma)
* Large, infiltrating tumors
* Extensive trauma
* Blindness with severe eye pain
* End-stage glaucoma
* Prophylaxis in sympathetic ophthalmia

## PREPROCEDURAL TEACHING

* Review the physician's explanation of the procedure and the reason for it; encourage the patient to ask questions and to discuss any fears or anxieties. Explain the need for informed consent for surgery and general or local anesthesia.

### Review of Preprocedural Care

* Review preprocedural tests.
  —Blood tests: to determine the status of electrolytes and show the presence of infection
  —Urine tests: to determine the presence of infection
  —Chest x-ray and electrocardiogram if indicated by age: to provide baseline and detect potential problems
* Inform the patient of the need to be NPO from the night before surgery.
* Discuss the need for a shower and shampoo with bactericidal soap the night before surgery.

### Review of Postprocedural Care

* Explain that the physician will implant a temporary artificial globe (conformer) made of Teflon or plastic, which is inserted to maintain orbit shape until a permanent ocular prosthesis can be made (usually 10-14 days after enucleation).

- Discuss the need for a pressure dressing for 2-3 days postoperatively to minimize swelling and prevent bleeding.
- Explain that diet and activity will be progressed as tolerated after the first postoperative day.
- Explain that touching and rubbing the orbit or tightly squeezing the eyelid is to be avoided because these actions can cause injury and infection.
- Explain that some pain is normal after surgery and will be controlled with analgesics. However, advise the patient to report the presence of headache or sharp pain, which could indicate hemorrhage, infection, or broken sutures.
- Tell the patient not to lie on the operative side but rather to lie supine or with head elevated 30 degrees to minimize intraorbital pressure.
- Advise the patient to avoid stooping, bending, lifting heavy objects, straining with bowel movements, and coughing or sneezing with a closed mouth, since these may cause bleeding.

## SIDE EFFECTS/COMPLICATIONS

- Hemorrhage
- Shock
- Infection
- Abscess formation
- Meningitis

## HOME CARE

- Give both the patient and the caregiver *verbal* and *written* instructions. Provide them with the name and telephone number of a physician or nurse to call if questions arise.
- *Warning signs*
  —Review the signs and symptoms that should be reported to a physician or nurse.
    Purulent drainage or bleeding
    Swelling of the orbit
    Pain
    Persistent orbital redness
    Fever
- *Special instructions*
  —Explain the importance of not rubbing, touching, or bumping the orbit or wearing eye makeup without the consent of the physician.

—Discuss the need for cleaning the lid and demonstrate how to remove drainage by gently sweeping the cotton ball from the inner to the outer aspect of the lid, using a new cotton ball with each sweeping motion. Permit time for a return demonstration.

—Review care of the eye socket. Discuss how to care for, insert, and remove an artificial eye if used.

—Explain the need to wear an eye shield or patch to keep the socket clean until the prosthesis is fitted. Demonstrate application of the shield.

—Discuss the need to protect the vision in the remaining eye. Advise the patient to wear safety glasses for protection and to have regular follow-up eye examinations.

—Explain that the conformer for the eyeball may become dislodged but that this is not a serious problem and that the conformer need not be reinserted.

- *Medications*
  —Explain the purpose, dosage, schedule, and route of administration of any prescribed drugs, as well as side effects to report to the physician or nurse.

  —Explain the importance of good handwashing before administering ophthalmic medications.

- *Activity*
  —Remind the patient that with the loss of one eye, the field of vision is limited and depth perception changes. Discuss the need to exaggerate head movement to attain a full visual field. Advise using caution during activities until the patient adjusts to the loss.

## FOLLOW-UP CARE

- Stress the importance of regular follow-up visits to the physician and ocular prosthetist. Make sure the patient has the necessary names and telephone numbers.
- Discuss the importance of wearing a Medic-Alert band and carrying an information card that identifies the presence of an ocular prosthesis.

# Epididymitis

—Epididymitis: inflammation of the epididymis, which may be caused by infection of the prostate, chemicals, or trauma. It may also result from long-term indwelling catheters or prostate surgery. Epididymitis usually affects only one side of the scrotum but may affect both. It is sometimes confused with torsion of the testis.

## CAUSES/CONTRIBUTING FACTORS

- Men under 35 years
  —Sexually transmitted diseases such as gonorrhea, syphilis, *Chlamydia* infection
- Men over 35 years
  —Abnormality of the urinary tract
  —Straining to urinate
  —After urologic procedures
  —Strenuous exercise
  —Mumps

## SIGNS/SYMPTOMS

- Early
  —Heavy feeling in the scrotum
  —Painful urination
  —Scrotal pain and swelling
- Acute stage
  —Scrotum reddened, warm to touch, swollen (one side or both)
  —Extreme pain that may radiate to the groin or flank
  —Nausea, vomiting
  —Fever
  —Possible urethral discharge

## COMPLICATIONS

- Hydrocele
- Orchitis, prostatitis, urethritis, cystitis
- Fibrosis of area
- Sterility

## DIAGNOSTIC TESTS

- Describe each procedure, its purpose, and the normal feelings or sensations that are likely, as well as any preprocedural and postprocedural care.
    —Blood studies
        White blood cell count: to check for infection
    —Urine studies
        Urinalysis: to check for infection
        Culture: to identify bacteria
        Culture of urethral discharge: to check for sexually trans-mitted diseases
    —Testicular radionuclide scan: to rule out torsion of the testis
    —Doppler stethoscope: to rule out torsion of the testis

## TREATMENT

*Medical*
- Therapy
    —Bed rest with elevation of the scrotum and application of ice packs to decrease swelling
- Drugs
    —Antibiotics
    —Analgesics
    —Spermatic cord block for extreme pain

## HOME CARE

- Give both the patient and the caregiver *verbal* and *written* instructions. Provide them with the name and telephone number of a physician or nurse to call if questions arise.
- *General information*
    —Review the disease, discussing causes and contributing factors.
- *Warning signs*
    —Review the signs and symptoms that should be reported to a physician or nurse.
        Increasing pain
        Swelling
        Scrotal area hot to touch
        Urethral discharge
- *Special instructions*
    —Advise the use of comfort measures: ice packs; elevation of scrotum; loose, lightweight clothing; scrotal support while walking.

—Stress the importance of notifying all sexual partners if the inflammation is due to sexually transmitted disease.
* *Medications*
   —Explain the purpose, dosage, schedule, and route of administration of any prescribed drugs, as well as side effects to report to the physician or nurse.
* *Activity*
   —Discuss the need to maintain rest and to avoid exercise, sexual activity, or other strenuous activity during a period of inflammation and swelling.

**FOLLOW-UP CARE**

* Stress the importance of regular follow-up visits to the physician and for laboratory examinations. Make sure the patient has the necessary names and telephone numbers.

**REFERRALS**

* Refer the patient to appropriate supportive services if sterility is suspected.

# Epilepsy
## (Seizure Disorder, Convulsions)

—**Epilepsy: a chronic neurologic disorder characterized by repeated occurrence of any of various forms of seizures. Some seizure disorders have a familial tendency. The seizures, or convulsions, are paroxysmal episodes in which sudden discharge of abnormal electrical brain activity produces involuntary muscle contractions, resulting in disturbances in consciousness, behavior, sensation, and autonomic functioning. For half the reported cases there is no specific known cause.**

**CLASSIFICATION**

* Partial: seizures arising from localized area of the brain, causing specific symptoms
   —Motor (Jacksonian)

—Sensory (simple partial)
—Psychomotor

- Generalized: seizures causing generalized electrical abnormality in the brain
  —Tonic-clonic (grand mal)
  —Absence (petit mal)
  —Myoclonic
  —Akinetic
  —Atonic

## CAUSES

- Idiopathic (no specific cause)
- Brain tumor
- Vascular anomalies
- Trauma
- Infections: encephalitis, meningitis
- Metabolic disturbances: hypoglycemia, hypocalcemia
- Fever
- Toxins

## PRECIPITATING FACTORS

- Drug withdrawal/noncompliance
- Fatigue, lack of sleep
- Flashing lights
- Certain sounds, noises, odors

## SIGNS/SYMPTOMS

- General
  —Involuntary recurrent muscle movements
  —Jerking, patting, rubbing
  —Sudden contractions of muscle groups
  —Fluttering of eyelids
  —Facial jerking
  —Lip smacking
  —Movements confined to one area or spreading from one side to the other
  —Head and eyes deviating to the side
- Specific
  —Tonic-clonic: lasts 2-5 minutes
  　　Tonic phase: body stiffens
  　　Clonic phase: alternates between muscle spasm and relaxation

Other signs
- ○ Tongue biting
- ○ Incontinence
- ○ Dyspnea, apnea
- ○ Cyanosis
- ○ After seizure: postictal sleep

—Petit mal: lasts 5-30 minutes

Change in consciousness (absence)

Blinking, rolling of eyes, blank stare

## COMPLICATIONS

- Physical injury
- Aspiration
- Respiratory impairment
- Status epilepticus

## DIAGNOSTIC TESTS

- Describe each procedure, its purpose, and the normal feelings or sensations that are likely, as well as any preprocedural and postprocedural care.
  - —Computed tomography scan
  - —Magnetic resonance imaging
  - —Skull roentgenogram
  - —Echoencephalogram
  - —Cerebral angiography
  - —Electroencephalogram
  - —Urine screening
  - —Serum chemistry/screen (hypoglycemia, increased blood urea nitrogen, alcohol)
  - —History and neurologic examination

## TREATMENT

*Medical*

- Drugs
  - —Anticonvulsant
    - Carbamazepine (Tegretol)
    - Phenytoin (Dilantin)
    - Phenobarbital (Luminal)
    - Primidone (Mysoline)
    - Ethsuximide (Zarontin)
    - Mephenytoin (Mesantoin)

Trimethadione (Tridione)
Valproic acid (Depakote)
Clonazepam (Klonopin)
Diazepam (Valium)
Methsuximide (Cleotin)

*Surgical*
- Excision of epileptogenic focus
- Excision of underlying cause (e.g., brain tumor)

## HOME CARE

- Give both the patient and the caregiver *verbal* and *written* instructions. Provide them with the name and telephone number of a physician or nurse to call if questions arise.
- *General information*
  —Explain the type of seizure disorder involved, causes, and possible precipitating factors.
- *Special instructions*
  —Explain the course of action to take during and after a grand mal seizure.

    Assist the patient and family to recognize and record prodromal symptoms or auras. Prevent or break the fall; ease the person to the floor.

    Stay with the person during the seizure.

    Protect the head by clearing the surrounding area and padding the floor.

    Note the time and type of seizure activity.

    Do not restrict movement.

    Do not place anything in the person's mouth.

    After the seizure, turn the person to the side to prevent aspiration. Loosen tight clothing. Call the physician and report the activity.

    Reassure and reorient the person.

    Maintain a quiet environment.

  —Explain the course of action to take during and after a petit mal seizure.

    Remain with the patient. Do not startle or attempt to awaken the patient.

    Be aware that there are no prodromal symptoms and that the patient will resume normal activity once the seizure passes.

—Advise a female patient that seizure activity may increase or decrease during menses or pregnancy. Stress the importance of planning all pregnancies. Discuss the risks associated with pregnancy: seizures may cause fetal death and antiepilepsy drugs are associated with birth defects. Provide birth control information and encourage questions.

—Assist the patient to identify and avoid stimuli that precipitate seizure activity (e.g., flashing lights, loud music).

- Advise the patient to lower water heater temperature to avoid scalding during a shower or bath if a seizure occurs.
- Teach stress management and progressive relaxation techniques to control excessive stress or emotional excitement that might trigger seizures.
- *Medications*

  —Explain the purpose, dosage, schedule, and route of administration of any prescribed drugs, as well as side effects to report to the physician or nurse.

  —Stress the importance of taking the prescribed medication regularly and on schedule and not discontinuing the medication without a physician's guidance. Explain that missing a dose can precipitate seizure activity many days later.

  —Explain that medications cannot be taken prn and that lack of seizure activity does not mean that the drug is unnecessary.

  —Stress that abrupt withdrawal of antiepilepsy medication can cause seizures and that discontinuing these medications is the most common cause of status epilepticus.

  —Discuss that the need for medications to prevent seizures may be lifelong.

  —Discuss with the patient methods to help the patient remember to take medication, to monitor the drug supply, and to reorder medications 2 weeks before running out.

  —Discuss side effects of medication that should be reported to the physician or nurse.

      Bruising, bleeding, jaundice
      Nausea, vomiting
      Ataxia
      Diplopia
      Nystagmus
      Dizziness

—Instruct the patient to notify the physician or nurse of any significant weight loss or gain because the medication dosage may need to be changed.

—Stress the need to avoid alcoholic beverages and over-the-counter medications with alcohol, aspirin, or antihistamines without first consulting a physician, since these substances may affect the potency of antiepilepsy medication.

- *Activity*

  —Discuss with the patient the need to evaluate activities for the potential risks and to have a buddy when participating in high-risk activities (e.g., climbing, bicycling, swimming).

  —Stress the need to continue with normal work and recreation routines as much as possible; assure the patient that activity may inhibit seizure activity.

  —Advise the patient to check state regulations about driving an automobile.

  —Advise the patient not to operate heavy or dangerous equipment until the patient is seizure free for the time specified by the physician or nurse.

- *Diet*

  —Stress the importance of a well-balanced diet with meals spaced throughout the day to avoid hypoglycemia. Avoid stimulants or depressants (caffeine or alcohol), since withdrawal from them may cause seizures.

**FOLLOW-UP CARE**

- Stress the importance of regular follow-up visits to ensure adequate medical management of the disease process. Make sure the patient has the necessary names and telephone numbers.
- Discuss with the patient the need for routine blood draws to determine that therapeutic levels of antiepilepsy medications are being maintained.
- Discuss the importance of wearing a Medic-Alert band and carrying an information card at all times.

**PSYCHOSOCIAL CARE**

- Discuss with the patient the nature of the seizure disorder and the need to adopt a positive attitude.
- Stress the importance of verbalizing feelings of shame, humiliation, anxiety, and fears regarding the seizure disorder.

- Encourage questions to clarify common fears and dispel myths about epilepsy.
- Emphasize the need to avoid overprotection.

# Erectile Dysfunction
## (Penile Impotency)

—**Erectile dysfunction: inability to produce an erection of the penis of sufficient duration and rigidity to engage in intercourse.**

## CONTRIBUTING FACTORS/RISK FACTORS

- Endocrine problems (diabetes mellitus)
- Congenital problems (e.g., Klinefelter's syndrome)
- Chronic heart disease
- Drugs (immunosuppressants associated with transplants)
- Chronic renal insufficiency
- Chronic renal failure
- Neurologic conditions or injury (multiple sclerosis, trauma, epilepsy)
- Arteriosclerosis
- Surgical procedures (prostatectomy, ileostomy, colostomy)
- Mechanical defects (priapism [painful erection], abnormal lateral curvature)
- Reversible risk factors
    —Medications: antihypertensives, antidepressants, alpha and beta blockers, some heart medications such as digoxin, diuretics, immunosuppressants, weight reduction drugs, anabolic steroids
    —Recreational drugs: cocaine, marijuana, amphetamines, opiates
    —Alcohol

## SIGNS/SYMPTOMS

- Inability to initiate erection
- Inability to attain erection
- Inability to sustain erection

## COMPLICATIONS

- Psychosocial implications (depression, marital problems)
- Following penile implants
  —Infection
  —Rejection of penile implant
  —Mechanical failure
  —Seepage of fluid from balloon (inflatable device) into sur-
  rounding tissue
  —Erosion of glans and urethra
  —Persistent penile pain (after 4 weeks)

## DIAGNOSTIC TESTS

- Describe each procedure, its purpose, and the normal feelings
  or sensations that are likely, as well as any preprocedural and
  postprocedural care.
  —Blood studies: to evaluate presence of hormones or glucose
  —Snap-gauge testing: to check for nocturnal erections; a
  pressure-sensitive rubbber band around the penis will break
  under the pressure
  —Penile blood pressure
  —Penile pulse recording
  —Dynamic infusion cavernosometry and cavernosography:
  to check blood flow in the blood vessels necessary for erection

## TREATMENT

*Medical*
- Therapy
  —Vacuum pump
- Drugs
  —Hormones: to stabilize the endocrine condition
  —Vasodilator injection (papaverine, prostaglandin E, phento-
  lamine): to correct vascular impotence

*Surgical*
- Prosthetic device
- Penile prosthesis implantation: semirigid or flexible rods
- Inflatable prosthetic device
- Revascularization of blood vessels
- Corrective surgery for mechanical defects

## PREPROCEDURAL TEACHING

- Review the physician's explanation of prosthetic implantation and the reason for it; encourage the patient to ask questions and to discuss any fears or anxieties.
- Discuss postoperative care after a prosthetic implantation.
  —Explain the possible need for a temporary urinary drainage tube and restrictive dressing.
  —Discuss the reason for elevating the scrotum and applying cold packs.
  —Stress the need to avoid erections.

## HOME CARE

- Give both the patient and the caregiver *verbal* and *written* instructions. Provide them with the name and telephone number of a physician or nurse to call if questions arise.
- *General information*
  —Explain the patient's particular disorder, contributing causes, and type of prescribed treatment.
  —Review the types of sexual dysfunction associated with prostate or testicular cancer and following bilateral orchiectomy or chemotherapy, radiation therapy, and hormonal therapy: reduced fertility, ejaculatory and erectile dysfunction.
  —Discuss actual or potential dysfunctional problems the patient may encounter. Explain that some problems may be reversible; for example, hormonal therapy in prostate cancer may affect libido and erectile function but changes may be reversible once treatment is complete, or sperm production may be decreased for an extended time after chemotherapy. Discuss possible strategies to deal with problems; for example, for permanent infertility, strategies include banking sperm before therapy is begun or using alternative fertilization procedures such as artificial insemination through donor sperm, electro-ejaculation stimulation with intrauterine insemination, or in vitro fertilization.
  —Discuss alternative expressions of sexuality: physical intimacy, hugging, kissing, massage.
  —Review the written protocol for the prescribed prosthetic device or therapy (prosthetic implantation, vascular therapy, mechanical device) as provided by the nurse specialist or physician.

- *Prosthetic implantation*
  —Explain the name and type of prosthesis implanted.
  —Review the signs and symptoms of problems with the prosthetic implant that should be reported to a physician or nurse.

  Infection: redness, swelling, warm to touch, tenderness, drainage

  Persistent penile pain

  Inability to urinate

  Any mechanical failure of the pump (no erection after pumping)

  Painful intercourse

  Urinary tract infection (see Pyelonephritis, p. 556)

  Erosion of glans or penis: painful sexual intercourse, reddened area over implant and tender to touch, thinning area over implant area or visibility of implant
  —Advise how and where to obtain supplies.
  —Explain the need to keep the incision clean and dry.
  —Explain the allowable time frame for the inability to urinate.
  —Discuss the need to avoid the use of tight or restrictive clothing initially.
  —Encourage the use of jockey briefs or loose-fitting trousers if the patient is bothered with an aroused penis.
- *Vascular therapy*
  —Discuss care associated with vascular therapy.

  Stress the importance of condoms if performing self-injection therapy and having intercourse with multiple partners. Discuss and provide instructions on safe sex practices.

  Demonstrate and explain how and where to inject drugs, such as papaverine.

  Explain the need to report priapism (painful, sustained erection) to the physician or nurse.
- *Mechanical devices*
  —Discuss care associated with mechanical devices.

  Reinforce the physician's or nurse specialist's explanation and demonstrate the external vacuum device operation.

  For a patient with an internal inflatable pump device, explain when to start inflating and the length of time to keep inflated. Reinforce the need to inflate the device (as instructed) before actual use to encourage fibrous formation around the sheath.

Encourage questions regarding devices; permit time and privacy to practice activating devices.

- *Medications*
  —Explain the purpose, dosage, schedule, and route of administration of any prescribed drugs, as well as side effects to report to the physician or nurse.

  Amyl nitrate ampoules: to suppress penile erections after surgery

  Papaverine: injected into the base of the penis to produce erection

  Stress the importance of the amount to be used and the frequency (as prescribed). Explain that certain medications (heart medications or antihypertensives) cannot be stopped without consulting a physician.

- *Activity*
  —Advise the patient to avoid sitting for long periods (over 2 hours).
  —Explain the need to avoid strenuous exercise, jogging, or sports for about 3 weeks or as ordered.
  —Tell the patient to avoid lifting anything over 10 pounds.
  —Advise the patient to avoid intercourse until all pain and swelling are gone, the incision is completely healed, or the physician gives approval (approximately 6 weeks).

- *Diet*
  —Explain that a regular diet or one prescribed by the physician should be followed.

## FOLLOW-UP CARE

- Stress the importance of regular follow-up visits with the physician, physical therapist, or rehabilitation therapist. Make sure the patient has the necessary names and telephone numbers.

## PSYCHOSOCIAL CARE

- Encourage verbalization of fears, anxiety, and embarrassment. Encourage questions from the partner.

## REFERRALS

- Refer the patient for sexual counseling and supportive counseling, including family planning and urology, as needed.

# Fecal Ostomy
## (Ileostomy, Colostomy)

—Fecal ostomy: a temporary or permanent opening into the bowel that allows fecal materials to be expelled at the skin surface. The opening onto the skin is called a stoma.

—Ileostomy: permanent ileostomy is removal of the colon and rectum and closure of the anus (proctocolectomy). The terminal ileum is brought through the abdominal wall, and an external pouch is worn. Continent ileostomy (Kock's pouch) is surgical removal of the rectum and colon with construction of an internal ileal reservoir, nipple valve, and stoma. Fecal waste collects in the nipple-valved pouch until the patient drains the pouch through the stoma with a catheter. No external pouch is worn. The internal pouch is emptied several times a day. The stoma is flat with the skin surface. The ileostomy effluent is liquid.

—Colostomy: surgical removal of the entire rectum and affected colon and closure of the anus; if the rectum is left intact, the colostomy may be temporary. The location of the stoma and the effluent consistency depend on the section of colon resected: ascending (liquid effluent), transverse (loose semiformed effluent), descending, or sigmoid colon (effluent close to normal).

## INDICATIONS
* Ileostomy
    —Ulcerative colitis
    —Small bowel obstruction
    —Polyposis
* Colostomy
    —Colon cancer
    —Diverticulitis
    —Fistula

## PREPROCEDURAL TEACHING
* Review the physician's explanation of the procedure and the type of ostomy. Describe how the ostomy will function, its lo-

cation, and the appearance and smell of fecal drainage. Use simple descriptions and illustrations.

- Describe and allow the patient to see equipment and supplies such as the pouch.
- Explain the stoma selection process, asking the patient's preference. Permit the patient to wear a stoma pouch over the area to ensure comfort at the selected site.
- Arrange for a visit from the enterostomal therapist and an ostomy patient from the United Ostomy Association.

### Review of Preprocedural Care

- Review preoperative procedures (see Abdominal Surgery, p. 3), including bowel preparation.
- Permit time for questions. Encourage verbalization and expression of fears and feelings regarding changes in body image, sexuality, and role function.

### SIDE EFFECTS/COMPLICATIONS

- Leakage under the appliance
- Signs of wound infection
- Electrolyte imbalance
- Dehydration
- Obstruction
- Prolapse
- Hemorrhage
- Stricture
- Retraction
- Necrosis

### HOME CARE

- Give both the patient and the caregiver *verbal* and *written* instructions. Provide them with the name and telephone number of a physician, nurse, or enterostomal therapist to call if questions arise. Use visual aids to assist in instruction and permit time for practice and return demonstration.
- *General information*
  —Describe the type and location of the ostomy created, reviewing indications. Explain that drainage depends on food ingested.
  —Explain that an ostomy requires special attention, including diet modifications and restriction and meticulous skin care.

- *Warning signs*
  —Review the signs and symptoms that should be reported to a physician or nurse.

    Infection of stoma: redness, purulent drainage, swelling, pain, warm to touch, fever

    Prolapse of stoma, bloody drainage, persistent diarrhea through stoma, excessive flatus, lack of fecal material, or change in usual pattern of elimination

    Ileostomy: inability to intubate stoma, abdominal distention, nausea, vomiting, abdominal pain, nipple valve dysfunction, incontinence of stool, flatus

- *Special instructions*
  —Discuss and demonstrate skin care around the stoma. Permit time for the patient or caregiver to return demonstrate and practice.

    Inspect the skin daily for signs of irritation or infection.

    Each time the pouch is changed, clean the skin with soap and water. Apply a skin barrier to the clean, dry skin before the new pouch is attached.

    Place a pectin-based wafer in the pouch.

    If a rash occurs, use a heat lamp or hair dryer to dry the skin.

    Sprinkle a small amount of powder (e.g., karaya, Stomahesive) on the skin, wipe off the excess, and blot with a skin sealant to seal the powder to the skin.

    Powder the skin after the pouch has been applied.

  —Demonstrate emptying of a fecal ostomy pouch. Explain that the pouch should be emptied when it is about one-third full. Provide time for the patient or caregiver to return demonstrate and practice.

    Have the patient sit on the toilet with the pouch between the legs, or sit on a chair with the pouch opening in the toilet.

    While holding up the end of the pouch, remove the clamp and let the contents of the pouch drain into the toilet. Putting some toilet paper on the surface of the water helps to prevent splashing.

    Squeeze the remaining contents out of the pouch.

    Hold up the end of the pouch and pour a cup of water into the pouch through the opening. Swish the water around to clean out the inside of the pouch. Do not get the stoma or the seal around the stoma wet.

    Use toilet paper to clean around the opening of the pouch. Clamp the pouch shut again.

—Demonstrate removal of an ostomy pouch. Permit time for the patient or caregiver to return demonstrate and practice.

Instruct the patient to change the ostomy pouch every 5-7 days. Gather the following equipment before beginning: adhesive solvent, gauze pads, powder (if desired), towel, and scissors.

While standing, hold the skin around the stoma taut and begin peeling off the adhesive square that holds the pouch to the skin. Peeling from top to bottom works best. If the pouch cannot be peeled off, use adhesive solvent to loosen the edges.

Wipe excess drainage around the stoma with gauze pads.

Wash the area around the stoma with soap and water. Dry thoroughly. Apply powder if the skin is irritated. Apply a skin barrier if desired.

—Demonstrate application of an ostomy pouch. Permit time for the patient or caregiver to return demonstrate and practice.

Peel back the paper from the adhesive faceplate.

Center the pouch opening over stoma, and press all around the faceplate to ensure that it is firmly attached to the skin.

Attach the belt if the patient wishes to wear it.

Press the air out of the pouch and clamp the bottom.

—Explain the emptying of a continent ileostomy (Kock pouch).

To remove stool and flatus, place a large-bore tube into the stoma several times a day.

- *Medications*
  —Explain the purpose, dosage, schedule, and route of administration of any prescribed drugs, as well as side effects to report to the physician or nurse.
- *Activity*
  —Encourage the patient to resume activities of daily living as soon as able.
  —Explain that regular exercise will build the patient's strength. Inform the patient of the need to avoid activities that cause abdominal strain (e.g., weight lifting) or contact sports (e.g., football, ice hockey).
  —Encourage questions regarding specific allowances and limitations for occupation, recreation, or activities.
  —Assure the patient than a preosteotomy life-style can be resumed once the stoma has healed. Provide examples and guidelines.
  —Explain that showers and baths are permissible because the

stoma will not be hurt by soap or direct water. The patient may wear a disposable/temporary pouch if concerned about leakage.

—Advise the patient to avoid wearing tight, constrictive clothing (e.g., girdle, belt) directly over the stoma.

—Suggest measures to take before traveling.

> Purchase enough ostomy supplies for the entire trip or find out where to buy supplies en route.
>
> If the usual pouch is reusable, purchase disposable pouches as a precaution.
>
> Carry supplies in hand luggage to prevent loss. For long air travel, arrange with the airline to have special meals ordered.
>
> Notify the physician about the travel and request prophylactic medication for diarrhea or constipation. If traveling to a foreign country, drink only potable water.

—Discuss the effect an ostomy may have on the patient's sexual activity. Provide information and encourage counseling if the patient or partner is unable to discuss sexuality.

> The presence of an osteotomy usually does not interfere with sexual function, except that men with bladder or rectal cancer may have temporary or permanent impotence.
>
> Pregnancy is possible but should be planned. The female patient should talk with a physician or nurse before becoming pregnant and should be given information regarding contraception.
>
> Sexual activity may resume when the stoma is healed and the patient and partner are ready.
>
> Verbalization and communication between the patient and partner are important.
>
> The stoma cannot be injured by close physical contact.
>
> The pouch should be emptied before intercourse. The patient may wish to use a pouch cover.

- *Diet*
  —Review dietary restrictions (see below) for preventing stoma blockage and diarrhea, flatus, and odor. Provide written information and refer the patient to a dietitian for additional information and counseling.
  —Encourage fluid intake to maintain fluid and electrolyte balance, especially on hot days or during bouts of diarrhea. Advise the patient to avoid use of laxatives and diuretics, which increase fluid loss.

—Instruct the patient to avoid gas-producing foods such as broccoli, cabbage, beans, onions, and radishes. When eating such foods, the patient should use a product such as Beano to reduce gas formation.

—Suggest that the patient prevent odor by avoiding eggs, cheese, and alcohol.

—For ileostomy, instruct the patient to buy odor-absorbing tablets to place in the ostomy bag or a commercial gas release valve.

—Explain how to prevent blockage of the stoma by avoiding high-fiber foods such as celery, lettuce, nuts, and corn.

—Inform the patient that diarrhea can be avoided by not eating highly spiced foods or raw fruits and vegetables (e.g., green beans, broccoli).

—Instruct the patient to have meals at regular times, to eat slowly and chew well, to have moderate-sized portions, and to try new foods in small servings in case they have ill effects.

—Explain that gas formation can be prevented by avoiding use of straws, gum chewing or chewing with the mouth open, and smoking.

**FOLLOW-UP CARE**

• Stress the importance of regular follow-up visits. Make sure the patient has the necessary names and telephone numbers.

**PSYCHOSOCIAL CARE**

• Permit time for emotional adjustment. Encourage the patient to ask questions and express feelings about the change in body image.

**REFERRALS**

• Provide referrals for enterostomal therapy, home health, support groups, and the United Ostomy Association.

# Fixator Devices

—**Fixator devices: use of fixation devices to immobilize and repair damaged bones and joints and treat musculoskeletal conditions.**

—**External fixation:** surgical procedure used to immobilize and reduce complicated fractures and nonunion fractures. External fixation is also used in maintaining bones, in limb lengthening procedures such as the Ilizarov method, and in the treatment of other musculoskeletal disorders such as osteomyelitis. Stabilizing pins or wires are inserted into and through the bone and attached to an external metal frame. Fixation may be applied to the jaw, arm, leg, ribs, pelvis, fingers, or toes. External fixator devices are also used to increase use of the joint while maintaining immobilization of bone. Thus they permit earlier discharge to home because they hold unstable fractures in place while permitting the patient to ambulate.

—**Internal fixation:** surgical implantation of metallic pins, nails, screws, plates, rods, and other devices for immobilizing or repairing traumatized or damaged bones and joints. Open reduction with internal fixation can be performed on most bones except the skull and facial bones. Bones most frequently treated with this type of procedure include the arms, legs, forearms, thighs, and vertebral column. Internal fixation is used most frequently to repair fractured bones. Similar to external fixation, it permits the patient to be ambulatory, to be discharged earlier, and to regain independence relatively quickly.

## PREPROCEDURAL TEACHING

• Review the physician's explanation of the procedure and the reason for it; encourage the patient to ask questions and to discuss any fears or anxieties. Discuss the need for informed consent for surgery and anesthesia.

### Review of Preprocedural Care

• Review care before external fixation.
  —The skin of the affected extremity or operative site will be cleansed with bactericidal soap.
  —X-rays will be taken to determine the location of the repair.
  —Prophylactic antibiotic therapy will be prescribed.
• Review care before internal fixation.
  —The physician may order skin or skeletal traction before surgery to lessen muscle spasm.
  —Routine diagnostic studies will be ordered: complete blood

count, urinalysis, chest x-ray, electrocardiogram, and x-rays to determine location of repair.

—Bowel preparation with an enema may be ordered the night before.

—The skin will be cleansed with bactericidal soap.

—NPO status will be maintained from midnight the night before.

—An indwelling catheter may be ordered before surgery.

## Review of Postprocedural Care

• Review postprocedural care for external fixation.

—The patient will remain in the hospital 2-3 days.

—Routine postoperative procedures will be performed: frequent checks of neurovascular status and peripheral pulses, decreasing in frequency; application of ice to the incision site; elevation of the extremity on pillows; upper extremity in a sling; for lower extremity, patient instructed to use crutches with no weight bearing; the nuts on the fixator will be turned and tightened.

—Stress the importance of range-of-motion exercises, quadriceps setting, and gluteal contractions according to the location of the fracture.

—Explain that the fixator causes little pain and permits early ambulation.

—Instruct the patient in proper use of ambulatory aids (crutches, cane, walker).

—Inform the patient of the need to monitor the neurovascular status of the affected extremity: color, sensation, mobility, peripheral pulse, temperature.

• Instruct the patient in pin care: cleanse around each pin with hydrogen peroxide and rinse with normal saline, then dry; apply antibacterial agent around each pin.

• Review postprocedural care for internal fixation.

—The length of hospital stay varies with the specific operation.

—Routine postoperative procedures will be performed: frequent checks of vital signs, neurovascular status, and peripheral pulses in the first hour, decreasing in frequency thereafter; dressing and wound checks; possible presence of drainage tube in the wound.

—The patient will be instructed in the proper use of a cane, crutches, or walker with the ordered amount of weight bearing.

—The signs of neurovascular impairment of the affected extremity will be reviewed: persistent changes in color (pallor, cyanosis, redness), coolness, delayed capillary refill, paresthesias (numbness, tingling), inability to move distal areas.

—The patient will be taught range-of-motion exercises for the unaffected joints.

## SIDE EFFECTS/COMPLICATIONS

- External fixation
  —Infection
  —Delayed healing because of torque and twist
  —Refracture after pin removal
  —Nonunion
  —Muscle or nerve damage or injury
  —Compartment syndrome
- Internal fixation
  —Infection
  —Hemorrhage
  —Loss of reduction or dislocation
  —Pneumonia
  —Thrombophlebitis
  —Nonunion
  —Refracture

## HOME CARE

- Give both the patient and the caregiver *verbal* and *written* instructions. Provide them with the name and telephone number of a physician or nurse to call if questions arise.
- *General information*
  —Review the specific type of device ordered and specific care.
- *Warning signs*
  —Review the signs and symptoms of problems after external fixation that should be reported to a physician or nurse.

  Infection
  ○ Fever
  ○ Chills
  ○ Redness
  ○ Swelling
  ○ Purulent drainage at pin sites
  Pin migration: tenting of the skin on the pin, which signals movement of the pin or infection

Neurovascular impairment: pallor, cyanosis, coolness, tingling, numbness

—Review the signs and symptoms of problems after internal fixation that should be reported to a physician or nurse.

Infection: persistent redness, swelling, increasing pain, wound drainage, local warmth, foul odor from cast, sensation of burning within cast, drainage from cast, fever

Neurovascular impairment: pallor, cyanosis, coolness, tingling, numbness

- *Special instructions*
  - —External fixation

    Provide instruction on pin and fixator care: cleanse fixator with sterile water and cover each pin head with cork or rubber tip to prevent injury.

  - —Internal fixation

    Explain that presence of the internal fixator poses a risk for refracture and review preventive measures: safety in crutch walking, no weight bearing until ordered by the physician.

    Inform the patient that some nails, rods, or large plates may be removed within a year.

- *Medications*
  - —Explain the purpose, dosage, schedule, and route of administration of any prescribed drugs, as well as side effects to report to the physician or nurse.

- *Activity*
  - —Remind the patient to plan frequent rest periods.
  - —Review special instructions for a patient who has undergone external fixation.

    Stress the need to increase movements and weight bearing slowly to lessen tenderness and to permit muscles to regain strength. Instruct the patient not to use the external fixator as a handle or support for the extremity but to support the extremity with pillows, two hands, or a sling to prevent excessive stress on the pins.

    Advise the patient to elevate the extremity when sitting or lying down.

    Stress the importance of not changing or adjusting the fixator bars, since this can cause misalignment.

    Explain that showering is permitted but that swimming should be avoided because chlorine and salt can corrode metal.

**FOLLOW-UP CARE**

• Stress the importance of regular follow-up visits to ensure that the device is functioning properly and to maintain adequate immobilization of the fracture(s) (for external fixation). Maintain appointments with the physician for physical therapy until recovery is complete (for internal fixation). Make sure the patient has the necessary names and telephone numbers.

**F**

# Fractures

—**Fracture: a discontinuity or break in bone. Fractures occur when stress placed on the bone exceeds the bone's loading capacity. The majority of fractures occur as a result of trauma. Pathologic (spontaneous) fractures, which occur with minimal stress or trauma, affect bones weakened by disease (e.g., osteoporosis, cancer, Paget's disease). Fractures are described according to a number of characteristics, including the extent of soft tissue damage:**

—**Closed: the skin is intact**

—**Open: the skin is pierced**

—**Transverse, oblique, spiral, or linear: describes the line of the fracture**

—**Compression: describes the force of the fracture**

—**Comminuted: describes the number of pieces**

—**Displaced, angulated: describes the anatomic position of the distal fragment**

—**Intraarticular, extraarticular: describes whether the fracture involves the joint**

**SIGNS/SYMPTOMS**

- Fracture site
  —Pain, tenderness, edema
  —Skin open or closed
  —Pallor, coolness of surrounding tissues
  —Numbness, tingling
  —Restricted or limited mobility, decreased range of motion
  —Abnormal position of extremity; deformity
  —Limb shortening
  —Crepitus (movement of parts not normally movable)
  —Bleeding, hematoma
  —Bruising, blisters

**COMPLICATIONS**

- Malunion, delayed union, or nonunion of fracture
- Thrombophlebitis
- Fat embolism
- Compartment syndrome
- Infection
- Nerve compression
- Pseudoarthrosis
- Avascular necrosis
- Limb length discrepancy

**DIAGNOSTIC TESTS**

- Describe each procedure, its purpose, and the normal feelings or sensations that are likely, as well as any preprocedural and postprocedural care.
  —X-rays of the fracture
  —Magnetic resonance imaging: to evaluate complicated fractures
  —Arthroscopy: to identify intraarticular fractures
  —Bone scans
  —Computed tomography
  —Blood tests: complete blood count, electrolytes

**TREATMENT**

*Medical*

- Therapy
  —Immobilization of bone
  —Closed reduction

—Bed rest
—No weight bearing on affected bone (use of crutches, cane, walker)
—Ice applications
—Antiembolic stockings
—Application of cast, splint, traction, sling

• Drugs
—Analgesics
—Antibiotics for open fractures
—Muscle relaxants
—Sedatives

*Surgical*

• Open reduction with internal fixation
• Arthroplasty with replacement with prosthesis
• Total joint replacement for crush injuries
• Amputation for severe crush injuries
• Application of external fixator, such as Hoffman, Ilizarov, or Ace-Fischer device
• Microvascular surgery, such as replantation of an amputated body part and revascularization of crush, avulsion, and other soft tissue injuries

## HOME CARE

• Give both the patient and the caregiver *verbal* and *written* instructions. Provide them with the name and telephone number of a physician or nurse to call if questions arise.
• Provide instruction regarding specific treatments: cast care (see Cast Care, p. 155) and external fixator (see Fixator Devices, p. 304).
• *General information*
—Discuss and review the type of fracture, causes or contributing factors, and prescribed treatment.
—Explain the bone healing process.
• *Warning signs*
—Review the signs and symptoms that should be reported to a physician or nurse.
  Neurovascular impairment of affected extremity: numbness, tingling, decreased movement, coolness, pallor, redness, blueness, decreased capillary refill
  Infection: fever, increased pain, swelling at fracture site, purulent drainage from cast or dressing, foul odor from cast or dressing

Fat embolism: chest pain; fever; rash on abdomen, neck, arms, or axillae; anxiety

• *Special instructions*
—Stress the importance of turning and moving frequently to avoid skin breakdown; advise the patient to handle injured tissues gently by supporting the joint above and below the site.
—Review and demonstrate wound care.

• *Medications*
—Explain the purpose, dosage, schedule, and route of administration of any prescribed drugs, as well as side effects to report to the physician or nurse.

• *Activity*
—Explain the importance of maintaining immobility and not bearing weight on the injured limb as prescribed by the physician.
—Explain that the recovery program takes twice the amount of time spent immobilized, so it will take that amount of time to use the fractured limb or bear weight on it again (i.e., if 6 weeks was spent in a cast, it will take 6 more weeks to recover fully).
—Instruct the patient to elevate the extremity and apply ice bags as indicated.
—Instruct the patient in the use of ambulatory aids (crutch walking, cane, walker).
—Explain the importance of range-of-motion exercises to maintain function of unaffected joints. Teach exercises to maintain strength and facilitate resolution of inflammation: quadriceps, buttocks, and triceps setting exercises.

• *Diet*
—Emphasize the importance of a well-balanced diet high in vitamins, proteins, carbohydrates, and minerals to promote healing and prevent weight loss.
—Stress the need to eat foods high in calcium and vitamins A, B, C, and D to promote bone healing and avoid hypocalcemia.
—Encourage fluids to avoid constipation and maintain skin turgor (8-10 glasses per day).

**FOLLOW-UP CARE**

• Stress the importance of regular follow-up visits with the physician, physical therapist, or rehabilitation therapist. Make sure the patient has the necessary names and telephone numbers.

# Frostbite

—Frostbite: a localized injury to tissues and blood vessels caused by exposure to cold or freezing temperatures. Individuals at risk include the elderly, the homeless, infants and small children, debilitated and immobile patients, and patients with chronic illnesses (e.g., cardiac disease, diabetes, vascular disease). Frostbite is classified as either superficial (affecting skin and subcutaneous tissue, especially of the face, ears, and other exposed body parts) or deep (affecting the skin, subcutaneous tissue, muscle, tendon, and neurovascular structures).

## CAUSES/CONTRIBUTING FACTORS

- Lack of insulating body fat
- Lack of acclimatization to cold temperatures
- Wet or inadequate clothing
- Drug abuse
- Smoking
- Hunger, fatigue
- Excessive alcohol intake

## SIGNS/SYMPTOMS

- Superficial frostbite
  - —Burning
  - —Tingling
  - —Numbness
  - —Skin mottling
  - —White or grayish skin color
  - —Absence of capillary refill
- With thawing, area becomes:
  - —Flushed
  - —Edematous
  - —Painful
  - —Purplish
  - —Blistered within 24 hours
- Deep frostbite
  - —Hard and solid
  - —Cold

—Mottled
—Blue or gray after thawing
—Swelling of entire limb
—Blisters after several weeks

## COMPLICATIONS

* Vasospasm
* Hyperesthesia
* Infection
* Gangrene
* Amputation

## TREATMENT

*Medical*
* Therapy
  —Rapid rewarming via immersion in water at 28°-45° C (100°-112° F)
  —Protective isolation
  —Whirlpool baths three times a day at 32°-37° C (90°-98° F)
* Drugs
  —Immunologic agents (tetanus)
  —Plasma expanders
  —Antibiotics
  —Analgesics

*Surgical*
* Escharotomy: removal of dead tissue
* Sympathectomy: for severe vasospasm and pain
* Debridement: after retraction of viable tissue, done 13 weeks to 4 months after injury
* Fasciotomy: to decrease tissue swelling, thereby increasing circulation
* Amputation of nonviable extremity: may be done several months after injury

## HOME CARE

* Give both the patient and the caregiver *verbal* and *written* instructions. Provide them with the name and telephone number of a physician or nurse to call if questions arise.
* *General information*
  —Explain the disorder and factors that contributed to the problem.

—Prepare the patient for amputation if indicated (see p. 26).
- *Warning signs*
  —Review the signs and symptoms that should be reported to a physician or nurse.

    Persistent increasing pain

    Foul-smelling drainage

    Fever

    Swelling area
- *Special instructions*
  —Provide instruction and demonstrate the application of dry, sterile dressings to small, open areas.

  —Discuss the importance of protecting the extremity from temperature extremes and rapid changes in temperature because the tissue is sensitive to temperature changes and refreezing causes tissue loss.

  —Instruct the patient to avoid tight, constrictive clothing or pressure to an area that might decrease circulation.

  —Discuss preventive measures to avoid future episodes or re-injury of the frostbitten part: protective, multilayered, warm, nonconstrictive clothing; avoidance of cold temperatures, fatigue, and hunger.

  —Emphasize the importance of not smoking or using alcohol when exposed to cold.

  —Advise the patient that there may be long-term residual effects: increased sensitivity to cold, burning and tingling, and increased sweating.
- *Medications*
  —Explain the purpose, dosage, schedule, and route of administration of any prescribed drugs, as well as side effects to report to the physician or nurse.
- *Activity*
  —If lower extremities are affected, advise the patient to avoid weight bearing and provide instruction in the use of ambulatory aids.

  —Stress the importance of elevating the affected extremity.

  —Instruct the patient in range-of-motion exercises to prevent contractures.
- *Diet*
  —Avoid drinks that contain caffeine, which causes vasoconstriction: coffee, tea, cola.

**FOLLOW-UP CARE**

- Stress the importance of regular follow-up visits with the physician, physical therapist, or rehabilitation therapist. Make sure the patient has the necessary names and telephone numbers.

# Gangrene

—Gangrene: tissue necrosis or death usually resulting from decreased blood supply (ischemia), bacterial infection, and subsequent putrefaction. The extremities are most often affected, but gangrene can occur internally (e.g., in the intestines or gallbladder). Gangrene may be a complication of strangulated hernia, appendicitis, thrombosis or mesenteric arteries, infection, or diabetes mellitus. Gangrene may also follow a crush injury or acute obstruction of blood flow (e.g., vascular disease, tourniquet, or embolism). Gas gangrene is necrosis accompanied by gas bubbles in soft tissue. It is caused by the anaerobic, spore-forming, gram-positive rod *Clostridium perfringens* or another clostridial species and usually follows trauma or surgery.

**SIGNS/SYMPTOMS**

- Dry gangrene
  - —Affected extremity cold, dry, shriveled, black
- Moist gangrene
  - —Affected extremity or wound necrotic, putrid
- Gas gangrene
  - —Crepitation caused by carbon dioxide and hydrogen accumulation in necrotic tissues
  - —Severe localized pain, swelling, and discoloration
  - —Tissue necrosis and rupture
  - —Foul-smelling discharge
  - —Tachycardia, tachypnea, hypotension
  - —Fever
  - —Delirium

**COMPLICATIONS**

- Amputation

- Gas gangrene: rapidly fatal
- Moist gangrene: death if untreated

## DIAGNOSTIC TESTS

- Describe each procedure, its purpose, and the normal feelings or sensations that are likely, as well as any preprocedural and postprocedural care.
  —Laboratory studies
    Blood tests: white and red blood cell counts to show infectious process and hemolysis
    Anaerobic wound cultures and Gram's stain of wound drainage: to identify *C. perfringens*
  —X-rays: to document the presence of gas in tissues

## TREATMENT

*Medical* (for gas gangrene)
- Therapy
  —Hyperbaric oxygenation: to prevent multiplication of anaerobic bacteria
- Drugs
  —Intravenous antibiotics, usually high doses of penicillin
  —Antipyretics
  —Analgesics

*Surgical*
- Debridement of affected tissues and necrotic muscle
- Amputation

## HOME CARE

- Give both the patient and the caregiver *verbal* and *written* instructions. Provide them with the name and telephone number of a physician or nurse to call if questions arise.
- *General information*
  —Explain the disorder and contributing factors.
  —Prepare the patient for amputation if indicated (see p. 26).
- *Warning signs*
  —Review the signs and symptoms that should be reported to a physician or nurse.
    Recurrence of infection
    Vascular impairment (ischemia) of surrounding area: cool skin, pallor, blueness of skin, sudden swelling or severe pain

- *Special instructions*
  —Prepare the patient for debridement and discuss the reason for the procedure.
  —After debridement, discuss wound care and dressing changes.
    Inspect the wound daily.
    Use aseptic technique.
    Perform meticulous wound cleansing.
- *Medications*
  —Explain the purpose, dosage, schedule, and route of administration of any prescribed drugs, as well as side effects to report to the physician or nurse.
- *Activity*
  —Explain the need for rest to conserve energy, promote healing, and lessen stress on involved tissues.
  —Stress the importance of immobilizing the affected extremity to decrease the spread of purulent drainage.
  —Instruct the patient in range-of-motion exercises to maintain strength of muscles and joints and to prevent atrophy of tissues.
  —Teach the use of ambulatory aids when the patient is allowed out of bed.

**FOLLOW-UP CARE**
- Stress the importance of regular follow-up visits with the physician, physical therapist, or rehabilitation therapist. Make sure the patient has the necessary names and telephone numbers.
- Emphasize the importance of not smoking or using alcohol when exposed to cold.

# Gastrectomy and Gastrostomy

—**Gastrectomy: surgical removal of the entire or a portion of the stomach with anastomosis to the small intestine.**

—**Gastrostomy: surgically constructed stoma (ostomy) in the stomach for the insertion of a catheter for tube feedings, decompression, or drainage.**

## INDICATIONS

- Hemorrhage
- Intractable ulcers
- Esophageal disorders: carcinoma, stricture, atresia, trauma, dysphagia
- Perforation

## PREPROCEDURAL TEACHING

- See also Abdominal Surgery, p. 3.
- Review the physician's explanation of the procedure and the reason for it; encourage the patient to ask questions and to discuss any fears or anxieties. Explain the need for informed consent.

### Review of Preprocedural Care

- Explain and enforce NPO status before and after the procedure.

### Review of Postprocedural Care

- Review anticipated postoperative care, including the nasogastric tube, incisions, intravenous fluid and electrolyte therapy, and indwelling urethral catheter.
- Discuss anticipated postoperative body changes: gastrostomy and presence of gastrostomy tube.
- Discuss anticipated life-style modifications: eating pattern, altered feeding methods, diet modifications, and symptomatic relief of dumping syndrome.
- Demonstrate coughing, deep breathing, and splitting incision.
- Discuss the purpose of and demonstrate the use of the incentive spirometer.
- Encourage early ambulation.
- Provide explanation of stoma or catheter care, the initiation of tube feedings, or diet modifications.

## COMPLICATIONS/SIDE EFFECTS

- Dehydration
- Electrolyte imbalance
- Aspiration pneumonia
- Wound infection
- Hemorrhage or shock
- Atelectasis

## HOME CARE

- Give both the patient and the caregiver *verbal* and *written* instructions. Provide them with the name and telephone number of a physician or nurse to call if questions arise.
- *General information*
  —Review the explanation of the procedure and specific follow-up care.
  —Explain and discuss the relationships among the underlying disease, the need for gastrectomy or gastrostomy, contributing factors (e.g., smoking, alcohol, irritating foods or drugs, or stress), care, and treatment. Stress the importance of eliminating causative factors.
- *Wound/incision care*
  —Discuss and demonstrate proper wound management, dressing changes, and ostomy care: procedure, frequency, and inspection of skin integrity and stoma site.
- *Warning signs*
  —Review the signs and symptoms that should be reported to a physician or nurse.
      Retention and bowel obstruction: nausea, vomiting, abdominal distention, abdominal pain, abdominal rigidity
      Infection: fever, erythema, pain, tenderness, purulent drainage, foul odor, warmth at the site
      Weight loss or failure to gain weight
      Diarrhea
      Dumping syndrome: abdominal fullness, cramping, nausea, vomiting, diarrhea, diaphoresis, fatigue, tachycardia, dizziness, palpitations
      For gastrostomy: change in color of stoma from normal bright red, change in color, consistency, or amount of gastric drainage; peristomal skin irritation
- *Special instructions*
  —Assist the patient in obtaining appropriate devices, such as ostomy appliances, sterile dressings, and tube feedings and feeding pump.
  —For patient with gastrectomy, discuss symptomatic relief of dumping syndrome.
      Assist the patient to plan a low-carbohydrate, high-fat, high-protein diet.
      Instruct the patient to eat small, frequent meals and to avoid taking liquids with meals.

Instruct the patient to asssume a recumbent position after meals.

—After gastrotomy, discuss and demonstrate the preparation and administration of tube feedings, including amount and frequency.

Instruct the patient to sit upright during feeding and for 1 hour after feeding to prevent reflux into the esophagus or backflow into the gastrostomy tube.

For continuous tube feedings, see p. 638.

—Teach care of the gastrostomy tube and provide written instructions.

Wash area gently with soap and water.

Rinse well and pat dry.

Apply skin barrier as needed.

Reapply dressings and appliance.

Securely tape gastrostomy tube to the skin to prevent stress and accidental dislodgment.

Change the tube every 2-3 days.

If a gastrostomy tube is permanent, explain that it may eventually be removed and inserted only for feedings; tell the patient to protect the stoma with a small gauze pad.

- *Medications*
  —Explain the purpose, dosage, schedule, and route of administration of any prescribed drugs, as well as side effects to report to the physician or nurse.
  —Stress the importance of taking iron supplements as ordered for the treatment of iron deficiency anemia.
  —Explain and demonstrate vitamin $B_{12}$ injections for the treatment of pernicious anemia, if ordered. Demonstrate medication preparation and administration via the gastrostomy tube.
- *Activity*
  —Encourage the patient to discuss allowances and limitations with respect to occupation, recreation, and activities.
  —Instruct the patient to gradually resume activities of daily living but to avoid heavy lifting ($>$10 pounds), pushing, or pulling.
  —Instruct the patient to weigh and record weight every 2-3 days.
- *Diet*
  —Refer the patient for a dietary consultation.
  —Provide the patient with a list of irritating foods and drugs to

avoid, including coffee, caffeine, spicy food, alcohol, aspirin, and ibuprofen.

—Emphasize the importance of not using alcohol or taking gastric-irritating drugs.

## FOLLOW-UP CARE

- Stress the importance of regular follow-up visits with the physician, dietitian, and enterostomal nurse. Make sure the patient has the necessary names and telephone numbers.
- Provide strategies for smoking cessation. Refer the patient to community resources for smoking cessation, if appropriate.

## PSYCHOSOCIAL CARE

- Encourage the patient to verbalize psychosocial concerns regarding body image, inability to consume food and drink orally, social value of mealtime, altered feeding methods, and life-style implications.
- Assist the patient and family to integrate the patient's altered feeding methods into social patterns of mealtime to prevent isolation.
- Encourage stress reduction techniques.

## REFERRALS

- Refer the patient to a social worker for psychosocial support, assistance with financial concerns over long-term feedings, and home health care support services.
- Refer the patient to Alcoholics Anonymous, if appropriate.

# Gastroenteritis

—**Gastroenteritis: inflammation of the stomach and small intestine, characterized by vomiting and severe diarrhea, leading to depletion of intracellular fluids. Gastroenteritis can occur in persons of all ages but is particularly dangerous in children, the elderly, and debilitated patients.**

## CAUSES/CONTRIBUTING FACTORS/RISK FACTORS

- Ingestion of contaminated food and water: bacteria *(Staphylococcus aureus, Salmonella, Shigella)*, viruses, or parasites
- Allergy or intolerance of specific foods; drug reactions
- Direct or indirect fecal-oral transmission from an infected person
- Poor sanitation conditions
- Crowded living conditions
- Travel to a foreign country

## SIGNS/SYMPTOMS

- Frequent diarrhea: may be mucoid or bloody
- Abdominal pain or cramping
- Nausea and vomiting
- Weight loss or failure to gain weight
- Anorexia
- Abdominal distention
- Fever
- Irritability
- Lethargy
- Dehydration: change in level of consciousness; loss of skin turgor, oliguria; dark, concentrated urine; dry mucous membranes; sunken eyes; no tears with crying; depressed anterior fontanels

## COMPLICATIONS

- Dehydration
- Electrolyte imbalance
- Hypovolemia or septic shock
- Death

## DIAGNOSTIC TESTS

- Describe each procedure, its purpose, and the normal feelings or sensations that are likely, as well as any preprocedural and postprocedural care.
  —Complete blood count with differential
  —Stool cultures: to detect pathogenic organisms, occult blood, mucus, or reducing substance
  —Serum antibody titers
  —Serum electrolytes

**TREATMENT**

*Medical*

- Therapy
  —Intravenous fluids and electrolyte therapy
  —NPO until rehydrated, then small, frequent amounts of clear liquids
- Drugs
  —Antibiotics

**HOME CARE**

- Give both the patient and the caregiver *verbal* and *written* instructions. Provide them with the name and telephone number of a physician or nurse to call if questions arise.
- *General information*
  —Explain and discuss gastroenteritis, causes and contributing factors, care and treatment, and prevention.
- *Warning signs*
  —Review the signs and symptoms that should be reported to a physician or nurse.
    Dehydration: change in level of consciousness, loss of skin turgor, oliguria, dark concentrated urine, dry mucous membranes, sunken eyes, no tears with crying, depressed anterior fontanels
    Continued diarrhea
    Increase in abdominal pain
    Fever
- *Special instructions*
  —Assist the patient or caregiver in obtaining appropriate supplies, such as oral glucose electrolyte solutions.
  —Teach the patient preventive measures.
    Wash hands before eating and after toileting.
    Thoroughly cook all meats, especially pork, and avoid recontamination with kitchen utensils after cooking.
    Refrigerate perishable foods: mayonnaise, potato or egg salad, cream-filled pastries.
    Drink pasteurized milk and chlorinated water. When traveling to areas with unprotected or untreated water supply, boil all water used in cooking, drinking, or making ice.
    Maintain foods at the appropriate hot or cold temperatures.
    Protect foods from fly and roach contamination.
  —Teach the patient that gastroenteritis is communicable while the organisms are present in the feces.

—Teach the patient and family that persons with *Shigella* infections should not handle food or provide child care until two successive fecal samples are free of the organism; instruct the patient to use disinfectant after toileting.

—Demonstrate proper disposal of contaminated materials.

—Discuss skin care for anal irritation.

Keep rectal area clean and dry.

Wash skin with mild soap and water after each stool, rinse well, and dry thoroughly.

Apply topical ointment as ordered.

Culture stool specimens from other family members and treat as appropriate.

- *Medications*
  —Explain the purpose, dosage, schedule, and route of administration of any prescribed drugs, as well as side effects to report to the physician or nurse.

- *Diet*
  —Instruct the patient to drink clear juices, bouillon, tea, and broth as tolerated.

  —Advise the patient to advance the diet from clear liquids to a soft, bland diet that includes bananas, rice, applesauce, toast, clear soup, soda crackers, and dry cereals, avoiding milk products, and then to a regular diet as stools continue to firm.

**FOLLOW-UP CARE**

- Stress the importance of regular follow-up visits. Make sure the patient has the necessary names and telephone numbers.

# Gastrointestinal Bleeding
## (Including Esophageal Bleeding)

—**Gastrointestinal bleeding: a complication of various gastrointestinal disorders in which ulceration of the mucosa has progressed to the vasculature; bleeding may be acute or chronic.**

**CAUSES/CONTRIBUTING FACTORS/RISK FACTORS**

- Peptic ulcer disease
- Erosive gastritis

- Esophageal varices
- Esophagitis
- Diverticular disease
- Cancer of the esophagus, stomach, or intestines
- Trauma
- Mallory-Weiss syndrome
- Blood dyscrasias

**SIGNS/SYMPTOMS**

- Hematemesis: bloody vomitus may appear red, dark red, brown, or black or have "coffee ground" characteristics
- Melena: black, tarry stools
- Hematochezia: passage of red blood through the rectum
- Occult blood in the stool
- Fatigue
- Pallor
- Nausea and vomiting
- Abdominal distention
- Abdominal cramping, tenderness, pain
- Diarrhea
- Fever, chills
- Dehydration
- With acute hemorrhage >500 ml, lightheadedness, syncope, diaphoresis, tachycardia, shock

**COMPLICATIONS**

- Hypovolemic shock
- Anemia
- Electrolyte imbalance
- Perforation
- Death

**DIAGNOSTIC TESTS**

- Describe each procedure, its purpose, and the normal feelings or sensations that are likely, as well as any preprocedural and postprocedural care.
    —Hemoglobin and hematocrit: to measure circulating erythrocytes and assess blood loss
    —Blood urea nitrogen: to detect digestion and absorption of blood proteins from the gastrointestinal tract
    —Electrolytes

—Esophagogastroduodenoscopy: to identify the cause and site of the hemorrhage

—Upper gastrointestinal barium study: to identify the cause and site of hemorrhage

—Stool specimen: to detect occult blood

## TREATMENT

*Medical*

• Therapy
  —Whole blood or packed red blood cell transfusions
  —Intravenous fluid replacement with normal saline and plasma expanders
  —NPO until bleeding subsides
  —Central venous pressure or Swan-Ganz catheter: to assess circulatory volume
  —Nasogastric tube: to aspirate blood and gastric contents
  —Gastric intubation with ice water or saline lavage: to control hemorrhage
  —Angiography with vasopressin infusion: to localize hemorrhage and promote vasoconstriction
  —Esophageal balloon tamponade: to help control hemorrhage

• Drugs
  —Antacids
  —Histamine receptor antagonists
  —Antiulcer drugs
  —Vasopressin
  —Analgesics

*Surgical*

• For esophageal bleeding
  —Endoscopic sclerotherapy
  —Portocaval or splenorenal shunt: to divert blood flow from the liver and thus reduce pressure
  —Ligation of bleeding esophageal varices
  —Esophageal tamponade

• For gastric bleeding
  —Partial gastrectomy
  —Vagotomy, excision of ulcer, pyloroplasty

• For intestinal bleeding
  —Bowel resection with anastomosis
  —Bowel resection with temporary colostomy
  —Exploratory laparotomy if source of hemorrhage is unknown

## HOME CARE

- Give both the patient and the caregiver *verbal* and *written* instructions. Provide them with the name and telephone number of a physician or nurse to call if questions arise.
- *General information*
  —Discuss the type of bleeding disorder, explaining the relationships among causative factors, disease process, care and treatment, and potential for recurrence.
  —Review the physician's explanation of scheduled medical procedures, permitting time to answer any questions.
  —Review the physician's explanation of surgical procedures as ordered: gastrectomy (see p. 318), bowel resection (see p. 108), and abdominal surgery (see p. 3).
- *Warning signs*
  —Review the signs and symptoms that should be reported to a physician or nurse.
    Epigastric distress on an empty stomach
    Pain with ingestion of food
    Anorexia, nausea, hematemesis, abdominal distention, abdominal fullness
    Weight loss
    Black or bloody stools
- *Special instructions*
  —Teach the patient how to monitor stools for blood and demonstrate stool occult blood test, if indicated.
  —Provide pain management, offering alternatives to medications: visualization, guided imagery, meditation, relaxation, and biofeedback.
  —Stress the importance of smoking cessation and complete abstinence from alcohol.
  —Advise the patient to avoid coughing, sneezing, lifting, straining during defecation, or vomiting. Discuss the need to take stool softeners as prescribed to prevent constipation.
- *Medications*
  —Explain the purpose, dosage, schedule, and route of administration of any prescribed drugs, as well as side effects to report to the physician or nurse.
  —Specify whether medications should be taken with food or require an empty stomach.
  —Advise the patient to avoid use of aspirin-containing medications and ibuprofen.

- *Diet*
  —Assist the patient to plan a diet high in vitamin K. Provide a list of specific foods high in vitamin K.
  —With associated advanced liver disease, advise the patient to plan a diet low in sodium, protein, and ammonia.
  —Instruct the patient to eat small, frequent meals, to chew food well, and to eat slowly.
  —Instruct the patient to drink water with meals.
  —Provide the patient with a list of irritating foods and drugs to avoid, including coffee, tea, caffeine, spicy foods, rough foods, citric acid juices, extremely hot foods or liquids, and alcohol.
  —Advise the patient to avoid milk because it sometimes contributes to increased gastric acid secretion.
  —Refer the patient to a dietitian for nutritional counseling.

**FOLLOW-UP CARE**

- Stress the importance of regular follow-up visits after surgery, even in the absence of overt symptoms. Make sure the patient has the necessary names and telephone numbers.

**REFERRALS**

- Refer the patient to Alcoholics Anonymous if appropriate.
- Refer the patient to community programs for alcohol and smoking cessation if appropriate.

# Glaucoma

—**Glaucoma: a disorder characterized by high intracellular pressure of the aqueous humor, leading to atrophy of the optic nerve (disc), visual field loss, death of the nerve fibers, and irreversible vision loss. Glaucoma results from the overproduction or inadequate drainage of aqueous fluid. With aqueous fluid buildup, increasing intraocular pressure blocks blood supply to the optic nerve and retina, causing tissues to become ischemic.**

## TYPES OF GLAUCOMA

- Primary glaucoma
  - —Open angle
    - Chronic, simple glaucoma
    - Most common form, affecting 90% of all people with glaucoma
    - May be familial, affects adults over 40 years of age
    - More common in persons with a history of myopia, diabetes, hypertension
    - Onset insidious and asymptomatic
    - Slow progression
  - —Closed angle
    - Acute: onset usually dramatic, rapid development of severe pain in eye(s)
    - Chronic: follows untreated acute attack of closed angle glaucoma; onset gradual and usually asymptomatic
- Secondary glaucoma
  - —Progressive blurring of vision
  - —Results from trauma, tumors, surgery, uveitis, drug therapy (e.g., corticosteroids)
- Congenital glaucoma
  - —Rapidly developing myopia

## SIGNS/SYMPTOMS

- Open angle
  - —Visual changes: decreased acuity especially at night, loss of peripheral vision, seeing halos
  - —Mild aching in eyes
  - —Dull headache in morning
- Closed angle
  - —Severe pain
  - —Visual changes: blurred vision, rainbows in artificial light, halos around lights
  - —Headache
  - —Nausea, vomiting
  - —Dilated pupil(s)
- Congenital glaucoma
  - —Decreased visual acuity
  - —Excessive tearing
  - —Photophobia

**COMPLICATIONS**

- Increased intraocular pressure
- Progressive visual impairment
- Blindness
- After surgery
  —Retinal detachment
  —Cataract development
  —Hemolytic glaucoma
  —Hemorrhage
  —Infection
  —Decreased visual acuity
  —Light sensitivity

**DIAGNOSTIC TESTS**

- Describe each procedure, its purpose, and the normal feelings or sensations that are likely, as well as any preprocedural and postprocedural care.
  —Tonometry: to measure intraocular pressure
  —Gonioscopy: to identify width of aqueous fluid drainage area, adhesions, trauma, and tumors; also differentiates open angle from closed angle glaucoma
  —Funduscopy: dilation of pupil to inspect the optic disc; identifies disc degeneration
  —Ophthalmoscopic examination: to identify increased cupping of the disc
  —Visual field studies: to identify blind spots and subsequent degeneration
  —Tonography: to measure how well aqueous humor flows

**TREATMENT**
**Open Angle Glaucoma**

*Medical*

- Drugs: to reduce intraocular pressure by decreasing aqueous humor production or to reduce the volume of intraocular fluid
  —Miotics
  —Synthetic epinephrine
  —Beta blockers

*Surgical*

- Laser trabeculoplasty: to create an opening and thus increase outflow of aqueous humor; done under local anesthetic on an outpatient basis

- Trabeculectomy: surgical filtering procedure to build a new channel for the aqueous humor; done as an inpatient procedure under general anesthetic

## Closed Angle Glaucoma (Acute)

*Medical*
- Drugs: to lower and control intraocular pressure so that surgery can be performed
  —Hyperosmotic agents
  —Carbonic anhydrase inhibitors (Diamox)
  —Narcotic analgesics
  —Miotics

*Surgical*
This is a medical emergency. If pressure is not relieved within a few hours, eye damage occurs. Surgery is performed once intraocular pressure is stabilized.
- Laser iridotomy: to create a channel for aqueous fluid flow; done on an outpatient basis
- Iridectomy: to create a fine hole in the periphery of the iris through which aqueous fluid can flow

## Secondary Glaucoma

- Medications or surgery depending on causative factor

## Congenital Glaucoma

*Surgical*
- Trabeculectomy
- Goniotomy: to ensure patency of the drainage system

## HOME CARE

- Give both the patient and the caregiver *verbal* and *written* instructions. Provide them with the name and telephone number of a physician or nurse to call if questions arise.
- *General information*
  —Explain the type of glaucoma, causes or contributing factors, and prescribed medical or surgical therapy.
- *Warning signs*
  —Review the signs and symptoms that should be reported to a physician or nurse.
    Severe pain in eye(s)
    Blurred vision
    Headache

        Halos or rainbows
        Tearing
        Nausea, vomiting

- *Special instructions*
  —Review the factors that increase intraocular pressure and should be avoided:
      Constrictive clothing around the neck or torso
      Constipation (straining)
      Exertion or lifting heavy objects
      Bending at the waist
      Sneezing or coughing (upper respiratory infection)
      Nausea, vomiting
  —Review postoperative care.
      Inform the patient of the need to wear an eye patch or sunglasses to avoid discomfort associated with light exposure.
      Advise the patient of the importance of follow-up visits to check intraocular pressure, which may increase temporarily after surgery.
      Explain the importance of not rubbing, squeezing, or touching the eye.
      Discuss the procedure for cleansing the eye.
      Review the signs and symptoms that may indicate infection or increasing intraocular pressure and should be reported to a physician: pain, redness, fever, drainage, decreased visual acuity, excessive lacrimation, marked photophobia, halos, sparks.
      Explain the importance of using glaucoma medication in the unoperated eye.
      Provide a detailed explanation of drug therapy, stressing the importance of compliance.
      Discuss the consequences of noncompliance, including optic nerve damage and blindness.
  —Review home safety precautions needed because of diminished peripheral vision.
      Turn the head to visualize either side.
      Use up and down head movements to judge stairs and oncoming objects and walk slowly.
      Reduce clutter (e.g., loose rugs, electrical cords, items on floor) to prevent falls.
      Be aware that seeing at night, in dim light, or at dusk will

be difficult because in diminished light miotic pupils do not dilate to admit more light to the retina.

Provide extra lighting in darkened areas and use extra caution when driving at night.

- *Medications*
  —Explain the purpose, dosage, schedule, and route of administration of any prescribed drugs, as well as side effects to report to the physician or nurse.
  —Stress the importance of taking drugs on schedule.
  —Teach the patient to label each eyedrop bottle and to write out schedules for administration (especially important for patients with minimal visual acuity, to whom all bottles look alike).
  —Teach the proper technique for administration of eyedrops or ointment. Allow time for return demonstration and practice.
  —Stress the importance of good handwashing technique before instilling drops or ointment to minimize risk of infection.
  —Explain that medications do not cure glaucoma but can control it.
  —Review side effects of medications to report:
     Miotics: blurred vision, diarrhea
     Timolol: fatigue, weakness, depression
     Diamox: numbness, tingling of extremities and lips, decreased appetite, nausea, impotence

## FOLLOW-UP CARE

- Stress the importance of regular follow-up visits. Make sure the patient has the necessary names and telephone numbers.

# Glomerulonephritis and Nephrotic Syndrome

—**Glomerulonephritis: inflammatory process involving the glomerulus that causes a problem in filtration of urine. Glomerulonephritis may occur as an acute or a chronic disease.**

—**Nephrotic syndrome: disorder characterized by a high concentration of protein in the urine that is caused by a filtration problem of the glomeruli. Nephrotic syndrome may occur in a number of diseases such as diabetes mellitus, as a reaction to drugs and allergens, or during pregnancy. The majority of cases, however, result from primary glomerulonephritis.**

## CAUSES/CONTRIBUTING FACTORS
* Immune system response
  —Systemic lupus erythematosus
  —Mixed connective tissue disease
  —Wegener's granulomatosis
  —Churg-Strauss syndrome
  —Polyarteritis nodosa
  —Goodpasture's syndrome
* Diabetes mellitus
* Hepatitis B
* Polycystic kidneys
* Essential hypertension
* Tuberculosis
* Vascular disease (affects the renal vein)
* Infections and infectious processes
  —Bacterial: *Streptococcus, Staphylococcus*
  —Syphilis
  —Malaria
  —Schistosomiasis
  —Mediterranean fever

## SIGNS/SYMPTOMS
* Urine: reddish brown, foamy
* Edema: extremities, periorbital, peritoneal, external genitalia

- Hypertension
- Shortness of breath on exertion, orthopnea
- Fatigue, malaise, lethargy
- Weight gain

**COMPLICATIONS**

- Renal failure
- Severe hypertension
- Renal vein thrombosis

**DIAGNOSTIC TESTS**

- Describe each procedure, its purpose, and the normal feelings or sensations that are likely, as well as any preprocedural and postprocedural care.
  —Blood studies: to evaluate kidney function
    Electrolytes
    Blood urea nitrogen
    Creatinine
    Protein
    Phosphates
    Cholesterol
    Albumin
  —Urine studies
    Urinalysis: to determine the presence of protein and blood
    Culture and sensitivity: to determine the presence and type of bacteria
    24-Hour study: for creatinine and protein
  —Radiographic tests: plain abdomen
  —Ultrasound: to determine the size of the kidney
  —Renal biopsy: to establish underlying disease

**TREATMENT**

*Medical*

- Therapy
  —Plasmapheresis: to remove immune complexes or antibodies
  —Dialysis: peritoneal or hemodialysis
  —Dietary: low sodium, low potassium, low protein (protein intake is based on glomerular filtration rate [GFR]; if GFR is decreased, protein intake is lowered; if GFR is normal, protein intake is increased)

- Drugs
  —Diuretics
  —Antihypertensives
  —Corticosteroids
  —Immunosuppressants
  —Antineoplastics
  —Plasma expanders

*Surgical*
- Bilateral nephrectomy
- Kidney transplant

**G**

## HOME CARE

- Give both the patient and the caregiver *verbal* and *written* instructions. Provide them with the name and telephone number of a physician or nurse to call if questions arise.
- *General information*
  —Explain the disease process and underlying cause.
- *Warning signs*
  —Review the signs and symptoms that should be reported to a physician or nurse.
      Weight increase >2 pounds in one day
      Change in urine color, amount, or froth
      Increased blood pressure
      Heart palpitations, dizziness, lightheadedness
      Progressive edema: puffy, swollen eyes
      Decreased urine output: <600 ml in 24 hours
- *Special instructions*
  —Explain the importance of daily weights: same time, same clothing, after urination, and before eating.
  —Demonstrate blood pressure measurement and discuss how often to perform it. Advise the patient on obtaining supplies for home blood pressure monitoring.
  —Instruct the patient on maintaining a written daily log of weight, vital signs, and intake and output.
  —Discuss the need to maintain good skin care of edematous body areas to prevent excoriation and skin breakdown (see Decubitus Ulcers, p. 230).
  —Advise female patients to avoid pregnancy. Provide information on contraception.

- *Medications*
  —Explain the purpose, dosage, schedule, and route of administration of any prescribed drugs, as well as side effects to report to the physician or nurse.
  —If the patient is taking immunosuppressants, stress the importance of avoiding persons with infections and upper respiratory infections. Discuss the need to report signs of infection: fever, fatigue, malaise.
- *Activity*
  —Encourage the patient to discuss allowances and limitations with respect to occupation, recreation, or activities.
  —Discuss the need to avoid fatigue, exercise to tolerance, and plan frequent rest periods.
- *Diet*
  —Refer the patient to a dietitian for a specific diet plan. Review dietary restrictions and provide a list of foods to avoid.
  —Explain how to read labels on cans and boxes for ingredients and sodium content. Instruct the patient to rinse canned foods in water to remove excess salt.
  —Discuss fluid restrictions. Explain that fluids may depend on how much urine is put out.

**FOLLOW-UP CARE**

- Stress the importance of regular follow-up visits, including blood pressure checks if the patient is not on a home monitoring program. Make sure the patient has the necessary names and telephone numbers.

# Gout

—Gout: a metabolic disorder in which urate salts are deposited in joints and other body tissues such as ear, cartilage, and kidneys. The urate crystals form masses called tophi, which are sharp and pointed and cause irritation and inflammation of the joints. While any joint may be affected, gout commonly (90%) affects the first metatarsal joint of the great toe, causing excruciating pain. The ankle, midfoot, and wrist are also frequently affected. Primary gout is a hereditary disease in which overproduction or decreased excretion of uric acid and urate salts leads to high levels of uric acid in the blood. Primary gout most commonly occurs in males over 30 years of age. Secondary gout is associated with other conditions in which uric acid is overproduced or retained, such as lead poisoning, use of thiazide diuretics, chronic renal disease, psoriasis, and chemotherapy.

## SIGNS/SYMPTOMS

- Joints inflamed, edematous, shiny, hot, painful
- Malaise
- Headache
- Increased temperature
- Chills
- Constipation
- Subcutaneous tophi: ear, joints, knuckles

## COMPLICATIONS

- Renal calculi
- Gouty arthritis
- Hypertension
- Infection

## DIAGNOSTIC TESTS

- Describe each procedure, its purpose, and the normal feelings or sensations that are likely, as well as any preprocedural and postprocedural care.
    —Laboratory tests
        Blood tests: uric acid, white blood cells, erythrocyte sedimentation rate
        Urine tests: uric acid levels to determine if the patient is an overexcretor or underexcretor of uric acid
    —Needle aspirations
        Joint fluid: to detect presence of urate crystals
        Tophaceous material: to identify urate crystals
    —X-rays: to document evidence of radiolucent tophi

## TREATMENT

*Medical*

- Therapy
    —During acute phase
        Joint rest

Complete bed rest with elevation of inflamed joint

Cold packs to the affected joint to decrease inflammation

—Low-purine diet

—Limitation of alcohol intake

• Drugs

—Nonsteroidal antiinflammatory drugs (NSAIDs)

—Uricosuric agents (e.g., probenecid): to increase excretion of urate salts

—Allopurinol: to decrease serum uric acid

—Antiinflammatory agents (colchicine)

—Corticosteroids, analgesics, antipyretics

*Surgical*

• Excision of gouty tophi when they erode through the skin or cause mechanical impairment

• Joint replacement

## HOME CARE

• Give both the patient and the caregiver *verbal* and *written* instructions. Provide them with the name and telephone number of a physician or nurse to call if questions arise.

• *General information*

—Describe the disease process, underlying causes, and contributing factors.

• *Warning signs*

—Review the signs and symptoms of possible kidney stones that should be reported to a physician or nurse.

Severe pain in the flank, side, lower back, suprapubic area, groin, labia, or scrotum

Urinary retention

Nausea

Vomiting

• *Special instructions*

—Instruct the patient in checking urine pH using a test tape; if pH is <6.0, advise the patient to increase fluid intake and avoid high-purine foods.

—Describe home care of inflamed joints during an acute attack.

Complete bed rest with elevation of the affected joint with pillows

Ice applications to inflamed joints

As inflammation subsides, need for rest periods to avoid fatigue

Bed cradle to keep linens off joint; advise the patient where to obtain equipment

Avoidance of weight bearing

—Teach range-of-motion exercises of joints, and instruct the patient to increase these exercises as inflammation decreases to avoid disuse syndrome.

—Explain that gout cannot be cured but can be controlled with medication.

- *Medications*

—Explain the purpose, dosage, schedule, and route of administration of any prescribed drugs, as well as side effects to report to the physician or nurse.

—Review specific drug therapies. Explain that the type of treatment depends on whether the patient overexcretes or underexcretes uric acid.

Colchicine: instruct the patient to notify the physician or nurse when pain subsides or when nausea, vomiting, abdominal cramping, or diarrhea occurs. Explain that the drug is usually stopped when symptoms occur

Uricosuric agents: stress the importance of drinking 2-3 liters of fluid per day unless contraindicated to prevent the development of kidney stones

Alkalinizing agents (sodium bicarbonate): to maintain urinary pH above 6.0 and thus prevent kidney stone formation

—Explain the need to avoid diuretics, low-dose aspirin, and nicotinic acid because these can increase serum uric acid.

- *Diet*

—Discuss the need to restrict intake of purines, which are metabolic precursors to uric acid. Advise the patient about foods that are high in purine: anchovies, liver, sardines, kidneys, sweetbreads, lentils.

—Instruct the patient to avoid alcoholic beverages, especially beer and wine.

—Discuss the need to decrease weight if obese. Refer the patient to the dietitian for a low-calorie diet plan for weight reduction.

## FOLLOW-UP CARE

- Stress the importance of regular follow-up visits. Make sure the patient has the necessary names and telephone numbers.

# Guillain-Barré Syndrome

—**Guillain-Barré syndrome: an acute syndrome characterized by widespread inflammation or demyelination of the peripheral nerves. Guillain-Barré syndrome is also known as acute idiopathic polyneuritis, acute polyradiculoneuropathy, and postinfectious polyneuritis. It is thought to be an autoimmune disease triggered by recent infection. Over half of affected persons have had a nonspecific infection (e.g., upper respiratory or gastrointestinal infection) 10-14 days before the onset of symptoms. The onset is rapid, and the symptoms are generally reversible.**

## CAUSES/CONTRIBUTING FACTORS
- Upper respiratory infection
- Infectious mononucleosis
- Cytomegalovirus infection
- Herpes zoster
- Influenza A
- *Mycoplasma* infection
- Mumps
- AIDS
- Lyme disease
- Lymphoma (especially Hodgkin's)
- Serum sickness
- Postsurgical
- Inoculation for swine flu

## SIGNS/SYMPTOMS
- Symmetric muscle weakness beginning in the legs and ascending rapidly (in a few days) to the arms
- Weakness accompanied by paresthesia, pain
- Paralysis of upper extremities (partial or complete); quadriplegia
- Reduced reflexes, then loss of deep tendon reflexes
- Bilateral facial and oropharyngeal paresis
- Difficulty swallowing
- Urinary retention
- Respiratory muscle paralysis
- Blood pressure fluctuation

## COMPLICATIONS

- Aspiration, atelectasis
- Pneumonia
- Thrombophlebitis
- Pulmonary embolus
- Respiratory failure
- Ileus, gastric dilation
- Gastrointestinal bleeding
- Septicemia
- Autonomic dysfunction, arrhythmias, postural hypertension
- Chronic inflammatory demyelinating polyradiculoneuropathy

## DIAGNOSTIC TESTS

- Describe each procedure, its purpose, and the normal feelings or sensations that are likely, as well as any preprocedural and postprocedural care.
    - Cerebrospinal fluid sampling: protein initially decreased (15-45 mg), then increased as high as 600 mg
    - Electromyography: reduced nerve conduction velocity at peak of illness
    - Pulmonary function tests: decreased

## TREATMENT

*Medical*
- Therapy
    - Intensive care admission
        - Cardiac monitoring
        - Arterial blood gas monitoring
        - Mechanical ventilation and respiratory support
    - Plasmapheresis (blood exchange)
    - Chest physiotherapy
    - Nutritional maintenance (intravenous or nasogastric feedings)
    - Physical therapy

*Surgical*
- Tracheostomy for prolonged ventilatory support as indicated

## HOME CARE

- Give both the patient and the caregiver *verbal* and *written* instructions. Provide them with the name and telephone number of a physician or nurse to call if questions arise.

- *General information*
  —Review the explanation of the disorder, causes, and residual neurologic effects.
- *Warning signs*
  —Review the signs and symptoms that should be reported to a physician or nurse.
    Difficulty breathing
    Increased weakness
    Numbness
- *Special instructions*
  —Instruct the caregiver to inspect the patient's skin daily for signs of irritation or breakdown if the patient is on bed rest (see Decubitus Ulcers, p. 230).
  —Encourage open verbalization regarding fear of permanent disability, changes in body image, loss of function (temporary or permanent), and dying.
  —Stress the importance of avoiding persons who have infections, especially upper respiratory infections.
  —Assist the patient to obtain any adaptive devices (e.g., splints, wheelchair, or walker) and provide instruction on use.
  —Demonstrate proper transferring technique from bed to chair and from chair to toilet.
- *Medications*
  —Explain the purpose, dosage, schedule, and route of administration of any prescribed drugs, as well as side effects to report to the physician or nurse.
  —Stress the need to check with a physician before taking any over-the-counter medications.
- *Activity*
  —Encourage the patient to discuss allowances and limitations with respect to resuming work, recreation, and other activities.
  —Explain the need to resume activities slowly, exercising to tolerance level and then stopping.
  —Explain the importance of maintaining planned rest periods.
  —Stress the need for independence and socialization; advise self-care and eating with the caregiver.
  —Explain the need for diversional activities (television, reading, listening to the radio).

—Teach the patient and caregiver necessary exercises and ask for a return demonstration.

Speech exercises

Active or passive range-of-motion exercises with massage of all extremities

Exercises that increase strength and mobility of fingers (squeeze toys, clay, balls)

—Refer the patient for specific home therapy exercises.

—Discuss the importance of warm baths to alleviate pain and stiffness.

• *Diet*

—Advise a high-calorie, high-protein diet, cautioning the patient to progress from soft to solid food if facial weakness is present.

—Explain the need to have eating utensils and food arranged so the patient can manage them easily.

—Stress the importance of avoiding constipation.

Drink fluids to maintain intake at 2000 ml per day unless contraindicated.

Use stool softeners (as approved by physician).

Eat foods and fruits high in roughage.

**FOLLOW-UP CARE**

• Stress the importance of regular follow-up visits with the physician, physical therapist, and occupational therapist. Make sure the patient has the necessary names and telephone numbers.

**REFERRALS**

• Provide the patient with the following address to obtain patient education materials: Guillain-Barré Syndrome Foundation International, P.O. Box 262, Wynnewood, PA 19096, (610) 667-0131.

# Head Trauma

—**Head trauma: any sudden impact, blow, or physical injury to the head that causes damage to brain tissue. Head** injuries are categorized as open, or penetrating, and closed, or blunt. Types of injuries include scalp injuries (lacerations, abrasions, hematomas), skull fractures (linear, depressed, basilar), concussions (temporary loss of consciousness after the brain strikes the skull; may last for a few days), and contusions (bruising of the brain tissue, disrupting neural function).

## CAUSES/CONTRIBUTING FACTORS/RISK FACTORS

- Trauma: motor vehicle accidents, falls
- Assaults: gunshot and stab wounds

## SIGNS/SYMPTOMS

- Periods of consciousness followed by unconsciousness
- Concussion
  —Amnesia: anterograde, retrograde
  —Headache
  —Nausea, vomiting
  —Dizziness
- Contusion
  —Mental changes: confusion, agitation, restlessness, delirium, stupor, coma
  —Posturing: decorticate or decerebrate
  —Sensorimotor disturbances: unilateral or bilateral; paresis or paralysis
  —Unequal pupils and uncoordinated eye movements
- Skull fractures
  —Drainage from ears and nose
  —Localized headache
  —Bilateral periocular ecchymosis (raccoon's eyes)
  —Hearing impairment

## COMPLICATIONS

- Cerebral edema
- Sensorimotor and neurologic deficits
- Increased intracranial pressure
- Intracranial hemorrhage
- Hematoma: subdural, epidural
- Brain herniation
- Seizures
- Brain damage

## DIAGNOSTIC TESTS

- Describe each procedure, its purpose, and the normal feelings or sensations that are likely, as well as any preprocedural and postprocedural care.
  —Skull x-rays: to visualize bone fragments and fractures
  —Cervical x-rays: to confirm or rule out cervical spinal injury
  —Computed tomography or magnetic resonance imaging: to assess hematoma or distortion of cerebral ventricles
  —Cerebrospinal fluid sampling: may be contraindicated with increased intracranial pressure
  —Cerebral angiography: to locate hematomas and displacement of vessels
  —Electroencephalogram: to assess for development of pathologic waves
  —Pneumoencephalogram: to assess for cerebral ventricular shift, distortion, or dilation
  —Cisternogram: to identify dural tear site with basal skull fractures
  —Serum electrolytes and osmolarity
  —Urine osmolarity
  —Arterial blood gases

## TREATMENT

*Medical*
- Therapy
  —Patent airway and adequate ventilation and oxygenation
  —Proper positioning with head of bed elevated to promote venous drainage and thus reduce intracranial pressure, cerebral edema, and congestion
  —Hypothermia blanket
  —Cervical collar
  —Cardiac monitoring
  —Rehabilitation
    Physical therapy
    Occupational therapy
    Speech therapy
    Bowel and bladder retraining
    Cognitive rehabilitation
  —Diet
    Immediate: NPO
    Later, total parenteral nutrition, intralipids, tube feedings, or progressive diet, depending on the patient's level of

consciousness, ability to swallow, and gastrointestinal tract functioning

Fluid restriction to decrease cerebral edema

—Intracranial pressure monitoring

—Hemodynamic monitoring: to assess fluid volume status

—Indwelling urinary catheter: to measure urinary output

—Nasogastric tube: to aspirate gastric contents and free air

- Drugs
  —Antiepilepsy drugs
  —Glucocorticoids
  —Osmotic diuretics
  —Antibiotics
  —Tetanus prophylaxis
  —Antipyretics
  —Analgesics
  —Sedatives
  —Antacids and $H_2$ blockers
  —Stool softeners
  —Neuromuscular blocking agents
  —Barbiturate coma therapy

*Surgical*

- Suturing: to repair superficial lacerations
- Craniotomy, craniectomy: to evacuate hematomas, control hemorrhage, remove bone fragments or foreign objects, debride tissues, or elevate depressed fractures
- Trephination (burr holes): to evacuate hematoma or insert intracranial monitoring devices
- Cranioplasty: to repair traumatic defects in the skull
- Ventriculostomy: to remove excess cerebrospinal fluid
- Ventricular shunting procedures: to drain cerebrospinal fluid and reduce intracranial pressure

## HOME CARE

- Give both the patient and the caregiver *verbal* and *written* instructions. Provide them with the name and telephone number of a physician or nurse to call if questions arise. Provide a head injury sheet to assist in instruction.
- *General information*
  —Explain and discuss types of head injuries, causes, contributing factors, care and treatment, residual effects, and prevention of further injury.

- *Wound/incision care*
  —Discuss and demonstrate the care of any lacerations or surgical incisions, if indicated.
    Wash area gently.
    Wear clean gloves and cover scalp wounds with gauze dressings.
- *Warning signs*
  —Review the signs and symptoms that should be reported to a physician or nurse.
    Infection from surgical incision: fever, erythema, tenderness, pain, warmth, purulent drainage
    Meningitis: fever, chills, malaise, back stiffness and pain, nuchal rigidity
    Neurologic changes: behavioral and personality changes, irritability, confusion, slurred speech
    Sensorimotor changes: incoordination, weakness in extremities, difficulty walking
    Increased intracranial pressure: altered level of consciousness, such as difficulty in waking patient or increased drowsiness; nausea and vomiting; seizures; worsening headache
    Visual abnormalities: blurred vision; diplopia; changes in visual field, depth, or perception
    Changes in cognitive ability, judgment, emotional control, orientation, memory, and concentration
    Leakage of cerebrospinal fluid: clear or bloody drainage from ear, nose, or throat; complaints of salty taste or frequent swallowing; presence of "halo ring" on pillowcase
    Respiratory distress
- *Special instructions*
  —If the patient is discharged home with a mild head injury for observation, instruct a responsible caregiver to stay with the patient for 24-48 hours. Tell the caregiver to awaken the patient every 2 hours the first night, asking name, where the patient is, and whether the patient can identify the caregiver. If unable to arouse the patient, the caregiver should notify the physician and return the patient to the hospital.
  —Teach seizure precautions, as indicated.
    Try to prevent or break a fall.
    Ease the patient onto the floor.
    Support and protect the patient's head.

Turn the patient to one side.

Remove surrounding furniture and any hard or sharp objects.

Loosen constrictive clothing around the neck.

Stay with the patient and call the physician immediately.

—Explain that possible residual effects (postconcussion syndrome), such as dizziness, headaches, and memory loss, may persist for up to 3-4 months after trauma.

—Explain that the patient may experience changes in personality, inappropriate social behavior, inappropriate affect, hallucinations, and altered sleep patterns after head injury.

—Assist the patient in obtaining assistive devices for ambulation or activities of daily living, as indicated.

—For concussion, advise the patient to avoid Valsalva maneuvers such as straining during defecation, vigorous coughing, nose blowing, or sneezing.

—Offer methods other than medications for dealing with pain: visualization, guided imagery, meditation, relaxation, biofeedback.

• *Medications*

—Explain the purpose, dosage, schedule, and route of administration of any prescribed drugs, as well as side effects to report to the physician or nurse.

—Stress the importance of avoiding over-the-counter medications without consulting the physician. Tell the patient not to take aspirin because of the risk of bleeding.

• *Activity*

—Encourage the patient to discuss allowances and limitations with respect to resuming work, recreation, and other activities.

—Encourage the patient in self-care activities as tolerated.

—Encourage decision making by the patient.

—Provide structured daily activities and routines with planned rest periods.

—Advise the caregiver to avoid overprotection. Assist the family and caregiver to identify and correct hazards in the home to prevent falls and injuries.

Remove all hazardous objects.

Maintain clear pathways.

Provide good lighting.

Provide the patient with proper shoes and glasses. Place objects within the patient's visual field.

Install assistive and safety aids such as ramps, rails, and shower chairs.

—Instruct the family and caregivers to supervise or assist with ambulation.

—Teach the family range-of-motion exercises and involve them in the exercise program.

—Instruct the patient to avoid alcohol, driving, smoking, use of hazardous appliances and machinery, contact sports, tub baths, and swimming until advised by a physician.

• *Diet*

—Advise the patient to chew food well and swallow slowly.

—Provide supplemental feedings, if ordered.

**FOLLOW-UP CARE**

• Stress the importance of regular follow-up visits with the physician, physical therapist, occupational therapist, and speech therapist. Make sure the patient has the necessary names and telephone numbers.

• Encourage the patient to obtain a Medic-Alert bracelet and identification card listing the diagnosis, medications, and treatment, if appropriate.

**PSYCHOSOCIAL CARE**

• Encourage the patient and caregivers to verbalize fears and concerns regarding head injury, disability, body and functional changes, and adaptation to the patient's residual deficits and mental and emotional sequelae.

**REFERRALS**

• Refer the patient to a social worker for further support and counseling.

• Assist the patient and caregivers to obtain referral to support groups, community resources, and home health support services.

• Provide referral to the following source of information: National Head Injury Foundation, 1140 Connecticut Avenue SW, Suite 812, Washington, DC 20036, (202) 296-6443 or (800) 444-6443.

# Heart Failure

—Heart failure: inability of the heart muscle to pump with enough force to meet the body's metabolic demands. In this chronic and progressive syndrome, impairment of heart function or heart failure may involve the right or left side of the heart or both sides. Symptoms depend on which side of the heart is failing; right-sided failure usually follows left heart failure.

## CAUSES/CONTRIBUTING FACTORS

- Coronary artery disease
- Myocardial infarction
- Valvular heart disease
- Congenital heart defects
- High blood pressure
- Cardiomyopathy
- Inflammatory heart disease

## SIGNS/SYMPTOMS

- Left-sided failure
  —Shortness of breath with exertion at rest or night
  —Orthopnea
  —Restlessness
  —Fatigue, weakness
  —Nocturia
- Right-sided failure
  —Dry cough
  —Edema: pretibial, ankle
  —Abdominal swelling (ascites)
  —Abdominal pain
  —Anorexia
  —Sudden weight gain

## COMPLICATIONS

- Pulmonary edema
- Dysrhythmias
- Thromboembolism
- Venostasis

## DIAGNOSTIC TESTS

- Inform the patient that several procedures may be done to aid in the diagnosis of this condition. Describe each procedure, its purpose, and the normal feelings or sensations that are likely, as well as any preprocedural and postprocedural care.
  —Blood tests: electrolytes, blood chemistry profile
  —Chest x-ray: to detect pulmonary congestion and an increase in heart size
  —Electrocardiogram
  —Echocardiogram
  —Multiple gated acquisition

## TREATMENT

*Medical*
- Drugs
  —Digitalis
  —Diuretics
  —Inotropic drugs
  —Vasodilators
  —Potassium replacements

*Surgical*
- Heart transplant for end-stage heart failure

## HOME CARE

- Give both the patient and the caregiver *verbal* and *written* instructions. Provide them with the name and telephone number of a physician or nurse to call if questions arise.
- *General information*
  —Explain the disease process, causes, and contributing factors.
- *Warning signs*
  —Review the signs and symptoms that should be reported to a physician or nurse.
    Decreased exercise tolerance
    Shortness of breath
    Dyspnea on exertion
    Paroxysmal nocturnal dyspnea
    Persistent cough
    Swelling of extremities
- *Special instructions*
  —Instruct the patient to take and record the pulse. Provide guidelines and rates to report.

—Instruct the patient to weigh daily at the same time, using the same scale, and wearing the same clothing, and to report a weight gain of 2-3 pounds in one day or 5 pounds in a week.
* *Medications*
    —Explain the purpose, dosage, schedule, and route of administration of any prescribed drugs, as well as side effects to report to the physician or nurse.
    —Discuss the need to take potassium supplements if non-potassium-sparing diuretics (thiazides, furosemide) are prescribed.
    —Discuss the need to avoid over-the-counter medications such as laxatives and cough medications, which may contain sodium.
* *Activity*
    —Assist the patient to identify activities that elicit symptoms or cause fatigue or shortness of breath.
    —Encourage activity as tolerated, but advise the patient to avoid strenuous activity that will put undue burden on the heart, such as heavy lifting, prolonged walking, carrying heavy suitcases, shoveling snow, changing a tire, and mowing the lawn.
    —Suggest energy-saving devices and techniques for activities of daily living.
    —Tell the patient to space activities with periods of rest and to stop and rest when tired.
    —Encourage questions regarding occupation or recreation.
    —Explain the need to avoid extremes in temperature or activities during days with high pollution.
    —Tell the patient to avoid situations that might cause colds, flu, or other infections.
* *Diet*
    —Explain the importance of maintaining the prescribed diet and fluid restrictions.
    —Discuss the need to avoid food high in sodium. A 3 g sodium diet, or in severe cases a 2 g sodium diet, may be prescribed. Explain the need to read food and drink labels for sodium content, to avoid commercially prepared foods, to wash all canned vegetables to remove sodium, and to eat foods high in potassium (bananas, orange juice) to replenish potassium lost from the use of diuretics.

**FOLLOW-UP CARE**

- Stress the importance of regular follow-up visits for medical and laboratory evaluation. Make sure the patient has the necessary names and telephone numbers.
- Emphasize the importance of not smoking, using tobacco products, or drinking alcohol.

**REFERRALS**

- Provide referrals for home health care or other supportive resources as needed.

# Hemolytic Anemia

—**Hemolytic anemia: a disorder in which the rate of erythrocyte destruction is greatly accelerated. Hemolytic anemia, which occurs as a result of an intracorpuscular (inherited) defect or extracorpuscular (acquired) factors, results in a shortened red blood cell life span. The bone marrow is unable to replace the destroyed red blood cells.**

**CAUSES/CONTRIBUTING FACTORS**

- Intracorpuscular defects
  —Deficiency in glucose 6-phosphate dehydrogenase
  —Hereditary spherocytosis
- Extracorpuscular factors
  —Trauma (burns, prosthetic valve replacement)
  —Chemical agents/medications
  —Immune response
  —Infections
  —Systemic diseases
  —Hemolytic reactions (blood transfusion)
  —Autoimmune disorders

**SIGNS/SYMPTOMS**

- Decreased urinary output
- Fluid loss or overload
- Nausea and vomiting

- Jaundice
- Fever and chills
- Weakness and fatigue
- Back or abdominal pain
- Headache

**COMPLICATIONS**

- Acute renal failure

**DIAGNOSTIC TESTS**

- Describe each procedure, its purpose, and the normal feelings or sensations that are likely, as well as any preprocedural and postprocedural care.
    —Laboratory studies
        Red blood cell count
        Reticulocyte count
        Red blood cell fragility
        Erythrocyte life span
        Fecal and urinary urobilinogen
    —Bone marrow biopsy
    —Ultrasound/gallbladder studies

**TREATMENT**

*Medical*
- Therapy
    —Blood component transfusion
- Drugs
    —Corticosteroids
        Prednisone
    —Osmotic diuretics
    —Sodium bicarbonate or lactate
*Surgical*
- Splenectomy if steroids fail to arrest red blood cell destruction

**HOME CARE**

- Give both the patient and the caregiver *verbal* and *written* instructions. Provide them with the name and telephone number of a physician or nurse to call if questions arise.
- *General information*
    —Explain and discuss the type of hemolytic disorder, causes, and contributing factors if acquired. Explain the underlying condition and prescribed treatment.

- *Special instructions*
  —Teach the patient to rate pain on a scale of 1-10 and to monitor pain levels. Assist the patient to identify precipitating factors. Discuss methods of relieving pain or discomfort.
- *Warning signs*
  —Review the signs and symptoms of hemolytic crisis that should be reported to a physician or nurse.
    Jaundice
    Shortness of breath
    Joint or abdominal pain
    Headache
    Vertigo
  —Stress the need to avoid factors that precipitate hemolytic crisis: infection, trauma, chemicals, toxic drug reactions.
- *Medications*
  —Explain the purpose, dosage, schedule, and route of administration of any prescribed drugs, as well as side effects to report to a physician or nurse.
  —Review the side effects of steroid therapy (see Steroid Therapy, p. 608).
- *Activity*
  —Encourage the patient to discuss allowances and limitations with respect to occupation, recreation, and activities.
  —Discuss the need to find a balance between activity and rest and to keep physical and emotional stress at a minimum.
  —Instruct the patient to decrease activities during crises or when symptoms appear.
- *Diet*
  —Discuss the need for a well-balanced diet that is rich in iron and protein.
  —Advise the patient to avoid fatty foods.
  —Teach the patient to take small, frequent meals.
  —Discuss methods to maintain hydration status; encourage daily fluids unless contraindicated. Instruct the patient to notify the physician or nurse if output decreases.

## FOLLOW-UP CARE

- Stress the importance of regular follow-up visits for medical and laboratory evaluation. Make sure the patient has the necessary names and telephone numbers.
- Discuss the need to wear a Medic-Alert bracelet and carry an information card if receiving long-term treatment.

# Hemophilia

—Hemophilia: a hereditary disorder characterized by impaired coagulability of the blood with a tendency to bleed. Hemophilia A (classic hemophilia) is caused by a deficiency of factor VIII and affects 80% of hemophilia cases. Hemophilia B results from deficiency of factor IX and affects 5% of cases. Both types of hemophilia are sex-linked genetic disorders. The disease affects males. Females are asymptomatic carriers, with a mother having a 50% chance of transmitting the disease to her son.

## SIGNS/SYMPTOMS

- Easy bruising
- Bleeding after minimal trauma
- Bleeding from mucous membranes, gastrointestinal tract, genitourinary tract
- Joint pain, swelling from bleeding into the joint (hemarthrosis)

## COMPLICATIONS

- Joint deformity
- Hemorrhagic shock
- Intracranial hemorrhage
- Peripheral neuropathy

## DIAGNOSTIC TESTS

- Describe each procedure, its purpose, and the normal feelings or sensations that are likely, as well as any preprocedural and postprocedural care.
    —Partial thromboplastin time
    —Bleeding time
    —Platelet count
    —Activated clotting time
    —Assays of factors VIII and IX

## TREATMENT

*Medical*

- Therapy
    —Factor transfusion (for hemophilia B)
    —Transfusion of fresh frozen plasma

—Cryoprecipitate (for hemophilia A)
—Treatment for the development of antibody inhibitors against the specific coagulation factor
—Plasmapheresis to remove the inhibitor
—Prothrombin complexes to bypass inhibitors
• Drugs
—Agents such as desmopressin (DDAVP) and aminocaproic acid (Amicar)
—Immunosuppressive agents

## HOME CARE

• Give both the patient and the caregiver *verbal* and *written* instructions. Provide them with the name and telephone number of a physician or nurse to call if questions arise.
• *General information*
—Explain and discuss with the patient the specific hemophilia disorder, its causes, and contributing factors.
• *Special instructions*
—Review the procedure in case of bleeding.
  Apply cold compresses and gentle direct pressure to the site.
  Elevate the affected part if possible.
  Seek medical attention promptly.
—Review precautions to prevent bleeding as appropriate.
  Use an electric razor.
  Avoid constipation.
  Use a soft-bristled toothbrush, and maintain good dental hygiene.
—Stress the importance of frequent assessment of joint function to allow rapid identification and treatment of hemophilic arthritis.
—Discuss the need to receive regular dental care.
—Stress the importance of informing all physicians and dentists of the bleeding disorder.
—Stress the importance of notifying the physician immediately of any injury to the head or the abdomen for evaluation and treatment of internal bleeding.
• *Medications*
—Explain the purpose, dosage, schedule, and route of administration of any prescribed drugs, as well as side effects to report to the physician or nurse.

—Caution the patient to avoid over-the-counter medications containing ibuprofen and aspirin components.

—Discuss the need for lifelong factor replacement.

—Teach the patient and significant others venipuncture and intravenous administration of factor products. Allow time for return demonstration and practice.

—Teach the patient and caregiver to keep blood factor concentrate and infusion equipment available at all times, even on vacation.

—Discuss the storage of fluids and the proper disposal of equipment.

—Review adverse reactions, such as bloodborne infection and factor inhibitor development.

—Discuss common side effects of factor and blood product infusion and management of possible symptoms.

> Flushing, headache, or tingling with factor replacement may be decreased by slowing infusion.
>
> Urticaria with cryoprecipitate or plasma may be relieved with diphenhydramine. Persons who have frequent reactions should receive antihistamine 4 minutes before factor infusion.
>
> Fever and chills resulting from plasma infusion may be decreased with acetaminophen.

—Review symptoms of anaphylaxis: rapid or difficult breathing, wheezing, hoarseness, stridor, and chest tightness.

—Teach the patient or caregiver to administer epinephrine and then to contact the physician immediately.

• *Activity*

—Encourage the patient to discuss allowances and limitations with respect to occupation, recreation, and activities.

—Stress the need to avoid contact sports (e.g., soccer, football) or activities that may pose a risk of falls or injury.

—Discuss the benefits of regular aerobic exercise, such as swimming, walking, and cycling.

## FOLLOW-UP CARE

• Stress the importance of regular follow-up visits for medical and laboratory evaluation. Make sure the patient has the necessary names and telephone numbers.

• Discuss the importance of wearing a Medic-Alert bracelet and carrying an information card; assist the patient to obtain them.

# Hemorrhoid

—Hemorrhoid: varicose veins in the anal canal or anorectal area. Hemorrhoids may occur proximal (internal) or distal (external) to the anal sphincter. Continuous increased abdominal pressure leads to the development and enlargement of hemorrhoids. Persistent, high downward pressures during defecation subject hemorrhoids to congestion, bleeding, prolapse, and thrombosis.

### CAUSES/CONTRIBUTING FACTORS
- Pregnancy
- Prolonged sitting or standing
- Straining during defecation
- Cirrhosis with portal hypertension

### SIGNS/SYMPTOMS
- Rectal itching
- Rectal bleeding
- Rectal or anal discomfort
- Constipation

### COMPLICATIONS
- Hemorrhage
- Infection

### DIAGNOSTIC TESTS
- Describe each procedure, its purpose, and the normal feelings or sensations that are likely, as well as any preprocedural and postprocedural care.
  - Rectal examination
  - Proctoscopy or sigmoidoscopy: to confirm the diagnosis and rule out carcinoma or inflammatory disease

### TREATMENT
*Medical*
- Therapy
  - Heat application
  - Sitz baths

- Drugs
  —Stool softeners
  —Topical anesthetics
  —Steroid preparations

*Surgical*

- Sclerotherapy: injection of sclerosing agent between and around hemorrhoid to cause tissue shrinkage
- Rubber band ligation (internal hemorrhoids): to cause tissue necrosis and sloughing of hemorrhoids
- Cryosurgery: freezing of hemorrhoids
- Laser removal
- Hemorrhoidectomy

## HOME CARE

- Give both the patient and the caregiver *verbal* and *written* instructions. Provide them with the name and telephone number of a physician or nurse to call if questions arise.
- *General information*
  —Review any explanation about treatment and specific follow-up care.
  —Explain and discuss the development of hemorrhoids, causes or contributing factors, care treatment, and potential for recurrence.
- *Warning signs*
  —Review the signs and symptoms that should be reported to a physician or nurse.
      Frequent, unrelieved urge to defecate
      Constipation or lack of bowel movement
- *Special instructions*
  —Discuss measures to prevent the development or enlargement of hemorrhoids.
      Eat a diet high in fiber to promote regular bowel movements and soft stools.
      Drink plenty of fluids, up to 2-3 liters per day, unless contraindicated.
      Use stool softeners and bulk laxatives to prevent constipation.
      Perform daily mild exercise to enhance peristalsis and promote elimination.
      Defecate promptly after the urge so that pressure in the rectum will be prevented.

Avoid prolonged sitting (including on the toilet), squatting, or standing.

Avoid straining during defecation, which could increase discomfort and pressure on the affected area.

—Advise the patient to sit on thick foam pillows or pads and to avoid air or rubber doughnuts because they spread the buttocks apart.

—Discuss the procedure for using sitz baths after bowel movements to relieve discomfort and for cleansing.

Use warm sitz baths for brief periods to avoid hypotension secondary to vasodilation of pelvic blood vessels.

Discontinue sitz bath when feeling dizzy or faint.

—Stress the importance of perianal cleanliness at all times. Explain to the patient that proper hygiene helps prevent infection.

—Instruct the patient to wipe gently after a bowel movement. Encourage the use of moist perineal wipes.

—Discuss and demonstrate the use of cold compresses to reduce congestion and edema when hemorrhoids are inflamed.

—Provide and demonstrate the use of warm compresses to promote circulation.

—Advise the patient to abstain from anal intercourse until healing is complete.

• *Medications*

—Explain the purpose, dosage, schedule, and route of administration of any prescribed drugs, as well as side effects to report to the physician or nurse.

—Advise the patient to use topical anesthetics, astringents, and prescribed antiinflammatory preparations.

**FOLLOW-UP CARE**

• Stress the importance of regular follow-up visits for medical and laboratory evaluation. Make sure the patient has the necessary names and telephone numbers.

# Hemorrhoidectomy

—**Hemorrhoidectomy: surgical excision of hemorrhoids that do not respond to other therapies.**

## PREPROCEDURAL TEACHING

- Review the physician's explanation of the procedure and the reason for it; encourage the patient to ask questions and to discuss any fears or anxieties. Explain the need for informed consent.

### Review of Preprocedural Care

- Explain that the procedure may be performed on an outpatient basis.

### Review of Postprocedural Care

- Discuss postoperative care, including pain management, rectal packing, and bowel elimination.
- Inform the patient that early ambulation will be encouraged to promote peristalsis.
- Explain that a postoperative bowel movement will be encouraged to prevent complications such as anal strictures. Tell the patient that the first postoperative bowel movement will be stimulated by a stool softener. Warn the patient that the movement will be painful and may cause dizziness.

## SIDE EFFECTS/COMPLICATIONS

- Hemorrhage
- Infection
- Anal strictures or stenosis

## HOME CARE

- Give both the patient and the caregiver *verbal* and *written* instructions. Provide them with the name and telephone number of a physician or nurse to call if questions arise.
- *General information*
  —Review any explanation about the procedure and specific follow-up care.
  —Explain and discuss the development of hemorrhoids, causes or contributing factors, care, treatment, and potential for recurrence.
- *Warning signs*
  —Review the signs and symptoms that should be reported to a physician or nurse.
    Infection: fever, purulent drainage, redness, swelling, warmth, tenderness
    Increased rectal bleeding (more than two saturated pads in 8 hours)

Frequent, unrelieved urge to defecate

Urinary retention

Constipation or lack of bowel movement

- *Special instructions*
  —Discuss and demonstrate rectal packing or perianal dressing: procedure, frequency, and signs to report.
  —Assist the patient in obtaining appropriate supplies, such as dressings and perineal pads to protect clothing from postoperative oozing.
  —Advise the patient to sit on thick foam pillows or pads and to avoid air or rubber doughnuts because they spread the buttocks apart.
  —Stress the importance of perianal cleanliness at all times. Explain to the patient that proper hygiene helps prevent infection. Instruct the patient to wipe gently after a bowel movement. Encourage the use of moist perineal wipes.
  —Advise the patient to abstain from anal intercourse until healing is complete.
  —Warn the patient to anticipate some bleeding 8-12 days postoperatively when sutures begin to dissolve.

**FOLLOW-UP CARE**

- Stress the importance of regular follow-up visits. Make sure the patient has the necessary names and telephone numbers.

# Hepatitis, Viral
## (Hepatitis A and Hepatitis B)

—**Hepatitis, viral: inflammation of the liver caused by hepatitis viruses. Viral hepatitis may lead to liver damage, necrosis, and failure.**

### CAUSES/CONTRIBUTING FACTORS/RISK FACTORS

- Hepatitis A (infectious)
  —Ingestion of food, water, or shellfish contaminated with hepatitis A virus
  —Direct fecal-oral transmission

—Travel to underdeveloped countries
—Poor sanitation
- Hepatitis B (serum)
  —Exposure to blood, secretions, or body fluids contaminated with hepatitis B virus via direct or indirect contact with infective source
  —History of intravenous drug use
  —History of accidental exposure to contaminated needles or blood, body fluids, or secretions
  —History of blood transfusion
  —History of multiple sexual partners or homosexual contact
  —History of household contact with an infected person
  —Perinatal transmission

## SIGNS/SYMPTOMS

- Anorexia
- Malaise
- Tenderness and pain in the right upper quadrant
- Jaundice
- Clay-colored stools
- Dark urine
- Nausea and vomiting
- Diarrhea
- Headache
- Scleral icterus
- Fever (hepatitis A)
- Pruritus (hepatitis B)
- Urticaria (hepatitis B)
- Muscles or joint aches (hepatitis B)

## COMPLICATIONS

- Fulminant hepatitis
- Chronic hepatitis infection
- Hepatic coma

## DIAGNOSTIC TESTS

- Describe each procedure, its purpose, and the normal feelings or sensations that are likely, as well as any preprocedural and postprocedural care.
  —Serum antigen or antibody tests: to detect the antigen or antibodies and to indicate the course of the disease and immune status

—Serum enzymes and serum bilirubin: to indicate liver dysfunction

—Complete blood count: to detect the presence of infection

—Prothrombin time: to assess clotting function

—Stool specimen analysis: to detect the presence of hepatitis A in stool

—Urinalysis: to reveal elevation of urobilinogen in the presence of infection

—Liver biopsy: for pathologic examination of liver tissue

## TREATMENT

*Medical*

- Therapy
  —Bed rest with a gradual return to normal activities as symptoms subside
  —Dietary therapy
  —Diet as tolerated
  —Small, frequent, low-fat, high-carbohydrate feedings
  —Parenteral or enteral feedings if oral intake is not tolerated
  —Prohibition of alcoholic beverages
  —Vitamin supplements
- Drugs
  —Antiinfective agents
  —Hepatitis A: immune globulin
  —Hepatitis B: hepatitis B vaccine
  —H$_2$ blockers
  —Antihistamines
  —Vitamin K

## HOME CARE

- Give both the patient and the caregiver *verbal* and *written* instructions. Provide them with the name and telephone number of a physician or nurse to call if questions arise.
- *General information*
  —Explain and discuss hepatitis, transmission, causes and contributing factors, care, treatment, and prevention.
  —Explain that the symptomatic infected patient and the carrier patient are infectious.

- *Warning signs*
  - —Review the signs and symptoms that should be reported to a physician or nurse
    - Altered level of consciousness: lethargy, somnolence, stupor, coma
    - Confusion and personality changes
    - Asterixis
    - Easy bruising; prolonged bleeding; blood in the vomitus, urine, or stool
    - Edema in the extremities or abdomen
    - Unexplained weight gain
- *Special instructions*
  - —Discuss the infectious nature of hepatitis A and B.
  - —Review necessary precautions for hepatitis A.
    - Tell the patient to wash hands thoroughly after toileting.
    - Instruct the family or caregiver to wear gloves if contact with feces is possible and to boil articles (e.g., linens, clothing) soiled by feces.
    - Instruct the patient not to prepare food for others during the symptomatic phase of the disease.
    - Instruct the patient not to share items, such as eating utensils, toothbrushes, or toys.
    - Refer close family members and friends for injection of gamma globulin.
  - —Review necessary precautions for hepatitis B.
    - Teach the patient and caregiver to exercise blood and body fluid precautions until the patient is free of HBsAg.
    - Advise the patient not to share razors or toothbrushes.
    - Tell the patient to use an electric razor and soft-bristled toothbrush to help prevent bleeding.
    - Advise the patient to handle cuts and lacerations cautiously.
    - Offer hepatitis B vaccine to the patient's close personal contacts. Advise the patient to avoid sexual activity during the acute stage of illness and ideally until HBsAg tests are negative or until the partner has received hepatitis B vaccine.
    - Explain to the patient that blood donation is no longer possible.
    - Stress the importance of informing other physicians, dentists, and health care workers of the hepatitis diagnosis.

Encourage caregivers to provide a separate bed and bathroom for the patient if possible.

—Discuss skin care.

Advise the patient to avoid using alkaline soaps and to use mild soaps.

Advise the patient to keep the skin moist with emollient lotions.

Encourage the patient not to scratch, but to apply pressure to the affected area.

Encourage the patient to keep nails trimmed and smooth and to use knuckles to relieve itching.

Suggest cool water showers or cool compresses for pruritus.

Encourage the patient to wear loose, soft clothing, such as cotton.

—Explain that jaundice will disappear as the disease resolves.

—Suggest wearing bright red or blue clothing to offset the jaundice.

• *Medications*

—Explain the purpose, dosage, schedule, and route of administration of any prescribed drugs, as well as side effects to report to the physician or nurse.

—Tell the patient to avoid using over-the-counter medications, especially aspirin or drugs containing aspirin.

• *Activity*

—Encourage the patient to discuss allowances and limitations with respect to occupation, recreation, or activities.

—Tell the patient to alternate planned rest periods with activities during the symptomatic phase.

—Provide diversional activities and socialization to promote social interaction during therapeutic isolation.

• *Diet*

—Advise the patient to avoid alcohol intake for up to 1 year after the attack.

—Offer small, frequent feeding of low-fat, high-carbohydrate foods.

—Encourage fluids up to 2 liters per day, unless contraindicated. Offer fruit juices and carbonated beverages.

—Instruct the patient to monitor and record daily weights and to report any sudden or steady decrease.

**FOLLOW-UP CARE**

- Stress the importance of regular follow-up visits and liver function tests. Make sure the patient has the necessary names and telephone numbers.
- For a patient with hepatitis B, instruct the patient to return for follow-up serologic tests in 1 or 2 months to determine if HBsAG is present.
- Assist the patient to obtain a Medic-Alert bracelet and information card listing the diagnosis, medications, and treatment.

**PSYCHOSOCIAL CARE**

- Encourage caregivers to verbalize feelings and concerns about precautions and adaptations for the disease process.
- Encourage the patient to verbalize concerns about body image related to jaundice.

**REFERRALS**

- Refer the patient to drug and alcohol treatment programs, if appropriate.

# Hernia and Herniorrhaphy

—**Hernia: a protrusion of an organ, usually the intestine, through an abnormal opening in the abdominal wall. A hernia may occur secondary to a congenital opening, abdominal wall weakness, increased abdominal pressure, or trauma. Hernias may occur at any age, in both males and females. Most hernias occur in the groin. Some examples of hernia are indirect inguinal, direct inguinal, femoral, and umbilical. A hernia may be reducible (returned to proper position spontaneously or by manual manipulation), incarcerated (trapped by the narrow neck of the opening), or strangulated (becomes gangrenous).**

—**Herniorrhaphy: surgical repair of an incarcerated or strangulated hernia.**

## INDICATIONS

- Incarcerated hernia
- Strangulated hernia

## PREPROCEDURAL TEACHING

- See also Abdominal Surgery (p. 3).
- Review the physician's explanation of the procedure and the reason for it; encourage the patient to ask questions and to discuss any fears or anxieties. Explain the need for informed consent.

### Review of Preprocedural Care

- Explain that an elective procedure may be performed on an outpatient basis; strangulated or incarcerated repairs require a hospital stay.

### Review of Postprocedural Care

- Discuss anticipated postoperative care, including pain management and incisions.
- Discuss and demonstrate splinting the incision during coughing or sneezing.
- Discuss the purpose of and demonstrate the use of the incentive spirometer.
- Encourage early ambulation.
- Explain that analgesics will be given for pain management.

## SIDE EFFECTS/COMPLICATIONS

- Infection
- Hemorrhage
- Impaired blood supply to the vas deferens

## HOME CARE

- Give both the patient and the caregiver *verbal* and *written* instructions. Provide them with the name and telephone number of a physician or nurse to call if questions arise.
- *General information*
  —Review any explanation about the procedure and specific follow-up care.
  —Explain and discuss the development of hernias, causes or contributing factors, care and treatment, and prevention.
- *Wound/incision care*
  —Discuss and demonstrate proper wound management and dressing changes: procedures, frequency, and signs to report.

- *Warning signs*
  —Review the signs and symptoms that should be reported to a physician or nurse.
    Infection: fever, pain, edema, erythema, warmth, purulent drainage, foul odor from the incision
    Abdominal distention, nausea, vomiting
    Hernia recurrence: firm, tender, globular, irreducible swelling in the groin
- *Special instructions*
  —Apply and demonstrate to the male patient scrotal support or ice packs to decrease scrotal edema and discomfort.
  —Assist the patient in obtaining appropriate supplies, such as sterile dressings.
- *Medications*
  —Explain the purpose, dosage, schedule, and route of administration of any prescribed drugs, as well as side effects to report to a physician or nurse.
    Analgesics
    Stool softeners
    Laxatives
- *Activity*
  —Encourage the patient to discuss allowances and limitations with respect to occupation, recreation, or activities.
  —Instruct the patient to avoid coughing, straining, stretching, constipation, heavy lifting (>10 pounds), strenuous exercise, and sports for 6 weeks.
  —Demonstrate splinting incision manually or with a pillow during coughing, sneezing, or hiccups.
  —Stress the importance of activity restrictions and splinting the incision for up to 6 weeks after surgery.
  —Demonstrate proper body mechanics for moving and lifting.
  —Advise returning to work in 2 weeks for desk workers and 6 weeks for heavy laborers.
  —Advise that sexual activity should be avoided for several weeks to avoid strain on the incision and discomfort to the scrotum, if edematous.
- *Diet*
  —Advise the patient to plan a high-fiber diet to help prevent constipation; provide the patient with a list of high-fiber foods.
  —Advise the patient to drink plenty of fluids, up to 2-3 liters per day, unless contraindicated.
  —Stress the importance of weight loss if the patient is obese.

**FOLLOW-UP CARE**

• Stress the importance of regular follow-up visits. Make sure the patient has the necessary names and telephone numbers.

• Stress the importance of smoking cessation to eliminate the smoker's cough as a contributing factor to hernia development.

**PSYCHOSOCIAL CARE**

• Encourage the verbalization of fears and concerns about altered sexual function secondary to impaired blood supply to the vas deferens.

**REFERRALS**

• Provide information and refer the patient to community resources for weight loss and smoking cessation, if indicated.

# Hip Replacement

—**Hip replacement: total hip replacement (arthroplasty) is removal of the hip joint (including femoral and acetabular sides) and its replacement with a prosthesis. Total hip replacement is performed when the joint has been severely affected by conditions that result in significant pain and dysfunction. Partial hip replacement involves replacement of only the femoral head with a prosthesis.**

**INDICATIONS**

• Total hip replacement
  —Osteoarthritis
  —Rheumatoid arthritis
  —Ankylosing spondylitis (Marie-Strumpell disease)
  —Legg-Calvé-Perthes disease
  —Severe hip trauma
• Partial hip replacement
  —Avascular necrosis of the head of the femur, caused by systemic steroid therapy, sickle cell anemia, and alcohol abuse
  —Fractures of the femoral head

## COMPLICATIONS

- Infection
- Neurovascular dysfunction
- Deep vein thrombosis
- Dislocation of the prosthesis
- Atelectasis
- Pneumonia
- Hemorrhage

## PREPROCEDURAL TEACHING

- Review the physician's explanation of the procedure and the reason for it; encourage the patient to ask questions and to discuss any fears or anxieties.

### Review of Preprocedural Care

- Explain that the patient will be admitted on the day of surgery or the night before and will remain in the hospital for 3-5 days.
- Review routine preoperative procedures.
  - Blood and urologic studies, type and crossmatch, chest x-ray, electrocardiogram
  - NPO from midnight the night before
  - Bowel preparation with enema the night before
  - Shower and shampoo the night before
  - Skin prep: cleansing with bactericidal soap and shave at operative site
- Explain that the hip will be x-rayed and measured to determine the size of the prosthesis.

### Review of Postprocedural Care

- Discuss the importance of exercises and teach the patient to perform them.
  - Coughing and deep breathing
  - Foot exercises (dorsiflexion and plantar flexion)
  - Gluteal and abdominal contractions and quadriceps setting
  - Range of motion of unaffected extremities
- Provide instruction on the use of ambulatory aids: crutches, cane, walker.
- Tell the patient that the diet will be NPO for the first 24 hours and then progress to a regular diet as tolerated.
- Explain that a drainage tube will be inserted to remove excess blood and fluid around the wound.

- Tell the patient that antiembolic stockings will be applied.
- Inform the patient that bed rest will be maintained for 24-48 hours and then the patient can get up with an ambulatory aid as prescribed by the physician.
- Discuss the importance of postoperative body position and measures to keep the hip from bending beyond 90 degrees and dislocating the prosthesis.
  —Use of continuous passive motion device
  —Use of knee immobilizer to prevent knee-hip flexion
  —Use of an abduction pillow to keep the legs apart and prevent them from turning inward (internal rotation)
- Explain that physical therapy will be started to strengthen muscles around the new hip, regain the hip's range of motion, and permit walking.

## HOME CARE

- Give both the patient and the caregiver *verbal* and *written* instructions. Provide them with the name and telephone number of a physician or nurse to call if questions arise.
- *General information*
  —Review any explanation about the procedure and specific follow-up care.
- *Wound/incision care*
  —Discuss and demonstrate proper care of the incision.
- *Warning signs*
  —Review the signs and symptoms that should be reported to a physician or nurse.
    Infection: fever; chills; redness; swelling; drainage from incision; deep, dull aching pain in operative area
    Deep venous thrombosis: pain or soreness in calf, redness, swelling along vein lines
    Neurovascular impairment: loss of sensation or movement of affected foot and leg, coolness, pallor, numbness, tingling in affected extremity
- *Special instructions*
  —Advise the patient to obtain self-help devices to limit hip bending: raised toilet seat, bath bench, long-handled grippers. Refer the patient to a medical supply store for purchase or rental.
  —Explain that the patient should avoid putting excess weight on the hip and should use a walker, then crutches, and then a cane until completely recovered.

—Stress the importance of participating in physical therapy to regain muscle strength and ensure adequate upper extremity strength for ambulating with a walker, crutches, or cane.

* *Medications*
—Explain the purpose, dosage, schedule, and route of administration of any prescribed drugs, as well as side effects to report to a physician or nurse.

* *Activity*
—Encourage the patient to discuss allowances and limitations with respect to occupation, recreation, or activities. For example, tennis and skiing are not recommended but golf and swimming may be permitted.
—Discuss restrictions and activities to avoid loosening or displacing the prosthesis.

> Avoid crossing the legs or ankles while standing, sitting, or lying.
>
> Sit with the feet 6 inches apart.
>
> When sitting, keep the knees below the hips; sit on a pillow to keep the hips higher.
>
> Avoid bending over at the waist. Use a long-handled shoehorn and sock aid to assist in putting on shoes and socks.
>
> Do not drive for approximately 3 months or until approved by physician.

—Discuss safety precautions be taken at home.

> Use handrails on stairs.
>
> Wear low-heeled shoes.
>
> Be sure floors are free of objects that could cause falls, such as throw rugs, electrical cords, and clutter. Avoid wet or waxed floors.

* *Diet*
—Encourage a diet high in protein, fiber, and vitamins to promote healing and prevent constipation.

## FOLLOW-UP CARE

* Stress the importance of regular follow-up visits with the physician and physical therapist until recovery is complete. Make sure the patient has the necessary names and telephone numbers.

# Hodgkin's Disease
(Hodgkin's Lymphoma)

—**Hodgkin's disease: a malignant disorder characterized by painless, progressive enlargement of the lymph node, lymphoid tissue, and spleen. Hodgkin's lymphoma is distinguished from malignant lymphomas by the presence of Reed-Sternberg cells, which proliferate and invade normal lymph tissue throughout the body. Hodgkin's disease occurs more frequently in young adults (15-38 years) and in men. If diagnosed in stage I or II, the disease is potentially curable.**

## RISK FACTORS
- Male, white
- History of infectious mononucleosis or immunodeficiency syndrome

## STAGING
  I. Single lymph node region
 II. Two or more nodes limited to one side of the diaphragm
III. Disease on both sides of the diaphragm, but limited to the lymph nodes and spleen
IV. Involvement of the bones, bone marrow, lung parenchyma, pleura, liver, skin, gastrointestinal tract, central nervous system, etc.

All stages are classified as A or B to describe the absence (A) or presence (B) of systemic symptoms.

## SIGNS/SYMPTOMS
- Painless, swollen lymph nodes (lymphadenopathy): usually cervical or supraclavicular (early sign)
- Fever, night sweats, weight loss, lethargy, malaise, anorexia, jaundice
- Edema or pain distal to swollen lymph nodes
- Splenomegaly
- Hepatomegaly

## COMPLICATIONS

- Cervical node enlargement: venous occlusion, neck edema, airway obstruction
- Mediastinal node enlargement: dyspnea, cough
- Inguinal node enlargement: dysuria, frequency, painful urination, low back pain
- Infection
- Fractures

## DIAGNOSTIC TESTS

- Describe each procedure, its purpose, and the normal feelings or sensations that are likely, as well as any preprocedural and postprocedural care.
  - —Staging procedure
    - Lymph node biopsy: to detect presence of Reed-Sternberg cells
    - Chest x-ray: to detect mediastinal or hilar lymphadenopathy
    - Bone marrow biopsy
    - Computed tomography scans: liver, spleen, and bone
    - Laparotomy
    - Lymphangiography
  - —Laboratory tests
    - Test for normocytic normochromic anemia
    - White blood cell count with differential
    - Alkaline phosphatase: increase indicates bone involvement

## TREATMENT

*Medical*
- Therapy
  - —Chemotherapy in combination with radiation therapy for stages III and IV
  - —Radiation therapy (stages I to III)
- Drugs
  - —Interferon, monoclonal antibodies: research on effectiveness being conducted

*Surgical*
- Laparotomy
- Splenectomy
- Autologous bone marrow transplantation: research on effectiveness being conducted

**HOME CARE**

- Give both the patient and the caregiver *verbal* and *written* instructions. Provide them with the name and telephone number of a physician or nurse to call if questions arise.
- *General information*
  —Explain and discuss Hodgkin's disease/lymphoma, its causes, and contributing factors.
  —Discuss staging of the disease and the impact that various stages may have on daily living.
- *Warning signs*
  —Review the signs and symptoms that should be reported to a physician or nurse.
    Persistent fever
    Weight loss
    Enlarged lymph nodes
    Malaise
    Decreased exercise tolerance
    Infection: cough, foul-smelling sputum, pain and burning with urination, frequency, urgency, hematuria, redness, swelling at wound site, drainage (foul smelling, containing pus, discolored)
- *Special instructions*
  —Discuss the importance of avoiding large crowds and persons suspected to have an active infection because chemotherapy decreases resistance to infection.
  —Stress the importance of avoiding trauma, which can cause bruising and bleeding. Thrombocytopenia commonly results from chemotherapy.
- *Medications*
  —Explain the purpose, dosage, schedule, and route of administration of any prescribed drugs, as well as side effects to report to the physician or nurse.
  —Explain the importance of following the chemotherapy regimen and reporting the side effects of therapy to the physician or nurse: sores in mouth or on tongue, anorexia, nausea, vomiting, malaise.
- *Activity*
  —Encourage the patient to discuss allowances and limitations with respect to occupation, recreation, or activities.
  —Discuss the need for planned rest periods. Stress the impor-

tance of avoiding overexertion. Teach stress reduction techniques.
- *Diet*
  —Stress the importance of a balanced diet to maintain nutrition.
  —Encourage small, frequent meals.
  —Discuss methods to maintain hydration, nutrition during periods of stomatitis, nausea, vomiting, anorexia associated with therapy: sip fluids all day, drink nectar juices, avoid spicy, hot, and citrus foods.

## FOLLOW-UP CARE

- Stress the importance of regular follow-up visits. Make sure the patient has the necessary names and telephone numbers.
- Emphasize the importance of planning radiation therapy and chemotherapy sessions and keeping appointments.

## REFERRALS

- Refer the patient to the American Cancer Society and local support groups as indicated.

# Hyperparathyroidism

—**Hyperparathyroidism: overactivity of one or more of the parathyroid glands. Excessive secretion of parathyroid hormone causes an increase of calcium that cannot be controlled by renal excretion or uptake in soft tissue or bones. Hyperparathyroidism is common in postmenopausal women and is classified as a primary or secondary disorder.**

## CAUSES/CONTRIBUTING FACTORS

- Primary hyperparathyroidism
  —Parathyroid adenoma
  —Cell hyperplasia
- Secondary hyperparathyroidism
  —Rickets
  —Chronic renal failure

—Osteomalacia
—Excessive intake of drugs: thiazide diuretics, calcium supplements

## SIGNS/SYMPTOMS

- Polyuria, polydipsia, kidney stones
- Abdominal pain, constipation, nausea, anorexia
- Fractures of ribs, spine
- Joint or back pain
- Depression, paranoia, mood swings
- Muscular weakness and atrophy

## COMPLICATIONS

- Gastric ulcers
- Skeletal problems
  —Pathologic fractures
- Renal disorder
  —Kidney stones
  —Urinary tract infection
  —Renal failure
- Pancreatitis
- Stupor/coma

## DIAGNOSTIC TESTS

- Describe each procedure, its purpose, and the normal feelings or sensations that are likely, as well as any preprocedural and postprocedural care.
  —Laboratory tests
    Total serum calcium: greater than 11 mg/dl
    Ionized calcium: increased
    Parathyroid hormone: increased
    Intact parathyroid hormone

## TREATMENT

*Medical*
- Therapy
  —Hydration: 2-3 liters per day
  —Low-calcium diet
- Drugs
  —Loop diuretics: to lower serum calcium levels
  —Phosphates, calcitonin, mithramycin: to inhibit bone reabsorption

*Surgical*
- Parathyroidectomy

**HOME CARE**

- Give both the patient and the caregiver *verbal* and *written* instructions. Provide them with the name and telephone number of a physician or nurse to call if questions arise.
- *General information*
  —Explain hyperparathyroid disease, including specific causes, contributing factors, and recurrence of symptoms of hypercalcemia.
- *Warning signs*
  —Review the signs and symptoms that should be reported to a physician or nurse.
  >Gastric problems: nausea, vomiting, abdominal pain
  >Musculoskeletal problems: tetany, bone tenderness, pain
  >Renal problems: decreased urine output, hematuria, dysuria, flank pain, kidney stones
- *Special instructions*
  —Advise the patient on the use of assistive devices (walker, cane) for ambulation as necessary.
  —Discuss pain management as indicated.
  >Teach the patient to rate pain on a scale and to describe pain so as to better monitor pain and analgesic effectiveness.
  >Encourage the patient to take pain medication on schedule rather than as needed.
  >Assist the patient in developing a plan for using alternative pain-relieving methods rather than relying on pain medication.
- *Medications*
  —Explain the purpose, dosage, schedule, and route of administration of any prescribed drugs, as well as side effects to report to the physician or nurse.
  —Explain the need to avoid over-the-counter drugs that contain calcium, such as antacids.
  —Advise the patient to avoid using enemas or laxatives.
- *Activity*
  —Encourage the patient to discuss allowances and limitations with respect to occupation, recreation, or activities.
  —Discuss the importance of proper body alignment and mechanics and the need to increase activity gradually according

to personal tolerance. If the patient has had pathologic fractures, advise the caretaker to assist with transferring from bed to chair and ambulation.

—Discuss safety measures to prevent accidents and injuries.

—Tell the patient to splint the ribs while coughing and turning to decrease pain and prevent further injury (pathologic fracture).

—Instruct the patient to monitor urine output and strain urine for kidney stones as indicated (see Urolithiasis, p. 666).

• *Diet*

—Explain the importance of maintaining adequate fluid intake (3000 ml per day) to reduce serum calcium unless contraindicated.

—Provide instruction on a low-calcium, low–vitamin D, high-fiber diet.

**FOLLOW-UP CARE**

• Stress the importance of regular follow-up visits. Make sure the patient has the necessary names and telephone numbers.

# Hypertension

—**Hypertension: blood pressure higher than 160/90 mm Hg. Blood pressure is the force that the heart muscle exerts as it pumps against the blood vessels. Normal blood pressure is 140/80 mm Hg. Borderline blood pressure is 140/90 mm Hg. Primary or essential hypertension is the most common form of hypertension, accounting for 90% of all cases. The cause is unknown, but certain risk factors are known to contribute to its presence. Secondary hypertension is high blood pressure related to some underlying disease such as renal disease, endocrine disease, or central nervous system disorders.**

**RISK FACTORS**

• Family history
• Age group: persons over age 50
• African-Americans have a higher incidence
• Obesity

- Stress
- Tobacco use: cigarettes, chewing tabacco
- Diet high in salt and saturated fats

**SIGNS/SYMPTOMS**

- Dizziness
- Fatigue
- Vertigo
- Palpitations
- Throbbing headache
- Nosebleed

**COMPLICATIONS**

- Malignant hypertension
- Stroke
- Myocardial infarction
- Kidney failure
- Heart failure

**DIAGNOSTIC TESTS**

- Describe each procedure, its purpose, and the normal feelings or sensations that are likely, as well as any preprocedural and postprocedural care.
  —Serial blood pressure measurements
  —Physical examination
  —Laboratory tests
  —Blood tests: potassium, blood urea nitrogen, and creatinine to assess kidney function
  —Urine tests: to assess kidney function for hypertension
  —Electrocardiogram
  —Chest x-ray
  —Intravenous pyelography: to detect kidney disease

**TREATMENT**

*Medical*

- Therapy
  —Low–saturated fat, low-salt diet; low-calorie diet for weight reduction
- Drugs
  —Diuretics
  —Beta blockers

—Calcium channel blockers
—Angiotensin-converting enzyme
—Antihypertensive agents

## HOME CARE

- Give both the patient and the caregiver *verbal* and *written* instructions. Provide them with the name and telephone number of a physician or nurse to call if questions arise.
- *General information*
  —Explain the disease process, contributing factors, and complications. Assist the patient to identify individual risk factors.
  —Explain what blood pressure is, its components, systolic and diastolic pressure, and interpretation of a blood pressure reading.
- *Warning signs*
  —Review the signs and symptoms that should be reported to a physician or nurse.
  - Headache (morning occipital)
  - Dizziness
  - Fatigue
  - Epistaxis (bloody nose)
  - Palpitations
- *Special instructions*
  —Explain that the goal of treating hypertension is one of lifestyle modification that includes diet, exercise, stress management, blood pressure self-monitoring, and regular medical follow-up.
  —Teach the patient how and when to take blood pressure measurements using home monitoring equipment if available. Instruct the patient to take blood pressure at the same time each day, to keep a record of blood pressure readings, noting any changes in diet or activities that might contribute to changes in pressure, and to report elevated blood pressure to the physician or nurse. Provide time for a return demonstration.
  —Discuss how stress contributes to hypertension. Assist the patient to identify stress-producing factors. Discuss methods of stress management: relaxation techniques, guided imagery, biofeedback.
  —Discuss the importance of avoiding all tobacco products. Explain that nicotine increases the heart rate and constricts blood vessels, which can cause blood pressure to rise.

—Discuss the need to prevent obesity. Explain that a 10- or 20-pound weight reduction may reduce blood pressure if the patient is overweight.

- *Medications*
  —Explain the purpose, dosage, schedule, and route of administration of any prescribed drugs, as well as side effects to report to the physician or nurse.
  —Emphasize the importance of taking medications on time and reporting side effects.
  —Instruct the patient not to stop taking medications if side effects occur without notifying the physician.

- *Activity*
  —Encourage the patient to discuss allowances and limitations with respect to occupation, recreation, or activities. Explain that isometric exercise, walking, jogging, swimming, bicycling, and aerobic exercise are permissible but weight lifting or any sport requiring muscle contractions should be avoided because they increase the work of the heart and raise blood pressure.
  —Discuss the benefits of regular exercise: eases the work of the heart, reduces stress, strengthens the heart muscle, helps to reduce or control weight, and reduces cholesterol levels. Explain that after aerobic exercise systolic pressure can be reduced 25% and that over time a regular aerobic exercise program can permanently lower at-rest diastolic pressure.

- *Diet*
  —Explain that salt causes fluid retention, which increases the pressure in the blood vessels. Tell the patient to avoid foods high in sodium (e.g., fast foods, canned goods), to read food labels for sodium content, and not to add salt to food while cooking or at the table.
  —Discuss the need to reduce or avoid foods high in saturated fats, such as butter, cream, foods high in animal fat (red meat, bacon, organ meats).
  —Refer the patient to the dietitian to assist in diet planning.
  —Explain the need to limit alcohol intake because alcohol raises blood pressure.

## FOLLOW-UP CARE

- Stress the importance of regular follow-up visits. Make sure the patient has the necessary names and telephone numbers.

**REFERRALS**

- Provide the patient with a list of hospital- or community-based resources for behavior modification.
- Give the patient literature on managing hypertension. Refer the patient to the American Heart Association for further information.

# Hyperthyroidism
(Graves' Disease)

—Hyperthyroidism: a clinical syndrome that causes tissues to be exposed to overproduction of thyroid hormones. The excessive production of thyroid hormones produces a state of hypermetabolism that is responsible for the symptoms. There are several varieties of hyperthyroidism, ranging in seriousness from mild to severe. Graves' disease (toxic diffuse goiter), the most common form, is more frequently seen in women than men during the third and fourth decades. The exact cause of Graves' disease is unknown, but it is believed to be an autoimmune disorder resulting from thyroid-stimulating immunoglobulins. Thyrotoxic crisis, or thyroid storm, is an acute manifestation of hyperthyroidism that is life threatening. Precipitating factors include stressful events such as surgery, trauma, and infection.

## SIGNS/SYMPTOMS

- Lid retraction and lag
- Proptosis
- Conjunctival irritation; lacrimation
- Characteristic bright-eyed, frightened, or startled look
- Increased systolic blood pressure, widening pulse pressure
- Increased body temperature and sweating
- Tachycardia
- Palpitations
- Weight loss

- Increased appetite
- Diarrhea
- Generalized muscle wasting and weakness
- Hyperactive deep tendon reflexes
- Tremors
- Restlessness, irritability
- Decreased concentration, memory
- Insomnia
- Labile emotions and manic behavior

## COMPLICATIONS

- Thyroid storm
  —Extreme restlessness
  —Confusion, delirium, disorientation
  —Stupor, coma
  —Marked tachycardia
  —Vomiting
- Dysrhythmias
- Pulmonary edema
- Shock

## DIAGNOSTIC TESTS

- Describe each procedure, its purpose, and the normal feelings or sensations that are likely, as well as any preprocedural and postprocedural care.
  —Laboratory tests
    Serum $T_4$ and $T_3$ and serum free $T_4$ and $T_3$: all increased
    Thyroid radioiodine uptake and scan: uptake increased in most patients with hyperthyroidism
    Thyroid-stimulating hormone: suppressed and does not respond to thyrotropin-releasing hormone
    Thyroid-stimulating immunoglobulins: present in Graves' disease

## TREATMENT

*Medical*
- Drugs
  —Thioamides: to inhibit thyroid hormone synthesis
    Propylthiouracil
    Methimazole (Tapazole)
    Oral cholecystographic agents (Ipodate)

—Beta-adrenergic blockers: to control symptoms of hyperthyroidism
—Iodides: to promote short-term inhibition of thyroid hormone synthesis
　　Potassium or sodium iodide (SSKI, Lugol's solution)
—Radioactive iodine ($^{131}$INaI or $^{125}$INaI: to destroy thyroid tissue)
—Glucocorticoids: to inhibit thyroid hormone secretion

*Surgical*
• Thyroidectomy

### Graves' Disease Ophthalmopathy

*Medical*
• Therapy
　—Irradiation of the orbit
　—0.5% Methylcellulose eyedrops for eye irritation and pain
• Drugs
　—Corticosteroids

*Surgical*
• Orbital decompression
• Correction of muscle imbalance

### Graves' Disease Dermopathy

*Medical*
• Drugs
　—0.2% Fluocinolone or other corticosteroid cream for palliative treatment of extensive bulbous or ulcerated lesions

### HOME CARE

• Give both the patient and the caregiver *verbal* and *written* instructions. Provide them with the name and telephone number of a physician or nurse to call if questions arise.
• Prepare the patient for thyroidectomy as ordered (see p. 630).
• *General information*
　—Explain hyperthyroidism and the effects of excessive thyroid hormones on body tissues. Review cause or contributing factors and prescribed treatments.
　—Explain thyroid storm, discussing precipitating factors, symptoms, and measures to take if a crisis is suspected.

- *Warning signs*
  —Review the signs and recurrent symptoms of hyperthyroidism (see above) that should be reported to a physician or nurse. Explain that many symptoms (e.g., nervousness) will decrease if treatment is followed.
- *Special instructions*
  —Discuss measures to manage ophthalmopathy or exophthalmos.

    Tell the patient to protect eyes from bright lights, corneal ulcerations, and infections; wear sunglasses or eye patches.

    Advise the patient to apply cool compresses to the eyes if irritated.

    Suggest that the patient apply lubricants as ordered to protect the cornea.

    Tell the patient to notify the physician or nurse of increased visual disturbances.
- *Medications*
  —Explain the purpose, dosage, schedule, and route of administration of any prescribed drugs, as well as side effects to report to the physician or nurse.

    Propylthiouracil: take medications with meals to avoid gastrointestinal distress

    Radioactive $^{131}$I: review signs and symptoms of hypothyroidism; discuss the need to avoid pregnant women, infants, and children for 1 week after treatment
  —Stress the importance of not using over-the-counter medications without checking with the physician or nurse.
  —Tell the patient to check all medication labels to see whether iodine is included.
- *Activity*
  —Encourage the patient to discuss allowances and limitations with respect to occupation, recreation, or activities.
  —Discuss with the patient the importance of planned rest and avoidance of excessive exercise.
  —Discuss measures to improve sleep patterns: avoid stimulants (diet, activities) before sleep, do not sleep during normal waking hours, develop regular sleep patterns.
- *Diet*
  —Discuss with the patient the need for a high-calorie, high-protein, high-carbohydrate diet until the patient's weight is stable.

**FOLLOW-UP CARE**

- Stress the importance of regular follow-up visits. Make sure the patient has the necessary names and telephone numbers.
- Instruct the patient to inform all health care providers about the medical condition.
- Discuss the need to wear a Medic-Alert bracelet.
- Inform a woman patient to notify the physician if menstrual irregularities occur or pregnancy is suspected. Advise pregnancy planning and provide contraceptive information.

**PSYCHOSOCIAL CARE**

- Explain that emotional outbursts are part of the disease process. Maintain a nonstimulating environment by controlling extraneous noise.

# Hypertrophic Cardiomyopathy

—**Hypertrophic cardiomyopathy: a heart muscle disorder resulting in impaired pumping of the heart. Other terms include idiopathic hypertrophic subaortic stenosis, asymmetric septal hypertrophy, and hypertrophic obstructive cardiomyopathy. A primary disease of the heart muscle, hypertrophic cardiomyopathy is characterized by thickening of the interventricular septum, hypertrophy of the left ventricle, and small ventricular cavities. The increase in muscle tissue can also affect the mitral valve. In hypertrophic cardiomyopathy, output may be low, normal, or high. Low heart output may lead to fatal heart failure.**

**CAUSES**

- Autosomal dominant trait resulting in abnormal heart structure

**SIGNS/SYMPTOMS**

- Dyspnea
- Chest pain
- Syncope
- Lightheadedness

## COMPLICATIONS

- Left ventricular failure
- Sudden death
- Arrhythmias: atrial and ventricular

## DIAGNOSTIC TESTS

- Inform the patient that several diagnostic procedures may be done to aid in diagnosis of the condition. Describe each procedure, its purpose, and the normal feelings or sensations that are likely, as well as any preprocedural and postprocedural care.
  —Chest x-ray: to determine heart size and detect signs of pulmonary congestion
  —Electrocardiogram: to detect ventricular dysrhythmias and heart enlargement
  —Echocardiogram: to detect thickening of the septum, abnormal motion of the aortic and mitral valves, and ventricular outflow
  —Radionuclide studies (thallium and technetium): to detect heart muscle thickening and the amount of blood the left ventricle may hold
  —Cardiac catheterization and angiography: to detect abnormal ventricular pressures and mitral insufficiency
  —Biopsy: to determine the structure of the heart muscle

## TREATMENT

*Medical*

- Therapy
  —Cardioversion for atrial fibrillation
- Drugs
  —Beta blockers: to reduce the work of the heart by reducing the amount of adrenaline that reaches the heart muscle; to slow the heart rate and relax heart muscle
  —Digitalis: indicated only in the presence of atrial fibrillation to strengthen and regulate the heart rhythm
  —Calcium channel blockers: to relax the arteries and thus reduce the amount of force the heart needs to pump against these arteries
  —Anticoagulants in the presence of atrial fibrillation

*Surgical*

- Ventricular myotomy: resection of the hypertrophic septum with mitral valve replacement

## HOME CARE

- Give both the patient and the caregiver *verbal* and *written* instructions. Provide them with the name and telephone number of a physician or nurse to call if questions arise.
- *General information*
  —Describe the nature of hypertrophic cardiomyopathy, explaining the limitation of the disease on life-style and the prognosis.
- *Warning signs*
  —Review the signs and recurrent symptoms that should be reported to a physician or nurse.
    Dyspnea
    Unusual fatigue
    Angina
- *Special instructions*
  —Explain the need to record daily weight to detect fluid retention. Tell the patient to report a sudden weight gain of 2-3 pounds in one day or 5 pounds in one week.
- *Medications*
  —Explain the purpose, dosage, schedule, and route of administration of any prescribed drugs, as well as side effects to report to the physician or nurse.
  —Caution the patient not to discontinue the use of beta blockers without notifying the physician. Abrupt discontinuation of a beta blocker may result in heart attack or sudden death.
- *Activity*
  —Stress the importance of avoiding isometric exercises and strenuous activities (e.g., competitive sports such as football and soccer, jogging, and weight lifting). Advise the patient to rest when tired and after heavy tasks.
  —Encourage discussion and questions regarding occupation, recreation, and activities.
- *Diet*
  —Discuss with the patient the need for a low-salt diet.

## FOLLOW-UP CARE

- Stress the importance of regular follow-up visits. Make sure the patient has the necessary names and telephone numbers.
- Encourage the caregivers to learn cardiopulmonary resuscitation because of the risk of sudden cardiac death. Assist with referral to hospital or community resources.

# Hypoparathyroidism

—Hypoparathyroidism: a deficiency of parathyroid hormone. Parathyroid hormone is necessary to maintain normal levels of serum calcium. A rare condition, hypoparathyroid disease may occur as the result of removal of or damage to the parathyroid glands (e.g., radiation or treatment with iodine-131).

## SIGNS/SYMPTOMS

- Personality disturbances: anxiety, depression, irritability
- Paresthesias, tetany, hyperreflexia
- Nausea, vomiting, diarrhea, abdominal pain
- Dry scaly skin, brittle nails, thin patchy hair

## COMPLICATIONS

- Cardiac arrhythmias
- Seizures
- Cardiac arrest

## DIAGNOSTIC TESTS

- Describe each procedure, its purpose, and the normal feelings or sensations that are likely, as well as any preprocedural and postprocedural care.
  —Serum tests
      Calcium: decreased
      Parathyroid hormone: decreased or absent
      Bicarbonate: decreased
      Phosphate: increased
  —Urine tests
      Calcium: decreased
      Phosphate: decreased

## TREATMENT

*Medical*
- Therapy
  —Dietary calcium supplement

- Drugs
  - —Vitamins
  - —Calcium replacement
  - —Phosphate binders

## HOME CARE

- Give both the patient and the caregiver *verbal* and *written* instructions. Provide them with the name and telephone number of a physician or nurse to call if questions arise.
- *General information*
  - —Explain and discuss hypoparathyroidism, its specific causes, and contributing factors.

**H**

- *Warning signs*
  - —Review the signs that should be reported to a physician or nurse.

    Hypocalcemia: tingling, emotional irritability, muscle stiffness, fatigue, palpitations, nausea and vomiting, abdominal pain

    Acute hypoparathyroidism: tetany (painful muscle spasms), irritability, tingling of fingers and around mouth

    Seizure activity: tremors, loss of consciousness, involuntary muscular contractions

- *Special instructions*
  - —Discuss the actions to take for seizure activity.

    Stay with the person.

    Avoid restraining or interrupting the behavior.

    Protect the head and clear surrounding areas.

    After the seizure, turn the head to the side to avoid aspiration.

    Record the activity, including the length of the seizure.

    Call the physician immediately.

- *Medications*
  - —Explain the purpose, dosage, schedule, and route of administration of any prescribed drugs, as well as side effects to report to the physician or nurse.
  - —Stress the importance of the continued need for calcium and vitamin D supplements and the reasons for the treatment.
  - —Instruct the patient to take calcium replacement medications on time to enhance the dietary intake of calcium.

- *Activity*
  —Discuss the need to exercise to tolerance, to alternate exercise with periods of rest, and to report increasing muscle weakness and fatigue.
  —Encourage the patient to discuss allowances and limitations with respect to occupation, recreation, and activities.
  —Discuss the potential for falls resulting from difficulty maintaining balance during the acute period. Inform the patient of the need for a safe home environment, and aid the patient in obtaining assistive devices or help in moving about as indicated.
- *Diet*
  —Encourage a high-calcium, high–vitamin D, low-phosphorus diet.
  —Discuss with the patient the need to maintain fluid balance, especially when nausea, vomiting, and diarrhea are present.

**FOLLOW-UP CARE**

- Stress the importance of regular follow-up visits. Make sure the patient has the necessary names and telephone numbers.

**PSYCHOSOCIAL CARE**

- Discuss with the patient and caregivers the need to decrease stressors.
- Discuss with the caregivers the symptoms of changes in mood or thought process that may require medical interventions.

# Hypothyroidism
(Myxedema)

—Hypothyroidism: the clinical sydrome caused by a deficiency in thyroid hormones. Hypothyroidism occurs most often in women between the ages of 30 and 60 years. Myxedema coma is a severe form of hypothyroidism that is often fatal. Precipitating factors include withdrawal of thyroid medication, severe stress, or infection. **Chronic autoimmune thyroiditis (idio-pathic hypothyroidism, Hashimoto's disease), the most common form of hypothyroidism, is generally believed to be an autoimmune disorder. Transient autoimmune thyroiditis is a pregnancy-related form that occurs 3-6 months post partum. Hypothyroidism may also follow radioiodine therapy, external neck radiation therapy, or postoperative thyroidectomy.**

## SIGNS/SYMPTOMS

- Decreased body temperature
- Dry, rough, scaly skin
- Puffy face, hands, and feet; periorbital edema
- Decreased blood pressure
- Bradycardia
- Decreased exercise tolerance
- Weight gain, constipation
- Anorexia
- Abdominal distention, myxedema ileus
- Nonspecific fatigue, weakness
- Delayed deep tendon reflexes
- Muscle aches and joint stiffness
- Intolerance to cold
- Slowed, slurred, monotonous speech
- Somnolence, lethargy
- Impaired memory, inattentiveness, slow cognition
- Loss of initiative
- Paranoia, depression, agitation
- Decreased libido

## COMPLICATIONS

- Myxedema coma
  —Hypothermia
  —Depressed respirations
  —Stupor advancing to coma
  —Cardiovascular collapse
  —Metabolic imbalances
- Ischemic heart disease: angina, myocardial infarction
- Heart failure
- Dysrhythmias
- Intestinal obstruction
- Anemia

## DIAGNOSTIC TESTS

- Describe each procedure, its purpose, and the normal feelings or sensations that are likely, as well as any preprocedural and postprocedural care.
  —Serum $T_4$ and $T_3$ and serum free $T_4$ and $T_3$: decreased
  —Serum thyroid-stimulating hormone levels: increased
  —Radioiodide uptake test: below normal uptake

## TREATMENT

*Medical*
- Therapy
  —Intravenous albumin and fluids
- Drugs
  —Synthetic thyroid hormones
     Levothyroxine sodium (Cytolen, Levoid, Levothyroid, Synthroid Sodium)
     Liothyronine sodium (Cytomel, Cytomine)
     Lotrix (Euthroid, Thyrolar)
  —Diagnostic agents
     Thyroid-stimulating hormone (Thytropar)
     Protirelin (thyrotropin-releasing hormone) (Relefact TRH, Thypinone)

## HOME CARE

- Give both the patient and the caregiver *verbal* and *written* instructions. Provide them with the name and telephone number of a physician or nurse to call if questions arise.
- *General information*
  —Explain hypothyroidism, including the effects of deficient thyroid hormones on body tissues and personality. Review causes and contributing factors, and tell the patient that the symptoms will subside with treatment.
  —Explain myxedema coma, the precipitating factors, and emergency measures to take if they are suspected.
- *Warning signs*
  —Review the signs and symptoms that should be reported to a physician or nurse.
     Hypothyroidism: puffy, masklike face; periorbital edema
     Myxedema coma: decreased exercise tolerance, lightheadedness, slowing pulse, difficulty breathing, decreasing temperature

Pulmonary infection: temperature above normal for patient; cold or flu symptoms

Urinary infection: burning, urgency, and frequent urination

- *Special instructions*
  —Explain the importance of avoiding infections.
- *Medications*
  —Explain the purpose, dosage, schedule, and route of administration of any prescribed drugs, as well as side effects to report to the physician or nurse.
  —Stress the importance of not discontinuing thyroid medication because the medication is essential for life and treatment is lifelong.
- *Activity*
  —Encourage the patient to discuss allowances and limitations with respect to occupation, recreation, and activities.
  —Discuss the importance of getting adequate periods of rest and of alternating periods of exercise with rest.
  —Advise avoiding extremely cold temperature until the condition is stabilized.
- *Diet*
  —Discuss with the patient the need for a high-fiber, low-calorie diet and adequate fluid intake to prevent constipation and promote weight loss.

**FOLLOW-UP CARE**

- Stress the importance of regular follow-up visits. Make sure the patient has the necessary names and telephone numbers.
- Advise the patient to inform all physicians (e.g., gynecologist, urologist) of the disease process.
- Discuss the need to wear a Medic-Alert bracelet.

**PSYCHOSOCIAL CARE**

- Discuss personality changes, explaining that slowness and lethargy will recede once treatment is started. Refer the patient to counseling as indicated.

# Hysterectomy, Radical

—**Hysterectomy, radical: surgical removal of the ovaries, tubes, uterus with the cervix, and parametrial tissue, along with lymph node dissection. The ovarian tissue is often preserved in premenopausal patients. Because of the extensiveness of the procedure, an abdominal approach is required.**

## INDICATIONS
- Chronic endometriosis
- Malignant neoplastic disease
- Leiomyomas

## PREPROCEDURAL TEACHING
- See Abdominal Surgery (p. 3) for general preoperative and postoperative instructions.
- Review the physician's explanation of the procedure and the reason for it; encourage the patient to ask questions and to discuss any fears or anxieties. Discuss the need for informed consent.

### Review of Postprocedural Care
- Explain that after surgery the patient will be maintained in a supine or low Fowler's position to prevent pelvic congestion.
- Discuss perineal care: sitz baths, heat lamps, ice packs.
- Inform the patient that an indwelling urinary catheter or suprapubic tube is required to avoid urinary retention.
- Explain that a nasogastric tube or rectal tube may be inserted to prevent abdominal distention.
- Explain that abdominal cramping with a moderate amount of drainage is expected and that the patient will have a perineal pad in place.

## SIDE EFFECTS/COMPLICATIONS
- Wound infection, dehiscence
- Hemorrhage
- Urinary retention
- Urinary tract infection
- Paralytic ileus

- Pneumonia
- Thrombophlebitis
- Constipation
- Pulmonary embolus
- Ureteral fistula, ureteral ligation

## HOME CARE

- Give both the patient and the caregiver *verbal* and *written* instructions. Provide them with the name and telephone number of a physician or nurse to call if questions arise.
- *General information*
  —Reinforce the patient's correct information about hysterectomy and provide factual information to correct any misconceptions. Common misconceptions about hysterectomy are that afterward a woman grows fat and flabby, develops facial hair, becomes wrinkled, old, and masculine, loses her mind, or becomes depressed and nervous. Normal concerns that should be discussed include fear of death, disfigurement, cancer, and loss of femininity and childbearing ability; pain; and changes in sexuality. Encourage the patient to verbalize her concerns with significant others.
- *Wound/incision care*
  —Instruct the patient to care for the incision with general cleanliness and daily bathing.
- *Warning signs*
  —Review the signs and symptoms that should be reported to a physician or nurse.
     Elevated temperature (>100° F [37.8° C])
     Incisional swelling
     Redness
     Purulent drainage
     Foul odor
     Vaginal bleeding (more than slightly bloody drainage)
     Abdominal pain
     Change in bowel habits
     Difficulty in urinating
- *Special instructions*
  —Tell the patient to avoid constipation by taking mild laxatives and stool softeners as necessary. Demonstrate care of the suprapubic catheter if the patient is discharged with one in place. Teach clean, intermittent self-catheterization as indicated.

—Explain that no intercourse, tampons, douching, or tub baths are allowed for 4-6 weeks or until permitted by the physician.

—Explain that menstruation will no longer occur.

• *Medications*

—Explain the purpose, dosage, schedule, and route of administration of any prescribed drugs, as well as side effects to report to a physician or nurse.

> Estrogen therapy if ordered
> Analgesic

• *Activity*

—Advise the patient of the importance of exercise and activity to tolerance.

—Tell the patient to avoid fatigue and plan rest periods.

—Explain that jarring activities, driving, and heavy lifting ($>10$ pounds) should be avoided for 4-6 weeks or as indicated by a physician.

—Advise the patient to avoid activities that increase pelvic congestion (e.g., dancing, horseback riding, sitting for long periods) until allowed to resume them by a physician.

## FOLLOW-UP CARE

• Stress the importance of regular follow-up gynecologic appointments. Make sure the patient has the necessary names and telephone numbers.

## PSYCHOSOCIAL CARE

• Explore the patient's fears and anxieties regarding changes in body image and sexuality: loss of uterus, fertility, femininity, or sexual functioning. Inform the patient that counseling for a sexually active woman and her partner is available and that she should discuss options with her physician or nurse.

# Implantable Cardioverter Defibrillator

—**Implantable cardioverter defibrillator: a self-contained device that monitors heart activity and treats ventricular tachy-**

cardia and ventricular fibrillation. The implantable cardio-verter defibrillator delivers electrical countershocks or rapid pacing in the presence of ventricular tachycardia or fibrilla-tion via electrodes that are surgically implanted into the heart.

## INDICATIONS

- Patients who have survived sudden cardiac death not associated with acute myocardial infarction
- Uncontrollable dysrhythmias
- History of multiple cardiac arrests
- Sustained ventricular tachycardia uncontrolled with antidys-rhythmia medications

## PREPROCEDURAL TEACHING

- Review the physician's explanation of the procedure and the rea-son for it; encourage the patient to ask questions and to discuss any fears or anxieties. Discuss the need for informed consent.

### Review of Preprocedural Care

- Review the implantation procedure, the type of device, and the recommended surgical approach: thoracotomy, sternotomy, sub-xiphoid, subcostal, or transvenous.
- Instruct the patient about the need to remain NPO after mid-night before the procedure.
- Review preprocedural tests: electrocardiogram, electrophysi-ologic study, and laboratory work, including blood type and crossmatch.
- Explain skin preparation of the chest and abdomen.

### Review of Postprocedural Care

- Discuss the use of the electrocardiogram and hemodynamic monitoring after the procedure.
- Discuss fear and anxiety about the device, discharges, possible malfunction, and underlying condition.

## SIDE EFFECTS/COMPLICATIONS

- Pneumothorax (collapsed lung)
- Bleeding
- Lead dislodgment
- Infection
- Atelectasis

- Pericarditis
- Malfunction of device

## HOME CARE

- Give both the patient and the caregiver *verbal* and *written* instructions. Provide them with the name and telephone number of a physician or nurse to call if questions arise. Use visual aids to assist in instruction.
- *General information*
  —Review any explanation about the procedure and device and any specific follow-up care.
- *Warning signs*
  —Review the signs and symptoms that should be reported to a physician or nurse.
    Infection (incision): redness, swelling, fluid, or purulent drainage, skin irritation, tenderness, warmth, fever
    More than one shock felt in 24 hours
    Symptoms associated with rhythm disturbances: dizziness, palpitations, loss of consciousness
- *Special instructions*
  —Review the procedure to follow when the device discharges inappropriately.
    Note symptoms and call the physician.
    If multiple discharges are given or the patient loses consciousness, call the physician, call the emergency number (911), or bring the patient to the emergency room.
  —Describe the sensations and feelings when the device delivers a countershock: a blow, thump, or "kick in the chest" that may last 1 second. Explain that the patient may be unconscious before receiving the shock.
  —Explain that someone touching the patient will not feel the shock or will feel only a tingle.
  —Instruct the patient not to wear tight, restrictive clothing, such as belts and girdles.
  —Stress the importance of avoiding the following:
    Strong magnets and magnetic fields, such as radio or television transmitting towers
    Spark plugs or running motor, such as a lawn mower or car
    Hand-held airport metal detectors
    Rough physical contact or dangerous sports

Large stereo speakers

Television that is in operation with the back off

Direct contact over alternators, such as in a running car engine

Diathermy, magnetic resonance imaging, or electrocautery

—Instruct the patient that contact with well-grounded home appliances, such as microwave ovens and hair dryers, is not harmful.

- *Activity*
  —Encourage the patient to discuss allowances and limitations with respect to occupation, recreation, or activities. Tell the patient to discuss occupational concerns with the physician.
  —Tell the patient that driving is not permitted for 6 months following surgery because of the potential loss of consciousness associated with dysrhythmias. The patient must be free of discharges for 6 months before driving is permitted.
  —Inform the patient that working at heights, swimming alone, or activities in which the patient or others could be injured if the patient loses consciousness should be avoided.
  —Instruct the patient to avoid heavy lifting (>10 pounds) for the first 6 weeks.
  —Tell the patient that sexual activity may be resumed as the patient tolerates.
  —Advise the patient to report any plans to travel alone or move.
  —Encourage the patient to engage in activities of daily living and exercises as tolerated.
  —Teach the pateint to check pulses during exercise. Inform the patient of the cutoff rate before discharge and tell the patient not to exceed that rate.
  —Explain that the life of the battery depends on the model used and the number of shocks delivered.

**FOLLOW-UP CARE**

- Stress the importance of regular follow-up visits to assess battery life and device function. Make sure the patient has the necessary names and telephone numbers.
- Encourage the patient to obtain a Medic-Alert bracelet and identification card listing the diagnosis and the device.
- Encourage the caregivers to learn cardiopulmonary resuscitation (CPR). Provide a list of community CPR instruction sites. Instruct the patient in cough CPR.

## PSYCHOSOCIAL CARE

- Encourage the patient and caregivers to verbalize fears and concerns about device function, possible malfunction, and the underlying condition.

## REFERRALS

- Refer the patient and caregivers to support groups for persons with implantable defibrillators.
- Refer the patient to community monitored exercise programs.

# Indwelling Catheter
(Foley, Suprapubic Catheter)

—**Indwelling catheter: catheter inserted through the urethra or through the abdomen (suprapubic) into the bladder to drain the urine into a drainage bag.**

## INDICATIONS

- Total incontinence
- Neurogenic bladder
- Inability to urinate because of enlarged prostate

## PREPROCEDURAL TEACHING

- Review the physician's explanation of the procedure and the reason for it; encourage the patient to ask questions and to discuss any fears or anxieties.
- Review catheter insertion.
  - Urethral approach: a thin flexible tube/catheter with a balloon is inserted through the urethra into the bladder. Once inserted, the balloon is inflated to prevent it from slipping out and is connected to a drainage bag. The catheter is taped to the thigh to prevent pulling.
  - Suprapubic or abdominal approach: the procedure may be done under local or general anesthetic and requires written consent. A urinary bladder catheter is inserted through the skin about 1 inch above the symphysis pubis and is sutured to the abdominal skin.

**Review of Postprocedural Care**

- Explain that the catheter is taped in place securely and a different site is used every day.
- Instruct the patient to keep the drainage bag below the level of the bladder.
- Explain that the abdominal dressing is changed every day; the area is cleansed with Betadine and sterile gauze is taped in place.

## SIDE EFFECTS/COMPLICATIONS

- Urinary tract infection
- Catheter obstruction
- Pyelonephritis
- Urinary tract stones
- Difficulty in urinating after removal
- Infection at site of insertion of suprapubic catheter

## HOME CARE

- Give both the patient and the caregiver *verbal* and *written* instructions. Provide them with the name and telephone number of a physician or nurse to call if questions arise.
- *General information*
  —Explain the underlying reason for the procedure.
- *Warning signs*
  —Review the signs, symptoms, and problems that should be reported to a physician or nurse.
    Lack of urine output longer than 4 hours (check for kinks)
    Infection: low back pain or flank pain; cloudy, foul-smelling urine; bloody urine; fever; chills; poor appetite; lack of energy; sediment in urine
    Persistent leakage around the catheter
    Pain, tenderness, or swelling around the catheter
    Break in the catheter
    Catheter falls out
- *Special instructions*
  —Explain that a *urethral catheter* may create the urge to urinate. Stress the importance of not trying to remove the catheter.
  —Explain that *urethral catheter* sites should be alternated daily (the inner thigh for women and the upper thigh or abdomen for men) and taped securely to prevent accidental pulling.
  —Instruct a patient with a *suprapubic catheter* to cleanse the "new" insertion site with a Betadine solution (if the patient

is not sensitive to iodine) and cover it with a gauze dressing. Crusting may be cleaned with a Q-tip and hydrogen peroxide and rinsed with water.

—Explain that a "seasoned" insertion site for a *suprapubic catheter* may be washed with unscented soap and water.

—Inform the patient that a *suprapubic catheter* may be taped to the abdomen if necessary.

—Instruct the patient to monitor and record urine output for amount and color of urine.

—Explain that the catheter should be connected to a drainage bag and the bag should be below the level of the bladder to prevent flow back into the bladder whether the patient is lying, sitting, or standing. Inform the patient that the drainage bag may be carried in a shopping bag while the patient is walking or the catheter may be connected to a leg bag.

—Discuss the types of drainage bags, and advise the patient where to obtain supplies.

Leg bag: usually used during the day. The tubing attaches directly to the catheter, and the bag holds about 500 ml (½ quart). Advise the patient to choose a bag that does not bulge when full. The leg bag is attached to the leg with cloth or Velcro straps or fits into a cloth sleeve. It should not show under clothing. Rubber straps should not be used, since they irritate the skin. The drainage valve or cap should be accessible and easily opened.

Drainage bag: a larger drainage bag is used for night and should hold about 1500 ml (1½ quarts). The bedside bag should have plenty of tubing to allow movement in bed. The bag should be placed on a stand below the level of the catheter. The drainage valve or cap should be accessible and easily opened.

—Demonstrate how to empty the drainage bag and tell the patient it should be emptied every 8 hours or when filled.

Hold the bag over the toilet.

Free the drain tip, loosen the clamp, and drain the bag into the toilet or collection container. Reclamp the tube and clean the tip of the drain tube with Betadine solution.

Do not touch the tip of the drain tube or let the drain tube touch the toilet or collecting container.

—Demonstrate how to change drainage bags.

Wash hands.

Wipe the connection with alcohol.

Protect the ends of the catheter and tubing with a clean gauze square when disconnecting the catheter and before reconnecting it to the drainage system.

—Explain that bags may be reused after careful cleansing.

Rinse the inside of the bag with soapy water and then rinse well with clear water. Fill the bag with one part vinegar to four parts water and soak the inside for 30 minutes.

Empty the bag and let it air dry.

Store in a clean, dust-free place until ready to use again.

—Stress the importance of perineal care and demonstrate.

Wash around the urethral catheter to prevent crusting. Wash with unscented soap and water twice a day and dry gently.

Wash around the rectal area with soap and water twice a day or after each bowel movement.

- *Medications*
  —Explain the purpose, dosage, schedule, and route of administration of any prescribed drugs, as well as side effects to report to a physician or nurse.
- *Activity*
  —Encourage the patient to discuss allowances and limitations with respect to occupation, recreation, or activities.
  —Explain that showering or bathing may be done on instructions from the physician (depending on the underlying reason for catheter placement).
- *Diet*
  —Inform the patient that the diet is regular or as prescribed by the physician according to the underlying condition.
  —Stress the importance of drinking 10-15 glasses of clear fluids and juices per day unless restricted by the underlying condition. Cranberry, plum, and prune juices help prevent urinary tract infection.
  —Inform the patient that caffeine and alcohol should be kept to a minimum.

**FOLLOW-UP CARE**

- Stress the importance of regular follow-up visits. Make sure the patient has the necessary names and telephone numbers.

**REFERRALS**

- Refer the patient for home health care as indicated.

# Iron Deficiency Anemia

—Iron deficiency anemia: an inadequate absorption or excessive loss of iron. Anemia is a common hematopoietic disorder, defined as a reduced red blood cell volume or a reduced concentration of hemoglobin. The general effects of anemia result from a deficiency of the oxygen-carrying mechanism, although some effects are related to varied pathogenetic factors.

## CONTRIBUTING FACTORS/RISK FACTORS

- Decreased dietary intake
- Blood loss (gastrointestinal bleeding)
- Chronic diarrhea
- Menstrual abnormalities
- Pregnancy
- Chronic disease (e.g., rheumatoid arthritis)

## SIGNS/SYMPTOMS

- Brittle hair and nails
- Dysphagia
- Sore mouth or tongue
- Fatigue
- Decreased ability to concentrate
- Cold sensitivity
- Menstrual irregularities
- Loss of libido
- Tachycardia
- Palpitations
- Tachypnea
- Exertional dyspnea
- Pale mucous membranes
- Pale nail beds
- Vertigo

## COMPLICATIONS

- Hemochromatosis (iron overdose)
- Infection

## DIAGNOSTIC TESTS

- Describe each procedure, its purpose, and the normal feelings or sensations that are likely, as well as any preprocedural and postprocedural care.
  —Blood count
  —Peripheral blood smear
  —Total iron-binding capacity
  —Reticulocyte count

## TREATMENT

*Medical*

- Therapy
  —Increased dietary intake of iron
  —Iron replacement (ferrous sulfate, ferrous gluconate)
  —Treatment of the cause

## HOME CARE

- Give both the patient and the caregiver *verbal* and *written* instructions. Provide them with the name and telephone number of a physician or nurse to call if questions arise.
- *General information*
  —Explain and discuss with the patient iron deficiency anemia, its causes, and contributing factors.
- *Warning signs*
  — Review the signs and symptoms that should be reported to a physician or nurse.
    Dyspnea
    Dizziness
    Palpitations
    Chest pain
    Headache
    Abnormalities in menstrual cycle
    Iron overdose: diarrhea, fever, stomach pain, nausea and vomiting
- *Special instructions*
  —Inform the patient that stools will appear dark or black as the result of iron replacement therapy. Discuss the importance of monitoring for blood loss in the stool when patients have gastrointestinal bleeding tendencies. Teach the proper use of guaiac tests.

- *Medications*
  —Explain the purpose, dosage, schedule, and route of administration of any prescribed drugs, as well as side effects to report to the physician or nurse.
  —Explain the need to avoid taking over-the-counter vitamins that may contain iron. Tell the patient to read labels and check with the physician.
  —Advise the patient to take oral iron with meals to maximize absorption. Advise the patient not to take iron with milk or an antacid, which could decrease absorption. Review the need to increase vitamin C intake, which can increase iron absorption.
  —Tell the patient to take liquid iron through a straw and to rinse the mouth afterward to minimize tooth staining.
- *Activity*
  —Encourage the patient to discuss allowances and limitations with respect to occupation, recreation, or activities.
  —Discuss the need to space activities to allow for frequent rest periods.
- *Diet*
  —Emphasize the importance of a well-balanced diet, especially iron intake, which is found in foods such as red meat, green vegetables, and raisins.
  —Discuss the benefits of eating six small meals spread throughout the day rather than trying to get all nutrition in three meals.
  —Discuss the need to increase liquids and fiber in the diet to prevent constipation, which is common with iron supplements.

**FOLLOW-UP CARE**
- Stress the importance of regular follow-up visits. Make sure the patient has the necessary names and telephone numbers.

# Laminectomy
## (Spinal Fusion, Diskectomy)

—Laminectomy: removal of a flat, bony portion of the vertebrae referred to as the lamina to access the intervertebral space for removal of protruding fragments of the ruptured disk or to remove the entire disk (diskectomy). The incision may be performed anteriorly or posteriorly in the cervical, thoracic, or lumbar region. Laminectomy is performed to relieve nerve root or spinal cord compression only after conservative treatment no longer alleviates pain.

—Spinal fusion: procedure done in conjunction with laminectomy, performed to stabilize the vertebrae. The procedure involves placing bone chips, obtained fom the iliac crest or a bone bank, over the unstable portion of the spine.

## INDICATIONS
- Ruptured disk (herniated disk)
- Trauma
- Displaced fracture
- Incomplete vertebral dislocation from rheumatoid arthritis or osteoporosis

## PREPROCEDURAL TEACHING
- Review the physician's explanation of the procedure and the reason for it; encourage the patient to ask questions and to discuss any fears or anxieties. Explain the need to obtain informed consent for surgery and anesthesia.

### Review of Preprocedural Care
- Explain that the incision will be between 1 and 3 inches long.
- Explain that the hospital stay is usually 3-5 days.
- Inform the patient of the need to be NPO from midnight the night before.
- Discuss routine blood and urine tests to detect signs of electrolyte imbalance or infection.
- Discuss the chest x-ray and electrocardiogram to evaluate signs of chronic disease.
- Inform the patient about skin preparation: cleansing the night before with bacterial soap and shaving the skin over the incisional area.
- Tell the patient that bowel preparation with an enema may be ordered the night before surgery.

**Review of Postprocedural Care**

- Explain that the patient will be NPO until the morning after surgery and then will be given clear fluids, advancing to a regular diet.
- Advise the patient that complete bed rest will be maintained until the evening of surgery, with turning from side to side every 2 hours. Explain that the patient will be allowed up at the bedside the evening of surgery and up to three times daily thereafter.
- Tell the patient that frequent checks of neurovascular status, peripheral pulses, and vital signs will be performed.
- Inform the patient that the first dressing change will be done after 24 hours.
- Discuss the need to deep breathe and cough every 2 hours.
- Inform the patient of the possibility of urinary retention. Tell a male patient that he may stand to void.
- For a patient with cervical laminectomy, explain that a neck brace and a nasogastric drainage tube may be used. Explain that the drainage tube will be removed in 1-2 days.
- Advise the patient that incisional pain will be mild to moderate and may include some radiation to the shoulders and occipital area (if cervical) or to the hips and buttocks (if lumbar). Tell the patient that nerve pain may not be relieved immediately after surgery.

**SIDE EFFECTS/COMPLICATIONS**

- Continued nerve compression pain
- Hoarseness (cervical)
- Bleeding, hemorrhage
- Spinal cord neurovascular damage
- Wound infection
- Urinary infection, retention
- Effects of anesthesia

**HOME CARE**

- Give both the patient and the caregiver *verbal* and *written* instructions. Provide them with the name and telephone number of a physician or nurse to call if questions arise.
- *General information*
  —Review any explanation about the procedure.

- *Wound/incision care*
  —Instruct the patient to keep the incision site clean and dry until sutures and staples are removed, which usually takes place within 10 days after discharge.
- *Warning signs*
  —Review the signs and symptoms that should be reported to a physician or nurse.
      Wound infection: fever, chills, redness, swelling, drainage of the incisional area
      Neurovascular impairment: increase or appearance of numbness (explain that some numbness as a sign of former nerve pressure may remain), tingling of extremities, coolness, pallor of extremities, increased pain
- *Activity*
  —Inform the patient that showering is usually not permitted until sutures or staples are out or until advised by the physician.
  —Provide instruction on good body mechanics.
      Use logrolling when getting in and out of bed to prevent back strain and twisting.
      Avoid sudden turning or twisting.
      Sit in straight-backed chairs; avoid soft chairs.
  —Tell the patient to avoid lifting and driving for 3-6 weeks or longer as prescribed by a physician.
  —Advise the patient to use a firm mattress (or plywood between the box spring and mattress).
  —Instruct the patient to resume activities gradually. Suggest beginning by walking around the house, progressing to longer walks outdoors. Advise the patient to wear shoes with good foot and ankle support.
  —For a patient with cervical laminectomy, explain the need to wear a neck brace as directed.
  —Encourage discussion with the physician as to any limitations on exercise, resumption of work, and recreational activities.
  —Discuss the importance of continuing with back exercises (see p. 89) as ordered and prescribed to increase muscle strength.
- *Diet*
  —Advise the patient that a regular diet high in protein and vitamins will aid wound healing, unless such a diet is contraindicated.
  —Explain the importance of avoiding weight gain. Refer the patient to a dietitian for diet management.

**FOLLOW-UP CARE**

- Stress the importance of regular follow-up visits. Make sure the patient has the necessary names and telephone numbers.

---

# Laryngeal Cancer

—Laryngeal cancer: cancer of the larynx (voice box). Laryngeal cancer occurs most commonly (60%) in the glottis (true vocal cords). Carcinoma of the supraglottic larynx (epiglottis, false cord) has a lower incidence. Ninety percent of cases of laryngeal cancer occur in men, with the highest incidence between 60 and 70 years. The death rate from laryngeal cancer is higher among blacks than whites. Squamous cell cancer of the glottic larynx is the classic smoker's cancer and generally occurs after decades of cigarette smoking. Cancer in situ may exist alone or in association with invasive disease. Malignancies of the supraglottis are usually in an advanced stage when diagnosed. Malignancy rarely develops in the subglottic larynx.

**RISK FACTORS**

- Cigarette smoking
- Alcohol abuse

**SIGNS/SYMPTOMS**

- Persistent hoarseness and other vocal complaints
- Aspiration on swallowing
- Dysphagia
- Foreign body sensation
- Unilateral sore throat
- Earache
- Neck mass (supraglottic)
- Dyspnea

**DIAGNOSTIC TESTS**

- Describe each procedure, its purpose, and the normal feelings or sensations that are likely, as well as any preprocedural and postprocedural care.
  - —Indirect mirror examination: to see the lesion on the larynx

—Direct laryngoscopy and biopsy: to see the lesion on the larynx and detect the presence of malignant cells

—Anterior laryngeal tomography: to detect subglottic extension of tumor

—Pulmonary function studies: to assess preoperative respiratory status

—Chest x-ray: to detect other pulmonary disease such as lung cancer

## TREATMENT

*Medical*
- Therapy
  —Radiation therapy: external beam
  —Chemotherapy
      Cisplatin
      5-Fluorouracil (5-FU)
      Adjuvant chemotherapy with methotrexate and 5-FU

*Surgical*
- Endoscopic laser excision: for small tumors
- Partial laryngectomy: removal of half or more of larynx
  —Supraglottic laryngectomy
  —Epiglottidectomy
  —Cordectomy
  —Anterior commissure resection
  —Vertical hemilaryngectomy
  —Frontolateral and extended frontolateral partial laryngectomy
  —Near-total laryngectomy
- Total laryngectomy: removal of larynx; voice permanently lost; tracheostomy performed
- Total laryngectomy with radical neck dissection: removal of larynx and surrounding lymph nodes, tissue, muscle, and blood vessels
- Reconstruction: skin flap

## HOME CARE

- Give both the patient and the caregiver *verbal* and *written* instructions. Provide them with the name and telephone number of a physician or nurse to call if questions arise. Use visual aids and permit time for return demonstration before discharge.
- For a patient who will undergo laryngectomy, see p. 418. Discuss the extent of the planned surgery and clarify any misconceptions.

- For radiation therapy, see p. 559; for chemotherapy, see p. 178.
- *General information*
  —Review the physician's explanation of the disease and the type of prescribed treatment: radiation therapy or surgery. Explain that treatment depends on the stage and site of the tumor.

## FOLLOW-UP CARE

- Stress the importance of regular follow-up visits. Make sure the patient has the necessary names and telephone numbers.

## REFERRALS

- If a patient is to undergo laryngectomy, arrange a meeting with a laryngectomy survivor before surgery.

# Laryngectomy

—**Laryngectomy: surgical removal of the larynx with or without neck resection to treat malignancies.**

## TYPES OF LARYNGECTOMY

- Partial laryngectomy: removal of half or more of the larynx
  —Supraglottic laryngectomy: hyoid bone, epiglottis, and false cords removed; negative effect on swallowing
  —Epiglottidectomy, cordectomy, anterior commissure resection
  —Vertical hemilaryngectomy: removal of one true cord, one false cord, arytenoid cartilage, one half thyroid cartilage; patient has hoarse but usable voice
  —Frontolateral and extended frontolateral partial laryngectomy
  —Partial laryngectomy laryngofissure: one vocal cord removed; patient has hoarse but usable voice
- Total laryngectomy: removal of larynx, hyoid bone, epiglottis, false and true cords, cricoid cartilage, two or three rings of trachea; patient has loss of voice as a result of trachealaryngectomy; swallowing is normal; procedure may be done with radical neck dissection

## PREPROCEDURAL TEACHING

- Review the physician's explanation of the procedure and the reason for it; encourage the patient to ask questions and to discuss any fears or anxieties. Discuss the need for informed consent for surgery and anesthesia.

### Review of Preprocedural Care

- Inform the patient that the skin will be cleansed with bactericidal soap or antiseptic solutions to remove bacteria.
- Discuss preprocedural tests: complete blood count and urinalysis to check for infection and bleeding.
- Tell the patient that NPO status must be maintained from midnight of the night before surgery.
- Provide preparatory instruction in suctioning (oral and tracheal) and wound care.
- Teach the patient to do own tube feedings.
- Review the use of a magic slate or paper and pencil, flash cards, or a communication board.
- Prepare the patient for permanent loss of speech if total laryngectomy is to be performed.
- Have a speech therapist visit the patient to discuss and plan for alternative means of speech.

### Review of Postprocedural Care

- Explain that the patient will be in the high Fowler's position to lessen edema, increase coughing and deep breathing, ease suctioning, and provide comfort.
- Explain that the patient will be given mechanical ventilation via a tracheostomy tube and that suctioning will be done frequently to maintain a clear airway for breathing.
- Discuss the importance of frequent deep breathing and coughing.
- Demonstrate the use of intermittent positive-pressure breathing devices and ultrasonic nebulization treatments.
- Explain the presence of pressure dressings and neck drainage tubes. Discuss the use of a nasogastric tube to assist with feedings (bolus or continuous drip based on patient tolerance).
- Explain that swallowing and speech rehabilitation will begin soon after surgery, with the need based on the type and extent of surgery.

## SIDE EFFECTS/COMPLICATIONS

- Hemorrhage
- Airway obstruction
- Infection
- Thoracic duct leakage
- Nerve injury

## HOME CARE

- Give both the patient and the caregiver *verbal* and *written* instructions. Provide them with the name and telephone number of a physician or nurse to call if questions arise. Use visual aids to assist in instruction.
- *General information*
  —Review any explanation about the procedure and any specific follow-up care.
- *Wound/incision care*
  —Instruct the patient and caregiver to inspect the incision site daily and to change the dressing using sterile supplies as demonstrated by the nurse.
- *Warning signs*
  —Review the signs and symptoms that should be reported to a physician or nurse.
    Infection of the stoma or incision: redness, drainage, pain, warm to touch, fever
    Dyspnea without exertion
    Difficulty swallowing
- *Special instructions*
  —Teach the patient to avoid voice strain and to whisper or use alternative methods of communication when the voice needs rest. If the voice is gone (total laryngectomy), have the patient work with a speech therapist to develop an alternative method of communicating.
- *Medications*
  —Provide pain management, encouraging the patient to use mild analgesics when possible (see Pain Management, p. 501).
- *Activity*
  —Remind the patient to plan frequent rest periods to avoid shortness of breath.
  —Assist the patient to begin self-care as soon as possible, including tracheostomy care (see p. 635) and taking food and fluids by mouth.

- *Diet*
  —Plan a diet with the patient and caregivers that will avoid the possibility of choking or aspirating. For example, the patient may initially receive tube feedings and progress to soft foods and liquids as the swallowing reflex returns.

## FOLLOW-UP CARE

- Stress the importance of regular follow-up visits. Make sure the patient has the necessary names and telephone numbers.

## PSYCHOSOCIAL CARE

- Encourage questions and verbalization of fear and anxieties regarding possible loss of the voice.

## REFERRALS

- Assist the patient to obtain referral services, supplies, and information about support groups from the Lost Cord Club/International Association of Laryngectomees, sponsored by the American Cancer Society.
- Arrange a reconstructive surgery consultation as needed.

# Leukemia

—Leukemia: malignant proliferation of abnormal immature white blood cells. These abnormal cells, which accumulate in the bone marrow, infiltrate body tissues and blood vessels and eventually cause malfunction by encroachment, hemorrhage, or infection. Acute leukemia, the most common type, affects children under 5 years of age and older adults. There are two forms: acute lymphocytic leukemia (ALL), which involves the lymphocytes and lymphoid organs, and acute myelocytic leukemia (AML), which affects adults over 65 years and involves the hematopoietic cells (granulocytes, erythrocytes, and platelets). In chronic leukemia the white blood cells produced are more mature and accumulate much more slowly. Chronic leukemia occurs in adults after age 20 and is classified as chronic lymphocytic leukemia (CLL) and chronic myelocytic (granulocytic) leukemia (CML).

## CAUSES/RISK FACTORS

- Idiopathic
- Chromosomal abnormality
- Overexposure to radiation, chemicals, drugs, or viruses

## SIGNS/SYMPTOMS

- Low-grade fever
- Pallor
- Chills
- Fatigue and weakness
- Gingivitis
- Easy bruising
- Nosebleeds
- Prolonged menstruation
- Acute indicators (crisis)
  —High fever
  —Diffuse petechiae
  —Bruising
  —Nosebleeds
  —Anorexia
  —Nausea and vomiting
  —Headaches
  —Visual disturbances
  —Weakness
  —Lethargy
  —Seizures

## COMPLICATIONS

- Hemorrhage
- Stroke, seizures
- Myocardial infarction
- Infection
- Organ failure (renal, liver)

## DIAGNOSTIC TESTS

- Describe each procedure, its purpose, and the normal feelings or sensations that are likely, as well as any preprocedural and postprocedural care.
  —White blood cell components elevated
      T cell (ALL)
      Blasts

Lymphocytes (ALL)
Auer rods (AML)
Phi bodies (AML)
—Reticulocytopenia
Normochromic (AML)
Normocytic
—Anemia
—Thrombocytopenia
—Prothrombin time and partial thromboplastin time: increased
—Serum copper: elevated
—Zinc: decreased
—Hypergammaglobulinemia (AML)
—Urine uric acid: elevated
—Bone marrow aspiration: proliferation of blast cells

## TREATMENT

*Medical*
- Therapy
  —Radiation therapy
    CLL: local irradiation of spleen lymph nodes
    CML: whole brain irradiation of leukopheresis
  —Blood and blood product transfusion
  —Fluid therapy
  —Chemotherapy
    ALL: vincristine sulfate, prednisone, and daunorubicin
      with or without L-asparaginase and methotrexate
    AML: daunorubicin hydrochloride, cytarabine, and thio-
      guanine
    CLL: chlorambucil or cyclophosphamide and prednisone
      to produce remission
    CML: busulfan and hydroxyurea (during stable chronic
      phase); daunorubicin, cytarabine, vincristine, prednisone,
      and thioguanine (during acute phase)
  —Analgesics

*Surgical*
- CML: splenectomy if destroying platelets; bone marrow transplantation

## HOME CARE

- Give both the patient and the caregiver *verbal* and *written* instructions. Provide them with the name and telephone number
  of a physician or nurse to call if questions arise.

- *General information*
  —Explain the particular leukemic disorder, possible causes, and precipitating factors.
  —Discuss disease progression and the possibility of exacerbations as well as remissions.
- *Warning signs*
  —Review the signs and symptoms that should be reported to a physician or nurse.
  
  Acute crisis: high fever, easy bruising, bleeding, lethargy, headaches, visual blurring
  
  Infection: high fever, cough, chills
  
  Bleeding: oozing of blood from gums and mucous membranes, ears, nose; bruising; petechiae
- *Special instructions*
  —Discuss measures for preventing infections.
  
  Avoid persons who are suspected of having infection.
  
  Avoid large crowds.
  
  Change air and furnace filters on a regular basis.
  
  Maintain good personal hygiene.
  
  Maintain good oral hygiene (brushing and flossing regularly; when mouth sores are present, use oral rinses and avoid brushing and flossing).
  —Discuss measures to take for bleeding.
  
  Apply direct pressure and ice to the area.
  
  Seek medical attention if unable to control the bleeding.
- *Medications*
  —Explain the purpose, dosage, schedule, and route of administration of any prescribed drugs, as well as side effects to report to the physician or nurse.
  —Discuss the side effects of particular chemotherapeutic agents and procedures for managing these symptoms (see Chemotherapy, p. 178).
- *Activity*
  —Encourage the patient to discuss allowances and limitations with respect to occupation, recreation, or activities.
  —Discuss the need to maintain activities as tolerated to prevent depression and physical debilitation.
  —Discuss bleeding precautions: use an electric razor and soft-bristled toothbrush; avoid activities that increase the risk of trauma or injury, such as contact sports and working with sharp tools and instruments.

—Encourage pacing of activities and the use of assistance to avoid overexertion.
* *Diet*
  —Explain the need for nutritious foods and liquids to 2500 ml per day.
  —Encourage the patient to continue normal eating patterns to enhance appetite.
  —Discuss alternative resources for delivery of meals to the home as appropriate (i.e., Meals on Wheels).
  —Teach the patient methods of maintaining nutritional intake during times of anorexia, nausea, vomiting, stomatitis, and other symptoms.

## FOLLOW-UP CARE

* Stress the importance of regular follow-up visits. Make sure the patient has the necessary names and telephone numbers.
* Discuss the importance of informing all medical and dental personnel of bleeding tendencies before any procedures (e.g., dental cleanings, injections).
* Instruct the patient to wear a Medic-Alert bracelet and carry an identification card with a list of medications at all times.

## PSYCHOSOCIAL CARE

* Encourage the verbalization of feelings and fears regarding the diagnosis.
* Discuss the need to maintain open communications with family, friends, the physician, and the nurse, to discuss needs and how they can be met.

## REFERRALS

* Encourage the use of formal cancer support and educational services: American Cancer Society, local cancer support groups.

# Liver Biopsy

—**Liver biopsy: percutaneous introduction of a needle into the liver to obtain tissue for pathologic examination and diagnosis of liver diseases.**

## INDICATIONS

- Abnormal liver function
- Cirrhosis
- Hepatitis
- Hepatomegaly or hepatosplenomegaly of unexplained origin
- Suspected malignancy of the liver
- Suspected systemic or infiltrative disease, such as sarcoidosis
- Routine evaluation for rejection in a transplanted liver

## PREPROCEDURAL TEACHING

- Review the physician's explanation of the procedure and the reason for it; encourage the patient to ask questions and to discuss any fears or anxieties. Discuss the need for informed consent.

### Review of Preprocedural Care

- Review preprocedural laboratory tests: type and crossmatch, prothrombin time, hemoglobin, hematocrit, and platelet count.
- Inform the patient of the need to be NPO for 4-8 hours before the biopsy.
- Explain that the patient will be asked to void before the biopsy.
- Discuss instructions for the patient during the biopsy.
  - —Instruct the patient to lie still during the biopsy. Local anesthetic will be administered.
  - —Instruct and coach the patient to hold his or her breath at the end of expiration to maximally elevate the liver.
  - —Stress the importance of sustaining expiration because failure to do so may result in puncture of the lung.

### Review of Postprocedural Care

- Explain that vital signs will be monitored, breath sounds will be auscultated for 6-8 hours, and the patient will be observed for complications.
- Inform the patient that sedatives and analgesics will be administered as ordered.
- Tell the patient that it will be necessary to lie on the right side for the first 6 hours to keep pressure on the site and remain on bed rest for 8-12 hours after the biopsy to minimize the risk of hemorrhage.
- Discuss the resumption of a normal diet.

## SIDE EFFECTS/COMPLICATIONS

- Hemorrhage
- Pneumothorax
- Peritonitis

## HOME CARE

- Give both the patient and the caregiver *verbal* and *written* instructions. Provide them with the name and telephone number of a physician or nurse to call if questions arise.
- *General information*
  —Review any explanation about the procedure and any specific follow-up care.
- *Warning signs*
  —Review the signs and symptoms that should be reported to a physician or nurse.
     Severe abdominal pain
     Abdominal distention and rigidity
     Rebound tenderness
     Nausea and vomiting
     Pallor
     Respiratory distress
     Fever
- *Medications*
  —Provide pain management, encouraging the patient to use mild analgesics when possible (see Pain Management, p. 501).
  —Advise the patient to avoid taking nonsteroidal antiinflammatory drugs (NSAIDs) and hepatotoxic medications.
  —Provide a list of NSAIDs and hepatotoxic medications to avoid.
- *Activity*
  —Instruct the patient to avoid strenuous activity or heavy lifting for the first day or as instructed.
- *Diet*
  —Advise the family or caregiver to provide assistance with eating as needed for 24 hours.
  —Explain that a regular diet can be resumed as prescribed by the physician for the underlying disease.

## FOLLOW-UP CARE

- Stress the importance of regular follow-up visits. Make sure the patient has the necessary names and telephone numbers.

# Lung Cancer
(Bronchogenic)

—Lung cancer: cancer of the lung, the leading cause of cancer-related deaths. Approximately 80% of lung tumors are linked to cigarette smoking. Contributing factors include exposure to carcinogenic substances and industrial air pollutants, genetic predisposition, and vitamin A deficiency. Types of lung cancer include non–small cell lung cancer, which is usually treated surgically and includes squamous cell (epidermoid), adenocarcinoma, and large cell undifferentiated, and small cell lung cancer, or oat cell cancer, which is aggressive but highly sensitive to chemotherapy and radiation therapy.

## SIGNS/SYMPTOMS
- Chronic cough
- Change in volume or odor of sputum
- Shortness of breath
- Dull chest pain
- Upper respiratory infection
- Fatigue
- Chest tightness
- Aching joints
- Later signs
  —Blood in sputum
  —Clubbing of fingers
  —Weight loss
  —Pleural effusion
  —Edema of neck and face
  —Paralysis of diaphragm
  —Hoarseness
  —Shoulder and arm pain or numbness

## COMPLICATIONS
- Superior vena cava syndrome
- Paraneoplastic syndromes: hypercalcemia, dermatomyositis, clubbed fingers, Cushing's syndrome, anemia, disseminated intravascular coagulation

## DIAGNOSTIC TESTS

- Describe each procedure, its purpose, and the normal feelings or sensations that are likely, as well as any preprocedural and postprocedural care.
    - —Bronchoscopy, mediastinoscopy, thoracentesis, and sputum cytology: to detect the presence of malignant cells
    - —Chest x-ray: to determine the size and location of the tumor
    - —Computed tomography scan and magnetic resonance imaging: to determine precise size and density and invasion or compression of blood vessels
    - —Tissue biopsy (scalene, supraclavicular node, bone marrow): to detect presence of malignant cells
    - —Pulmonary function tests: to determine impact of tumor on vital capacity
    - —Computed tomography, ultrasound scan, magnetic resonance imaging: to detect evidence of metastatic disease

## TREATMENT

*Medical*
- Therapy
    - —Radiation therapy
        External beam
        Interstitial/endobronchial bradytherapy with iridium-192
    - —Endobronchial laser therapy (photodynamic therapy)
    - —Sclerosis: treatment of pleural effusion
    - —Chemotherapy
        For advanced non–small cell lung cancer
        ○ VdP (vindesine, cisplatin)
        ○ VbP (vinblastine, cisplatin)
        ○ CAMP (cyclophosphamide, doxorubicin, methotrexate, procarbazine)
        ○ MVbP (mitomycin, vinblastine, cisplatin)
        ○ PtVP-16 (etoposide/VP-16, cisplatin)
        ○ CAP (cyclophosphamide, doxorubicin, cisplatin)
        ○ CBP (cyclophosphamide, bleomycin, cisplatin)
        ○ FOMi (5-fluorouracil, vincristine, mitomycin-C)
        For small cell lung cancer
        ○ CAV (cyclophosphamide, doxorubicin, vincristine)
        ○ CEA (cyclophosphamide, etoposide, doxorubicin)
        ○ CEV (cyclophosphamide, etoposide, vincristine)

○ EVAC (etoposide, vincristine, doxorubicin, cyclophosphamide)

Hansen's (cyclophosphamide, lomustine, vincristine, methotrexate)

Hansen's VP (cyclophosphamide, lomustine, vincristine, etoposide)

VP-16+P (etoposide, cisplatin)

—Biological response modifiers

—Monoclonal antibody KC4 for NSCLC

*Surgical*

• Indications

—Removal of limited primary or secondary tumor

—Extended resection for widespread disease

• Procedures

—Thoracotomy: surgical incision of chest wall, collection of biopsy specimen; limited pulmonary resection (segmental, wedge)

—Lobectomy: removal of lobe of lung and regional node dissection

—Pneumonectomy: surgical removal of an entire lung

—Extended resection: en bloc removal of portions of the chest wall, vertebral body, left atrium, and diaphragm

## HOME CARE

• Give both the patient and the caregiver *verbal* and *written* instructions. Provide them with the name and telephone number of a physician or nurse to call if questions arise.

• For surgery, see Thoracentesis, p. 625.

• For radiation therapy, see p. 559.

• For chemotherapy, see p. 178.

• *General information*

—Review the physician's explanation of the type of cancer and prescribed treatment. Use illustrations to identify the tumor's location.

—Encourage questions and verbalization of feelings and concerns about the disease prognosis and changes in life-style.

—Explain and outline prescribed treatment protocols, length of therapies, and expected outcomes and results.

—Stress the importance of not smoking or using tobacco products. Provide referral to smoking cessation programs as indicated.

- *Warning signs*
  —Review the signs and symptoms that should be reported to a physician or nurse.
    - Shoulder or arm pain
    - Difficulty in memory
    - Fatigue
    - Weight loss
    - Increased coughing or hemoptysis
- *Medications*
  —Explain the purpose, dosage, schedule, and route of administration of any prescribed drugs, as well as side effects to report to the physician or nurse.
- *Activity*
  —Discuss any limitations and restrictions necessary.
  —Discuss the importance of exercising to tolerance each day; alternate activities and periods of rest.
- *Diet*
  —Instruct the patient to eat a diet high in protein and calories.

## FOLLOW-UP CARE

- Stress the importance of regular follow-up visits. Make sure the patient has the necessary names and telephone numbers.

## REFERRALS

- Assist the patient to obtain referral services, such as the American Cancer Society and the American Lung Association, that can provide information, support groups, and equipment.

# Lupus Erythematosus, Systemic

—**Lupus erythematosus: systemic lupus erythematosus (SLE) is a chronic, autoimmune inflammatory disease of the connective tissues that produces biochemical and structural changes in skin, joints, and muscles. There is no characteristic clinical pattern. SLE usually involves multiple organs and is characterized by periods of exacerbation and remission. Women are 8 times more likely to have SLE than men and 15 times more likely in the childbearing years. SLE is most prevalent in**

Asians and African-Americans. Discoid lupus erythematosus (DLE) affects only the skin.

## RISK FACTORS

- Stress
- Streptococcal or viral infections
- Exposure to sunlight or ultraviolet light
- Immunization
- Pregnancy
- Abnormal estrogen metabolism

## SIGNS/SYMPTOMS

- Cutaneous lesions: raised, red, scaling rash on sun-exposed skin areas
- Facial erythema (butterfly rash)
- Fever
- Arthritis
- Mouth sores
- Light sensitivity
- Serositis (inflamed serous membranes)
- Anorexia
- Weight loss
- Malaise
- Fatigue
- Abdominal pain
- Irregular menstruation or amenorrhea

## COMPLICATIONS

- Stroke
- Cardiac arrest
- Renal failure
- Seizures
- Gangrene (fingers, toes)

## DIAGNOSTIC TESTS

- Describe each procedure, its purpose, and the normal feelings or sensations that are likely, as well as any preprocedural and postprocedural care.
    —Chest x-ray: pleurisy or lupus pneumonitis
    —Electrocardiogram: conduction defect, pericarditis
    —Electroencephalogram, brain scan, magnetic resonance imaging: to detect central nervous system involvement

—Renal biopsy: positive for renal disease

—Laboratory findings

    Serum complement (C3 and C4): decreased

    Complete blood count with differential: decreased red blood cells, white blood cells, and platelets

    Erythrocyte sedimentation rate: increased

    Electrophoresis: hypergammaglobulinemia

    Urine studies: positive for red blood cells, white blood cells, urine casts and sediment, and protein loss

    Lupus-specific blood tests

     ○ Antinuclear antibodies (anti-DNA, anti-Smith): positive

     ○ Anti–deoxyribonucleic acid: positive

     ○ Lupus erythematosus cell test: positive

## TREATMENT

*Medical*

- Drugs

  —Mild disease

    Nonsteroidal antiinflammatory drugs: aspirin for arthritis

    Corticosteroids: for skin lesions

    Antimalarials

  —Acute exacerbations

    Corticosteroids (prednisone)

    Cytotoxic agents (azathioprine, cyclophosphamide, methotrexate): to delay or prevent renal deterioration

    Antihypertensive drugs

    Warfarin: to prevent clotting caused by antiphospholipid antibodies

## HOME CARE

- Give both the patient and the caregiver *verbal* and *written* instructions. Provide them with the name and telephone number of a physician or nurse to call if questions arise.
- *General information*

  —Explain the disease process, causes, and precipitating factors. Stress the importance of avoiding factors that can trigger exacerbation.

- *Warning signs*

  —Review the signs and symptoms that should be reported to a physician or nurse.

    Fever

    Cough

Rash

Increase in chest, abdominal, muscle, or joint pain

- *Special instructions*
  —Explain that a woman with SLE can have a successful pregnancy, but pregnancies must be planned. Provide information and referrals for information about appropriate contraception.
  —Advise the patient to report any menstrual abnormalities.
  —Teach the patient to monitor for organ involvement.

    Renal: weight gain, hypertension

    Neurologic: personality changes, depression, drooping of eyelids, double vision

    Hematologic: bleeding (urine, stool, sputum)

    Skin: hair loss, petechiae, sores, pallor, bruising

    Immunologic: infection (fever, cough)

  —Teach skin care.

    Use only nonallergenic skin and hair care products.

    Avoid sun exposure; wear protective clothing (hats, long-sleeved shirts and blouses, pants) and use factor 15 sunscreen.

    Avoid hair dyes.

    Avoid fluorescent or ultraviolet lights.

  —Caution the patient to avoid infections by staying away from large crowds and persons known to have active infections.
  —Discuss the need for meticulous oral care to prevent infection.
- *Medications*
  —Explain the purpose, dosage, schedule, and route of administration of any prescribed drugs, as well as side effects to report to the physician or nurse.

    Corticosteroids (see Steroid Therapy, p. 608).

    Warfarin (see Anticoagulation Therapy, p. 42).

  —Advise the patient to avoid penicillin, sulfa, phenytoin, and oral contraceptives.
  —Warn against trying "miracle" drugs for arthritis without consulting the physician.
- *Activity*
  —Encourage the patient to discuss allowances and limitations with respect to occupation, recreation, or activities.
  —Encourage regular exercise to maintain range of motion and prevent contractures. Teach the patient to use heat packs to relieve joint pain and stiffness.
  —Stress the importance of avoiding physical exertion; discuss the need for planning regular rest periods and pacing activities.

—Encourage the use of assistive devices such as splints, walker, or cane, as indicated.
- *Diet*
  —Encourage a balanced diet with foods high in protein, vitamins, and iron to help maintain nutrition and prevent anemia.
  —Encourage small, frequent meals.

## FOLLOW-UP CARE

- Stress the importance of regular follow-up visits. Make sure the patient has the necessary names and telephone numbers.
- Discuss the importance of wearing a Medic-Alert bracelet and carrying an identification card at all times.

## PSYCHOSOCIAL CARE

- Stress the importance of avoiding emotional stress; discuss stress reduction methods: imagery, meditation, relaxation.

## REFERRALS

- Refer the patient to the Lupus Foundation of America and the Arthritis Foundation as indicated.

# Lyme Disease

—Lyme disease: an acute inflammatory disease transmitted by a tickborne spirochete via an animal vector (such as a deer). First described in 1975 in Lyme, Connecticut, the disease has been reported primarily in New York, New Jersey, and Connecticut but has also been reported in other states and sporadically in other countries. It can occur in all age groups. Flulike symptoms appear in recurrent episodes, lasting about 1 week and occurring at intervals from 1 to several weeks over a 2- to 3-year period. Other symptoms such as joint manifestations mimic diseases like arthritis. Lyme disease is also known as Lyme arthritis.

## SIGNS/SYMPTOMS

- Early stage
  —Spreading red, circular (target lesion) rash appearing at site of tick bites (axillae, thighs, groin)

—Flulike symptoms
  Headache
  Stiff neck
  Aches, pain
  Joint tenderness and swelling
  Fever, chills
  Nausea, vomiting
- Later stage
  —Palpitations, mild shortness of breath
  —Memory loss, confusion
  —Limb weakness, sensory loss
  —Bell's palsy
  —Arthritic symptoms
    Joint swelling
    Redness
    Limited movement

## COMPLICATIONS

- Arthritis
- Meningitis
- Encephalitis
- Cerebellar ataxia
- Cranial or peripheral neuropathies
- Cardiac: heart block, myocarditis, pericarditis

## DIAGNOSTIC TESTS

- Describe each procedure, its purpose, and the normal feelings or sensations that are likely, as well as any preprocedural and postprocedural care.
  —Serologic tests
    Enzyme-linked immunosorbent assay (ELISA): positive
    Indirect immunofluorescence assay: elevated
    Erythrocyte sedimentation rate: sometimes elevated
    Rheumatoid factor: negative

## TREATMENT

*Medical*
- Therapy (depends on symptoms and stage of illness)
  —Bed rest: to allow inflamed tissues to be rested and recover strength, especially with cardiac and neurologic involvement
  —Physical therapy: for muscle weakness, paralysis, arthritis

- Drugs
  —Antibiotics: oral in early stage, intravenous in later stage
  —Tetracycline in penicillin
  —Erythromycin
  —Analgesics, antipyretics: for pain and fever

## HOME CARE

- Give both the patient and the caregiver *verbal* and *written* instructions. Provide them with the name and telephone number of a physician or nurse to call if questions arise.
- *General information*
  —Explain the disease process and causes. Assist the patient to identify the possible site of the tick bite.
- *Warning signs*
  —Review the signs and symptoms of recurrence and complication that should be reported to a physician or nurse.
    Muscle weakness
    Altered mental functioning
    Excessive drowsiness
    Flulike symptoms
- *Special instructions*
  —Reinforce ways to prevent recurrence.
    Avoid tick-infested areas.
    Wear shirt tucked into pants and long pants tucked into boots when going into a wooded area.
    Apply insect repellent before going into the woods.
    Check body surfaces and clothing every 3-4 hours for ticks after being in the woods or infested areas.
    Remove tick immediately with tweezers or forceps, using a firm steady traction. Notify the physician or nurse of a tick bite.
    Detick dogs regularly to minimize tick population near residence.
- *Medications*
  —Explain the purpose, dosage, schedule, and route of administration of any prescribed drugs, as well as side effects to report to the physician or nurse.
  —Explain that antibiotic treatment will continue up to 20 days if symptoms persist.
  —Stress the importance of continuing medications as prescribed.

- *Activity*
    —Explain the need to avoid fatigue, to plan regular rest periods, and to maintain bed rest as ordered.
    —Instruct the patient in range-of-motion exercises to unaffected joints to maintain strength, but advise the patient to avoid overexertion.

**FOLLOW-UP CARE**

- Stress the importance of regular follow-up visits until recovery is complete.

---

# Lymphoma, Malignant
## (Non-Hodgkin's Lymphoma)

---

—**Lymphoma, malignant: neoplasms of the lymphoid tissues, which are classified by degree and differentiation of cellular content. Non-Hodgkin's lymphomas are characterized by spread to adjacent nodes and are likely to involve other organs. Non-Hodgkin's lymphoma is often widespread before detection. It affects adults 50 years of age and older and is more common than Hodgkin's lymphoma. The cause is largely unknown.**

**RISK FACTORS**

- Male, white, Jewish ancestry
- History of autoimmune disorders
- Immunosuppressant therapy (e.g., transplant patients)

**STAGING**

I. Single lymph node region
II. Two or more node regions limited to one side of the diaphragm
III. Disease on both sides of the diaphragm but limited to the lymph nodes or spleen
IV. Involvement of the bones, bone marrow, lung parenchyma, pleura, liver, skin, gastrointestinal tract, central nervous system, etc.

All stages are subclassified as A or B to describe the absence (A) or presence (B) of systemic symptoms.

**SIGNS/SYMPTOMS**

- Painless, swollen lymph nodes (lymphadenopathy): swelling and size fluctuate (early sign)
- Enlarged tonsils and adenoids
- Fever
- Night sweats
- Weight loss
- Lethargy
- Malaise
- Anorexia
- Edema or pain distal to swollen lymph nodes

**COMPLICATIONS**

- Cervical node enlargement: venous occlusion, neck edema, airway obstruction
- Mediastinal node enlargement: dyspnea, cough
- Inguinal node enlargement: dysuria, frequency, painful urination, low back pain
- Infections
- Fractures

**DIAGNOSTIC TESTS**

- Describe each procedure, its purpose, and the normal feelings or sensations that are likely, as well as any preprocedural and postprocedural care.
  - —Staging procedures
    Lymph node biopsy
    Chest x-ray
    Bone marrow biopsy
    Liver and spleen biopsy, scans
    Laparoscopy: to view peritoneal organs
    Computed tomography scans: bone, liver, spleen, abdomen
    Lymphangiography: to evaluate nodal involvement in abdomen and pelvis
  - —Laboratory tests
    Normocytic, normochromic anemia
    White blood cells with differential
    Erythrocyte sedimentation rate
    Hypercalcemia
    Alkaline phosphatase: increased (indicates bone involvement)

Copper: elevated
Lactate dehydrogenase: elevated
Antiglobulin (Coombs') test: positive
Hypoalbuminemia or hypergammaglobulinemia
Monoclonal immunoglobulin spikes

## TREATMENT

*Medical*
- Therapy
  —Radiation therapy for stages I, II, and III
  —Autologous bone marrow transplant: research being conducted to determine effectiveness
- Drugs
  —Chemotherapy in combination with radiation therapy for stages III and IV
  —Intrathecal chemotherapy if central nervous system involvement is present
  —Interferon, monoclonal antibodies: research being conducted as to effectiveness

*Surgical*
- Laparotomy
- Splenectomy

## HOME CARE

- Give both the patient and the caregiver *verbal* and *written* instructions. Provide them with the name and telephone number of a physician or nurse to call if questions arise.
- *General information*
  —Discuss non-Hodgkin's lymphoma, its possible causes, and contributing factors.
  —Discuss staging of the disease and the impact that various stages may have on daily living.
  —Discuss prescribed treatment (see Chemotherapy, p. 178, and Radiation Therapy, p. 559).
- *Warning signs*
  —Review the signs and symptoms of problems with the prosthetic implant that should be reported to a physician or nurse.
    Persistent fever
    Weight loss
    Enlarged lymph nodes
    Malaise

Decreased exercise tolerance

Infection (urinary tract, upper respiratory tract): cough, foul-smelling sputum, pain and burning with urination, frequency, urgency, hematuria, redness

- *Special instructions*
  —Discuss the importance of avoiding injury and trauma, which can cause bruising and bleeding.
  —Discuss the importance of avoiding large crowds and persons suspected of having an active infection.
- *Medications*
  —Explain the purpose, dosage, schedule, and route of administration of any prescribed drugs, as well as side effects to report to the physician or nurse.
  —Explain the importance of following the chemotherapy regimen and of reporting the side effects of therapy (e.g., sores in mouth and on tongue, anorexia, nausea, vomiting, malaise) to the physician or nurse.
- *Activity*
  —Encourage the patient to discuss allowances and limitation with respect to occupation, recreation, and activities.
  —Discuss the need for planned rest periods. Stress the importance of avoiding overexertion.
  — Teach stress reduction techniques.
- *Diet*
  —Stress the importance of a balanced, high-calorie, high-protein diet to maintain nutrition.
  —Encourage small, frequent meals.
  —Discuss methods to maintain hydration and nutrition during periods of stomatitis, nausea, vomiting, anorexia associated with therapy (sip fluids all day; drink nectar juices; avoid spicy, hot, and citrus-type foods).

## FOLLOW-UP CARE

- Stress the importance of regular follow-up visits for medical and laboratory evaluation. Make sure the patient has the necessary names and telephone numbers.
- Discuss the need to plan radiation therapy and chemotherapy sessions and to keep appointments.

## REFERRALS

- Refer the patient to the American Cancer Society and local support groups as indicated.

# Mitral Stenosis

—**Mitral stenosis: narrowing of the mitral valve because of calcification, fibrosis, or fusion of the leaflets.**

## CAUSES/CONTRIBUTING FACTORS/RISK FACTORS

- Rheumatic fever
- Female gender

## SIGNS/SYMPTOMS

- Shortness of breath with activity
- Weakness
- Fatigue
- Palpitations
- Angina
- Right ventricular failure (see Heart Failure, p. 352)
- Pulmonary edema

## COMPLICATIONS

- Atrial fibrillation
- Systemic embolism
- Bronchitis
- Pulmonary embolism
- Endocarditis
- Pulmonary hypertension

## DIAGNOSTIC TESTS

- Describe each procedure, its purpose, and the normal feelings or sensations that are likely, as well as any preprocedural and postprocedural care.
    - —Cardiac catheterization: to measure pulmonary and intracardiac pressures; to assess severity of the stenosis
    - —Chest x-ray: to show enlargement of the heart or pulmonary edema
    - —Echocardiography: to establish diagnosis and severity of the stenosis; to detect abnormal leaflet motion and enlargement of the left atrium

—Electrocardiogram: to reflect right ventricular hypertrophy or dysrhythmias

**TREATMENT**

*Medical*
- Drugs
  —Antibiotics
  —Diuretics
  —Digoxin
  —Beta blockers
  —Calcium channel blockers
  —Oral anticoagulants

*Surgical*
- Mitral commissurotomy
- Percutaneous mitral valve balloon valvuloplasty
- Mitral valvotomy
- Mitral valve replacement

**HOME CARE**

- Give both the patient and the caregiver *verbal* and *written* instructions. Provide them with the name and telephone number of a physician or nurse to call if questions arise. Use heart models or diagrams to assist in instruction.
- *General information*
  —Discuss the disease process, contributing factors, the cause of obstruction, and the signs and symptoms of disease progression. Show the patient the location of the affected valve and explain its role in the arterial circulation.
  —Instruct the patient for balloon angioplasty or surgery as recommended (see Valve Replacement, p. 671).
- *Warning signs*
  —Review the signs and symptoms that should be reported to a physician or nurse.
     Palpitations
     Chest pain
     Shortness of breath
     Dyspnea on exertion
     Swelling of ankles and feet
     Signs of emboli: syncope (faintness, muscle weakness, paresthesia, confusion)

- *Special instructions*
  —Explain the risk of endocarditis, discussing the causes and means of prevention. Tell the patient to alert the dentist or any other medical personnel (urologist, gynecologist) of valve disease.
  —Explain the importance of good oral hygiene and regular dental care. Explain the need for antibiotic prophylaxis before dental care and other invasive procedures (dilation and curettage, cystoscopy) for prevention.
  —Provide female patients with instruction regarding contraception and risk of pregnancy. Emphasize the importance of pregnancy planning. Tell the patient to avoid the use of estrogen-based contraceptives or intrauterine devices.
- *Medications*
  —Explain the purpose, dosage, schedule, and route of administration of any prescribed drugs, as well as side effects to report to the physician or nurse.
  —Provide specific instructions for a patient discharged with a prescription for anticoagulants (see p. 42).
- *Activity*
  —Stress the importance of avoiding strenuous activity (e.g., heavy lifting, pushing a car or changing a tire, engaging in competitive sports).
  —Encourage the patient to discuss allowances and limitations with respect to occupation, recreation, and activities.
  —Explain the need for moderate activity such as walking for conditioning.
  —Encourage frequent rest periods and avoidance of fatigue.
- *Diet*
  —Discuss the need to restrict salt intake to 3000 mg per day. Explain that further sodium restrictions may be necessary in the presence of heart failure.

## FOLLOW-UP CARE

- Stress the importance of regular follow-up visits for medical and laboratory evaluation. Make sure the patient has the necessary names and telephone numbers.
- Stress the importance of not smoking or using tobacco products. Provide information and referral to smoking cessation programs as necessary.

# Mitral Valve Insufficiency or Regurgitation

—**Mitral valve insufficiency or regurgitation: incomplete closure of valve that results when rigidity, calcification, and fusion of the valve leaflets with the chordae tendineae cause the leaflets to shorten and retract.**

## CAUSES/CONTRIBUTING FACTORS/RISK FACTORS
- Myocardial infarction
- Coronary artery disease
- Papillary muscle dysfunction
- Cardiomyopathy
- Inflammatory heart disorders
- Rheumatic fever
- Mitral valve prolapse
- Ruptured chordae tendineae or papillary muscle

## SIGNS/SYMPTOMS
- Pulmonary edema
- Fatigue
- Angina
- Palpitations
- Shortness of breath
- Anxiety

## COMPLICATIONS
- Heart failure
- Pulmonary hypertension
- Endocarditis
- Systemic emboli
- Pulmonary edema

## DIAGNOSTIC TESTS
- Describe each procedure, its purpose, and the normal feelings or sensations that are likely, as well as any preprocedural and postprocedural care.
  —Cardiac catheterization: to determine severity of insufficiency; to measure pulmonary and intracardiac pressures

- Echocardiography: to visualize the valves and determine the severity of the insufficiency
- Electrocardiogram; to detect evidence of past infarction and left ventricular hypertrophy; dysrhythmias
- Chest x-ray: to identify heart enlargement

## TREATMENT

*Medical*
- Drugs
  —Antibiotics
  —Digitalis
  —Oral anticoagulants
  —Vasodilators
  —Diuretics

*Surgical*
- Commissurotomy
- Valvuloplasty
- Valvotomy
- Mitral valve replacement

## HOME CARE

- Give both the patient and the caregiver *verbal* and *written* instructions. Provide them with the name and telephone number of a physician or nurse to call if questions arise.
- Use heart models or diagrams to assist in instruction.
- Instruct and prepare the patient for valve replacement as recommended (see p. 671).
- *General information*
  —Discuss the disease process and underlying and contributing factors. Show the patient the location of the affected valve.
- *Warning signs*
  —Review the signs and symptoms of disease progression that should be reported to a physician or nurse.
    Exertional dyspnea
    Orthopnea
    Paroxysmal nocturnal dyspnea
    Fatigue
    Palpitations
- *Special instructions*
  —Explain the risk of endocarditis, discussing the causes and means of prevention. Tell the patient to alert the dentist or

any other medical personnel (urologist, gynecologist) of valve disease.

—Explain the importance of good oral hygiene and regular dental care. Explain the need for antibiotic prophylaxis before dental care and other invasive procedures (dilation and curettage, cystoscopy) for prevention.

—Provide female patients with instruction regarding contraception and risk of pregnancy. Emphasize the importance of pregnancy planning.

—Stress the importance of not smoking or using tobacco products. Provide information and referral to smoking cessation programs as necessary.

- *Medications*
  —Explain the purpose, dosage, schedule, and route of administration of any prescribed drugs, as well as side effects to report to the physician or nurse.
- *Activity*
  —Stress the importance of avoiding strenuous activity.
  —Encourage the patient to discuss allowances and limitations with respect to occupation, recreation, and activities.
  —Explain the need for moderate activity.
  —Encourage frequent rest periods and avoidance of fatigue.
- *Diet*
  —Discuss the need to restrict salt intake. Explain that further sodium restrictions may be necessary in the presence of heart failure.

**FOLLOW-UP CARE**

- Stress the importance of regular follow-up visits. Make sure the patient has the necessary names and telephone numbers.

# Mitral Valve Prolapse

—**Mitral valve prolapse: a usually benign condition diagnosed in healthy people. One of the two mitral leaflets is displaced (prolapses) into the atrium during heart systole. In the majority of cases this does not impair valve closure. In rare cases** mitral regurgitation results. An estimated 2%-3% of the population has mitral valve prolapse. Most people are asymptomatic, although some report mild symptoms. The condition occurs in men and women 20-40 years of age but is more common in women.

## CAUSES
- A primary connective tissue abnormality
- A normal or abnormal variation

## SIGNS/SYMPTOMS
- Primarily asymptomatic
- Fatigue
- Palpitations
- Shortness of breath
- Panic attacks
- Anxiety
- Migraine (headache)
- Chest pain

## COMPLICATIONS
- Arrhythmias
- Mitral regurgitation
- Endocarditis
- Rarely sudden death

## DIAGNOSTIC TESTS
- Describe each procedure, its purpose, and the normal feelings or sensations that are likely, as well as any preprocedural and postprocedural care.
  - Echocardiogram: shows how the heart structures move, how large the heart chambers are, and the presence of valve deformities
  - Electrocardiogram: records how well the heart's electrical system is working; detects cardiac rhythm abnormalities and identifies cardac hypertrophy
  - Holter monitor or ambulatory electrocardiogram: to record the heart's activities as the patient follows a normal routine; correlates symptoms with actual cardiac events and the patient's activities
  - Treadmill electrocardiogram recording during exercise: to

identify the heart's response to exercise; to diagnose the cause of chest pain and identify cardiac arrhythmias
—Tilt table test: to check blood pressure and heart rate in an upright and prone position; to identify neurogenic cause of syncope

## TREATMENT

*Medical*
• Drugs
—Beta blockers: to slow heart rate and prevent headache
—Calcium channel blockers: to reduce workload of the heart

## HOME CARE

• Give both the patient and the caregiver *verbal* and *written* instructions. Provide them with the name and telephone number of a physician or nurse to call if questions arise.
• Use visual aids or heart models to help the patient understand the location of the mitral valve and its role in the heart function.
• *Warning signs*
—Review the signs and symptoms associated with this condition and the need to report any change in the condition to a physician or nurse.
• *Special instructions*
—Describe the condition and explain that in the majority of cases the diagnosis is based on a "clicking" sound heard during a routine examination. Tell the patient that the clicking sound alone is an otherwise asymptomatic person is usually benign and requires no treatment. Provide reassurance that the patient can expect to live a perfectly normal life.
—Instruct an asymptomatic patient that the disease is not life threatening and that symptoms are usually treated with beta blockers.
—Provide specific instruction for a patient with mitral regurgitation (see p. 445).
—Assist the patient to identify precipitating factors of palpitations, anxiety, or panic attacks.
—Suggest ways of reducing stress levels and practice relaxation techniques to prevent the occurrence of symptoms.
• *Activity*
—Inform the patient that full activity is permitted with no restrictions if the patient feels well and does not have significant mitral regurgitation.

- *Diet*
  —Explain that a regular diet can be followed but that patients with palpitations and anxiety should avoid caffeine beverages and use of tobacco products.

**FOLLOW-UP CARE**

- Explain to the patient the importance of notifying the dentist, urologist, and gynecologist of mitral valve prolapse only if prescribed by a physician. Generally, asymptomatic patients with simple prolapse are exempt from this notification, but emphasize that the patient should check with the physician for specific instructions. Make sure that the patient has the necessary phone numbers.

# Multiple Sclerosis
(Disseminated Sclerosis)

—**Multiple sclerosis: a chronic, progressive neurologic disease characterized by scattered demyelination of nerve fibers in the brain and spinal cord. Multiple sclerosis affects women slightly less often than men, with onset of symptoms commonly occurring between 20 and 40 years of age. The symptoms, severity, duration, and prognosis of multiple sclerosis vary. Remission and exacerbation of symptoms occur with multiple sclerosis. The exact cause is unknown.**

**CAUSES/CONTRIBUTING FACTORS/RISK FACTORS**

- Autoimmune processes
- Viral infection
- Allergic reactions to infections
- Familial tendencies
- Cool, temperate climates

**SIGNS/SYMPTOMS**

- Sensory impairment: numbness and tingling
- Loss of joint sensation and proprioception
- Loss of sense of position

- Fatigue, especially after a hot bath or shower
- Facial palsy
- Weakness of lower extremities
- Poor coordination: staggering gait, tremors, spasticity of extremities, ataxia (lack of muscle coordination)
- Dizziness
- Visual disturbances: diplopia, blurred vision, optic neuritis (pain with eye movement), decreased visual field, nystagmus, visual clouding
- Slurred speech
- Muscular spasms
- Difficulty chewing and swallowing
- Mental changes: mood swings, depression, euphoria, irritability, inattention, apathy, poor judgment
- Fecal or urinary incontinence or retention
- Impotence

## COMPLICATIONS

- Respiratory failure
- Neurologic deficits: paralysis
- Urinary tract infections
- Sexual dysfunction
- Contractures

## DIAGNOSTIC TESTS

- Describe each procedure, its purpose, and the normal feelings or sensations that are likely, as well as any preprocedural and postprocedural care.
    —Cerebrospinal fluid sampling: to evaluate levels of protein, oligoclonal bands of immunoglobulin G, gamma globulin, and lymphocytes in the cerebrospinal fluid
    —Magnetic resonance imaging: to reveal the presence of plaques and demyelination; the test of choice when multiple sclerosis is suspected
    —Computed tomography scan: to reveal the presence of plaques and demyelination
    —Positron emission tomography: to detect areas of altered cerebral glucose metabolism
    —Evoked potential studies: to evaluate the integrity of certain nerve pathways
    —Electroencephalogram: to assess for abnormal slowing of brain activity

## TREATMENT

*Medical*
- Therapy
  —Physical therapy
  —Occupational therapy
  —Rehabilitation
  —Bowel and bladder retraining
  —Speech therapy
  —Nutritional counseling
  —Counseling, including sexual counseling
  —Bed rest during acute exacerbation
  —Assistive devices: braces, walkers, wheelchairs, splints
  —Plasmapheresis: to remove antimyelin antibodies; provides short-term improvement only
- Drugs
  —Antiinflammatory agents
  —Pituitary hormones
  —Corticosteroids
  —Muscle relaxants
  —Smooth muscle relaxants or stimulants
  —Beta-adrenergic blockers
  —Antianxiety and antidepression agents
  —Immunosuppressive agents

*Surgical*
- Peripheral nerve block with rhizotomy or contralateral thalamotomy

## HOME CARE

- Give both patient and caregiver *verbal* and *written* instructions. Provide the name and telephone number of a physician or nurse to call if questions arise. Use visual aids in instruction.
- *General information*
  —Explain and discuss the development of multiple sclerosis, causes or contributing factors, care, and treatment.
  —Discuss factors that exacerate the symptoms of multiple sclerosis, and emphasize the importance of avoiding them.
    Overexertion
    Extreme hot and cold temperatures, such as with bath water or weather
    Fever
    Emotional stress
    High humidity

Pregnancy

Infections

- *Warning signs*
  —Review the signs and symptoms that should be reported to a physician or nurse.

  Disease progression: memory deficits, confusion, disorientation, scanning speech (slow speech with pauses between syllables)

  Urinary tract infection: urinary frequency, urgency, retention, or incontinence; suprapubic distention; pain or burning with urination; malodorous urine; cloudy or bloody urine; fever; chills; flank pain

  Flu or cold symptoms: fever, chills, fatigue

- *Special instructions*
  —Advise the patient to regulate bath water temperature because of the loss of sense of temperature.

  —Stress the importance of avoiding persons with upper respiratory infections.

  —Assist the patient in obtaining appropriate devices, such as assistive aids for ambulation and self-care. Assist the patient to identify and correct hazards in the home: remove small scatter rugs, arrange furniture to provide a clear pathway, provide rails for support, provide a ramp for wheelchairs.

  —Refer the patient to a bladder retraining program. Teach intermittent self-catheterization and Credé maneuver.

  —Suggest incontinence pads or garment protectors for incontinence. Advise the patient to establish regular bowel routines.

  —Advise the patient to avoid constipation.

- *Medications*
  —Explain the purpose, dosage, schedule, and route of administration of any prescribed drugs, as well as side effects to report to a physician or nurse.

  For corticosteroids and adrenocorticotropic hormones: perform and record daily weights; take medication with food, milk, or buffering agents; avoid aspirin or caffeine while taking these medications; do not discontinue medication abruptly; assist patient to plan a diet high in potassium and low in sodium; provide a list of specific foods that are high in potassium and low in sodium; report anorexia, nausea, muscle weakness (signs and symptoms of potassium deficiency), abrupt weight gain, and black, tarry stools to the physician or nurse.

**M**

For baclofen or dantrolene (muscle relaxants): take medications with food, milk, or buffering agents; avoid activities that require alertness; for patients with diabetes mellitus, monitor blood glucose levels and adjust insulin dosage as needed; advise the family to provide assistance and support for ambulation initially after the patient takes medication; advise the patient to avoid exposure to the sun and to use sunscreens when exposure is unavoidable; report fever, jaundice, dark urine, clay-colored stools, and pruritus (signs and symptoms of hepatitis) and severe diarrhea to the physician or nurse.

For cholinergic and anticholinergic agents: suggest sugarless gum or hard candy to relieve mouth dryness; advise slow position changes to prevent dizziness and fainting.

—Stress the importance of not taking over-the-counter medications without consulting the physician.

- *Activity*
  —Encourage the patient to discuss allowances and limitations with respect to occupation, recreation, or activities.
  —Encourage the patient to resume activities of daily living, work, chores, and recreational activites as tolerated and to take regular rest breaks.
  —Stress the importance of avoiding fatigue and overwork.
  —Provide diversional activities with planned rest periods.
  —Advise the family or caregiver to assist with activities of daily living but to allow independence as much as possible.
  —Teach the family or caregiver to support the patient when ambulating.
  —Teach the patient to walk with a wide base.
  —Instruct the patient to perform stretching exercises and range-of-motion exercises to reduce muscle spasms and tightness.
  —Demonstrate range-of-motion exercises to the family or caregiver and instruct them to assist the patient with exercises.
  —Instruct the patient and caregivers on proper skin care and positioning if the patient is confined to bed or wheelchair.
  —Advise the patient that sleeping in a prone position may help decrease spasms in hips and knees.
- *Diet*
  —Assist the patient to plan a high-fiber diet or a soft, semisolid diet as ordered.
  —Encourage the patient to drink plenty of fluids, up to 3 liters per day, unless contraindicated.

**FOLLOW-UP CARE**

- Stress the importance of regular follow-up visits with the physician and physical, occupational, and rehabilitation therapists. Make sure that the patient has the necessary phone numbers.
- Assist the patient to obtain a Medic-Alert bracelet and identification card listing diagnosis, medications, and treatment.

**PSYCHOSOCIAL CARE**

- Encourage the patient to maintain socialization with significant others.
- Encourage the patient to verbalize anxiety and concerns related to disease, disability, body image changes, and feelings of powerlessness, grief, and loss.
- Encourage caregivers to verbalize concerns related to disease, disability, and effect on life-style.

**REFERRALS**

- Refer the patient to a social worker for further support and counseling.
- Refer the patient for psychotherapy.
  - —Males: for sexual dysfunction, primarily impotence, caused by multiple sclerosis
  - —Females: for birth control and reproductive counseling, since pregnancy may exacerbate symptoms
- Refer to home health or custodial care services, if indicated.
- Assist the patient and caregivers to obtain referral to community resources, local support groups, and the National Multiple Sclerosis Society, 733 3rd Ave., Third Floor, New York, NY 10017, (212) 986-3240.

# Muscular Dystrophy

—**Muscular dystrophy: a hereditary, degenerative neuromuscular disease characterized by chronic, progressive wasting and weakness of the voluntary muscles. In muscular dystrophy, defective muscle cells leak proteins and other molecules. Muscle fibers undergo degenerative changes and are replaced** by connective and fatty tissues, which make muscles appear hypertrophic or pseudohypertrophic (varying in size). The different types of muscular dystrophy vary in the age at onset, rate of symptom progression, and clinical manifestations. The types include Duchenne (pseudohypertrophic); limb-girdle; facioscapulohumeral; myotonic; and Becker. Muscular dystrophy occurs more commonly in males than females and affects both children and young adults.

## SIGNS/SYMPTOMS

- Hypertrophied muscles
- Progressive, bilateral weakness of voluntary muscles
- Difficulty walking, running, or climbing stairs
- Waddling gait
- Difficulty raising from supine position
- Lordosis
- Weakness of facial, neck, oropharyngeal, shoulder, or pelvic girdle muscles
- Mental retardation

## COMPLICATIONS

- Neuromuscular deficits
- Cardiac failure
- Respiratory failure

## DIAGNOSTIC TESTS

- Describe each procedure, its purpose, and the normal feelings or sensations that are likely, as well as any preprocedural and postprocedural care.
    —Serum creatine kinase: to detect marked elevation
    —Electromyography: to detect myopathic changes
    —Muscle biopsy: to detect degenerative and myopathic changes
    —Electrocardiogram: to detect changes in cardiac musculature as disease progresses

## TREATMENT

*Medical*
- Therapy
    —Physical therapy
    —Assistive devices, such as ambulation aids
    —Muscle stretching and resistive exercises

## HOME CARE

- Give both the patient and the caregiver *verbal* and *written* instructions. Provide them with the name and telephone number of a physician or nurse to call if questions arise. Use visual aids in instruction.
- *General information*
  —Explain and discuss the progression of muscular dystrophy, causes, management of progressive disabilities, and steps to take to prevent them. Explain that there is no cure for muscular dystrophy; interventions are supportive.
- *Warning signs*
  —Review the signs and symptoms that should be reported to a physician or nurse.
    Difficulty chewing or swallowing
    Cardiac or respiratory distress
- *Special instructions*
  —Assist the patient in obtaining appropriate devices, such as aids for ambulation and self-care activities.
  —Assist the patient to identify adaptations in the home environment, such as bed trapezes, handrails, raised toilet seats, and widened doorways and ramps for wheelchairs.
  —Instruct the patient and family on proper skin care and positioning, if the patient is confined to a bed or wheelchair.
  —Provide instruction in pain management techniques to deal with chronic pain: visualization, guided imagery, meditation, relaxation, and biofeedback.
- *Medications*
  —Explain the purpose, dosage, schedule, and route of administration of any prescribed drugs, as well as side effects to report to a physician or nurse.
- *Activity*
  —Encourage the patient to discuss allowances and limitations with respect to occupation, recreation, or activities.
  —Stress the importance of performing stretching and resistive exercises to preserve range of motion, prevent or minimize contractures, decrease atrophy, and promote mobility.
  —Instruct the patient to avoid moving a joint beyond the point of resistance.
  —Instruct the patient to avoid applying force; movements should be gentle and slow.

—Instruct the patient to stop exercises when feeling pain.

—Teach the patient to avoid factors that increase spasticity: fatigue, tightening of muscles, maintaining a position too long, cold temperatures.

—Explain that physical inactivity may contribute to weight gain.

• *Diet*

—Assist the patient to plan a balanced diet with fruits, vegetables, milk, poultry, and fish.

—Advise smaller, frequent meals.

## FOLLOW-UP CARE

• Stress the importance of regular follow-up visits with the physician and physical, occupational, and rehabilitation therapists. Make sure that the patient has the necessary phone numbers.

• Assist the patient to obtain a Medic-Alert bracelet and identification card listing diagnosis, medications, and treatment.

## PSYCHOSOCIAL CARE

• Assist the patient to establish realistic goals and identify alternative methods for communication and mobility when physical disabilities increase.

• Encourage the patient to verbalize anxiety and concerns related to disease, disability, loss of mobility, body image changes, and feelings of grief.

• Encourage caregivers to avoid overprotectiveness.

• Encourage decision making and promote independence in the patient.

• Encourage caregivers to verbalize concerns related to disease, disability, and effect on their life-style.

## REFERRALS

• Refer the patient to a social worker for further support and counseling, if appropriate.

• Assist the patient and caregivers to obtain referral to community resources, local support groups, home health care, custodial care services, and the Muscular Dystrophy Association.

• Refer the patient and caregivers to genetic counseling so that familial carriers of the gene can be identified and affected infants can be identified in utero via amniocentesis.

# Myasthenia Gravis

—Myasthenia gravis: an autoimmune neuromuscular disease that produces sporadic but progressive weakness exacerbated by exercise and improved by rest and anticholinergic drugs. Myasthenia gravis is a chronic disorder that follows an unpredictable course of recurring exacerbation and remission. No cure is known. Myasthenia gravis occurs as a result of loss of the acetylcholine receptors at the postsynaptic neuromuscular junction. Although it may occur at any age, between 20 and 40 years females are more commonly affected and after 50 years men are more commonly affected.

## SIGNS/SYMPTOMS

- Eye muscles
  - —Ocular palsy
  - —Ptosis (unilateral or bilateral)
  - —Diplopia
- Facial muscles
  - —Masklike expression and mobility (weakness) of face
  - —Weak voice that may fade to a whisper
  - —Dysphagia
  - —Choking
  - —Aspiration, impaired swallowing
  - —Drooling
  - —Nasal speech
- Neck muscles
  - —Head bobbing up and down
- Respiratory muscles
  - —Shallow respirations
  - —Breathlessness
  - —Respiratory weakness
- Other muscles
  - —Stress incontinence
  - —Anal sphincter weakness
  - —Sexual impairment

- *Myasthenic crisis:* rapid or significant worsening of ocular, bulbar, and generalized weakness; urgent threat is to the respiratory system; may require mechanical ventilatory support
  —Respiratory distress
  —Tachycardia
  —Tachypnea
  —Generalized muscular weakness
  —Extreme fatigue
  —Anxiety
  —Restlessness
  —Irritability
  —Facial weakness
  —Dysphagia
  —Inability to chew
  —Elevated temperature
  —Ptosis
  —Speech impairment
  —Hypertension
- *Cholinergic crisis:* secondary to overmedication in relation to muscular requirement; may mimic myasthenic crisis; *only* cholinergic crisis will produce excessive drooling and twitching or cramping of muscles
  —Respiratory distress
  —Vertigo
  —Blurred vision
  —Sweating
  —Lacrimation
  —Salivation
  —Anorexia
  —Dysarthria
  —Dysphasia
  —Abdominal cramps, diarrhea
  —Nausea and vomiting
  —Muscular spasms or cramps
  —Generalized muscle weakness
  —Dyspnea and wheezing
  —Bradycardia
  —Hypotension

**COMPLICATIONS**

- Myasthenic crisis and cholinergic crisis
- Aspiration of secretions, choking
- Pneumonia
- Respiratory failure

**DIAGNOSTIC TESTS**

- Describe each procedure, its purpose, and the normal feelings or sensations that are likely, as well as any preprocedural and postprocedural care.
    - —Edrophonium (Tensilon) test: injection produces a sudden improvement in muscle function; also used to differentiate a myasthenic crisis from a cholinergic crisis (worsens if crisis is cholinergic)
    - —Electromyography: to differentiate nerve disorders
    - —Nerve conduction studies: to measure the speed at which electrical impulses travel along a nerve
    - —Chest x-ray or computed tomography scan: to identify a thymoma

**TREATMENT**

- Appropriate health care is usually on an outpatient basis, with the inpatient setting used for myasthenic or cholinergic crisis. Medical management of myasthenia gravis is difficult and best handled by a specialist in that field. It is important to be alert for myasthenic crisis and cholinergic crisis, which may often be quite difficult to differentiate, and which can be made dramatically worse by overmedication.
- Establish an accurate neurologic and repiratory baseline: tidal volume, vital capacity, and inspiratory force.

*Medical*

- Therapy
    - —Plasmapheresis: done before thymectomy, during a respiratory crisis, or as an adjunct treatment to reduce drug dosages
- Drugs
    - —Anticholinesterase
    - —Corticosteroids
    - —Pituitary hormones

*Surgical*

- Thymectomy
- Tracheostomy

## HOME CARE

- Give both the patient and the caregiver *verbal* and *written* instructions. Provide them with the name and telephone number of a physician or nurse to call if questions arise.
- *General information*
  —Discuss and describe the disease process and factors that can exacerbate symptoms: infection, stress, and surgery.
- *Warning signs*
  —Review the signs and symptoms of impending myasthenic or cholinergic crisis (see above; primarily increased muscle weakness, respiratory distress, difficulty talking and chewing) that should be reported to a physician or nurse.
- *Special instructions*
  —Assure the patient that an experienced patient with myasthenia gravis is often the best judge of his or her treatment requirements.
  —Advise and assist the patient in obtaining necessary supportive equipment and devices as the disease advances (e.g., suctioning equipment, adaptive devices).
  —Advise the patient to use an eye patch over the affected eye or a frosted lens to improve vision if diplopia persists.
  —Instruct the patient with ptosis to apply artificial tears to keep the corneas moist and free of abrasions.
- *Medications*
  —Explain the purpose, dosage, schedule, and route of administration of any prescribed drugs, as well as side effects to report to a physician or nurse.
  —Teach the patient to recognize adverse effects of anticholinesterase drugs: headache, weakness, sweating, abdominal cramps, nausea, vomiting, excessive salivation, and bronchospasm.
  —Teach the patient to recognize adverse effects of corticosteroids: decreased or blurred vision; increased thirst; frequent urination; rectal bleeding, burning, and itching; restlessness; depression.
- *Activity*
  —Advise the patient to plan daily activities to coincide with energy peaks, which usually occur in the morning or after a nap.
  —Stress the importance of rest periods throughout the day.
  —Advise the patient to avoid strenuous exercise, stress, infection, needless exposure to the sun or cold weather, and exposure to people with infections (e.g., upper respiratory infections).

—Explain that periodic remissions, exacerbations, and day-to-day fluctuations are common.

• *Diet*

—Teach the patient that as swallowing becomes more difficult, soft, semisolid foods (applesauce, mashed potatoes) instead of liquids will lessen the risk of choking and eating warm (not hot) foods can ease swallowing. Instruct the patient to eat slowly, cut food into small pieces, and chew thoroughly.

—Advise the patient to avoid alcohol because it increases weakness.

## FOLLOW-UP CARE

• Stress the importance of regular follow-up visits. Make sure that the patient has the necessary phone numbers.

• Assist the patient to obtain a Medic-Alert bracelet and identification card listing diagnosis, medications, and treatment.

## PSYCHOSOCIAL CARE

• Stress the importance of psychologic support. Encourage the patient to verbalize concerns, fears, and feelings about the disease process.

## REFERRALS

• Provide information on home health referrals as indicated.

• Encourage contact with a national support group and provide the following address for the patient to obtain printed materials and other forms of family support information: Myasthenia Gravis Foundation, 222 So. Riverside Plaza, Suite 1540, Chicago, IL 60606, (312) 258-0522. The Muscular Dystrophy Association is the umbrella organization for myasthenia gravis research and can provide materials and clinical services. Their address is: Muscular Dystrophy Association, 3300 E. Sunrise Drive, Tucson, AZ 85718-3208, (800) 572-1717.

# Myelogram

—Myelogram: study in which contrast material is injected through a lumbar or cisternal puncture to visualize the spinal canal and nerve roots. Myelography aids in the diagnosis of spinal stenosis or obstruction within the spinal canal caused by a ruptured or herniated nucleus pulposus. The entire canal from lumbar to cervical area can be examined. The *myelogram* is a roentgenographic procedure in which a needle is inserted into a disk space below the spinal cord and 2-15 ml of spinal fluid is removed. A contrast solution or air is injected and distributed to the various tissues and structures to be examined, and x-rays are taken frequently. Flow of the solution depends on the tilt of the table and patient position. With the needle in place, the patient is placed in the prone position on a tilt table with the head down. A foot support and shoulder brace or harness keeps the patient from sliding. Fluoroscopy shows flow of the contrast solution. The procedure takes 45 minutes and requires that the patient be positioned on the stomach on a tilt table to permit flow of the dye. In a *computed tomography myelogram* a water-soluble contrast material is instilled into the subarachnoid space. Films are taken at the time of contrast injection and followed by computed tomography scan of the appropriate regions. This procedure is particularly useful in cervical spondylosis in which magnetic resonance imaging may not demonstrate detail of an osteophyte or herniated disk.

## INDICATIONS

- Severe back pain
- Localized signs and symptoms of spinal cord injury or disease

## PREPROCEDURAL TEACHING

- Review the physician's explanation of the procedure and the reason for it; encourage the patient to ask questions and to discuss any fears or anxieties. Explain the need for informed consent.

### Review of Preprocedural Care

- Identify any possible allergies, particularly to iodine.
- Verify the list of current medications; tell the patient to stop anticoagulants at the appropriate time as determined by the physician.
- Review laboratory tests: complete blood count, prothrombin time/INR if the patient has previously received anticoagulation therapy.
- Explain the need to avoid phenothiazines, tricyclic antidepres-

sants, central nervous system stimulants, and amphetamines, which could decrease the seizure threshold.

- Inform the patient of the need for NPO status for food and fluids for 4 hours before the procedure.
- Discuss the type of contrast material that will be used and explain that a patient receiving water-soluble contrast should be well hydrated.
- Inform the patient that baseline vital signs and neurologic assessment will be performed.
- Explain that the patient will be tilted into an up-and-down position on a table so that the dye can properly fill the spinal canal and provide adequate visualization of the desired area.
- Instruct the patient to empty the bladder and bowel before the procedure.
- Explain the importance of lying still during the procedure.

**Review of Postprocedural Care**

- Explain that after the procedure the patient will be closely monitored for 24 hours or until discharge for signs of meningeal irritation or seizure activity.
- Tell the patient that vital signs and neurologic status will be checked every 30 minutes for 2 hours, every 60 minutes for the next 2 hours, and every 4 hours for the next 24 hours.
- Discuss the need for proper positioning after the procedure.
  —If air myelography is done, the patient is positioned with the head lower than the trunk to prevent air from gravitating to the cerebral space and causing headaches. This position should be maintained for 48 hours to allow absorption of the air. Then the head is elevated.
  —If water-soluble contrast is used, the patient is positioned upright at a 30-45 degree angle for 12 hours, then bed rest upright or flat is maintained for 12 hours.
  —If oil-based contrast is used, the patient is kept flat for 8-12 hours.
- Explain that there will be pain at the puncture site.

**SIDE EFFECTS/COMPLICATIONS**

- Headache
- Herniation of the brain
- Meningitis
- Seizures

- Allergic reaction to iodinated dye: mild flushing, itching, urticaria, life-threatening anaphylaxis

**HOME CARE**

- Give both the patient and the caregiver *verbal* and *written* instructions. Provide them with the name and telephone number of a physician or nurse to call if questions arise.
- *General information*
  —Review the physician's explanation of the procedure and any initial findings.
- *Warning signs*
  —Review the signs and symptoms that should be reported to a physician or nurse.
    Meningeal irritation: fever, stiff neck, occipital headache, photophobia
    Nausea and vomiting
    Severe headache
    Change in level of consciousness
    Seizure activity
- *Special instructions*
  —Advise the patient to lower the bed to the flat position to relieve a headache; inform the patient that mild analgesics may be ordered for persistent pain.
  —Advise the patient not to take phenothiazines for nausea and vomiting; these agents can increase symptoms of toxicity.
  —Explain the need to increase fluid intake to enhance excretion of the dye and to replace cerebrospinal fluid, if not contraindicated.

# Myocarditis

—**Myocarditis: an inflammatory process of the myocardium affecting portions or all of the heart muscle. It may be acute or chronic and affects persons of any age. Recovery is usually complete, but the disease may cause myofibril disarray, leading to ventricular failure. Myocarditis may be uncomplicated and self-limiting.**

## CAUSES

- Viral infections
- Bacterial infections
- Rheumatic fever
- Postcardiotomy syndrome
- Radiation therapy
- Chemical poisons, such as alcohol
- Parasitic infections

## SIGNS/SYMPTOMS

- Fatigue
- Dyspnea
- Palpitations
- Fever
- Chest pain

## COMPLICATIONS

- Dilated cardiomyopathy
- Arrhythmias
- Thromboembolism

**M**

## DIAGNOSTIC TESTS

- Describe each procedure, its purpose, and the normal feelings or sensations that are likely, as well as any preprocedural and postprocedural care.
    —Blood tests
        Cardiac enzymes
        Elevated antibody titers
        Elevated cardiac isoenzymes
        White blood cells
        Erythrocyte sedimentation rate
    —Cultures: throat, stool
    —Electrocardiogram
    —Endomyocardial biopsy

## TREATMENT

*Medical*

- Therapy
    —Treatment of underlying infection
    —Bed rest: to decrease myocardial oxygen demand

## HOME CARE

- Give both the patient and the caregiver *verbal* and *written* instructions. Provide them with the name and telephone number of a physician or nurse to call if questions arise.
- *General information*
  —Review the disease process, explaining the cause and prescribed treatment. Explain that medical treatment is aimed at treating underlying cause and preventing and treating complications.
- *Warning signs*
  —Review the signs and symptoms that should be reported to a physician or nurse.
    Chest pain that persists and is unrelated to exertion
    Shortness of breath at rest, on exertion, or at night
    Swelling of feet or ankles
    Palpitations
- *Medications*
  —Explain the purpose, dosage, schedule, and route of administration of any prescribed drugs, as well as side effects to report to a physician or nurse.
  —Review the symptoms of digitalis toxicity if the patient is discharged with a prescription for digitalis.
- *Activity*
  —Instruct the patient to restrict activities and to resume normal activities slowly or as directed to reduce work of the heart and promote healing.
  —Tell the patient to take regular rest periods during the day.
  —Stress the importance of avoiding physical exertion and competitive sports.
  —Advise the patient not to exercise or do demanding physical activities when a cold, flu, or other infection is present.
- *Diet*
  —Instruct the patient to follow a low-salt diet, especially if the patient has signs of heart failure.

## FOLLOW-UP CARE

- Stress the importance of regular follow-up visits. Make sure that the patient has the necessary phone numbers.

# Nephrectomy

—**Nephrectomy: surgical removal of part or all of a kidney.**
*Radical nephrectomy,* **usually done for a malignant tumor, is**
**removal of the entire kidney, surrounding tissue and fat, ad-**
**renal gland, part of the ureter, and the lymph nodes.**

## INDICATIONS

- Malignant tumor
- Polycystic kidney disease
- Donation of a kidney
- Trauma
- Large stones
- Hydronephrosis
- Congenital deformity
- Chronic pyelonephritis
- Vascular disease or narrowed renal arteries

## PREPROCEDURAL TEACHING

- Review the physician's explanation of the procedure and the reason for it; encourage the patient to ask questions and to discuss
  any fears or anxieties. Explain the need for informed consent
  for surgery, anesthesia, and blood transfusion.

### Review of Preprocedural Care

- Explain that hospital admission may be on the day of surgery.
- Review the preoperative tests that may be performed.
  - Chest x-ray and electrocardiogram
  - Blood tests: complete blood count, electrolytes, coagulation
    studies, tissue compatibility tests
  - Urine studies: urinalysis, culture and sensitivity, creatinine
    clearance
  - Intravenous pyelography
  - Urogram
  - Renal angiography (see box on p. 470)
- Inform the patient that a cleansing enema (e.g., Fleet) will be
  performed the night before the procedure.
- Discuss the need for a shower and shampoo with bactericidal

---

**RENAL ANGIOGRAPHY**

Renal angiography evaluates the status of both kidneys. Under local anesthesia a small catheter is inserted through a needle in the groin and is threaded up to the renal artery under fluoroscopy. Contrast medium is injected while x-ray pictures are obtained. The patient may feel a flushing sensation, a "funny taste" in the mouth, or nausea when the contrast is injected, but the symptoms pass quickly. After removal of the catheter, a pressure dressing is applied and a sandbag is placed. The patient must lie still for several hours before being allowed to leave. Further instructions include no heavy lifting (>10 pounds) and no strenuous exercise for several days. The test is performed on an outpatient basis.

---

soap (Safeguard, Dial, Hibiclens) the night before or morning of the procedure.
- Explain that the skin over the abdomen and flank may be shaved before surgery.
- Explain the need for NPO status from midnight of the night before.
- Review the possibility of renal angiography (see above) before surgery to decrease bleeding during and after surgery.

**Review of Postprocedural Care**
- See posteroperative care under Abdominal Surgery, p. 3.
- Tell the patient that the hospital stay after surgery will be 3-5 days.
- Stress the importance of turning, coughing, and deep breathing.
- Discuss the purpose of the incentive spirometer and demonstrate its use.
- Explain the purpose of wearing thigh-high elastic compression stockings and alternating pressure stockings while in bed.
- Emphasize the importance of getting out of bed (usually the second day) and moving about.
- Explain that drainage tubes may be needed after surgery and

describe the various possibilities: chest tube, nasogastric tube, urinary drainage tube from bladder, nephrostomy tube from kidney through flank, Penrose drain, or Jackson-Pratt drain from incisional area.

- Explain the need for frequent dressings soon after the procedure.
- Inform the patient that the urine will be blood colored (bright red) but will become normal appearing in several days.
- Discuss the need for pain relief medication and antibiotics.

## SIDE EFFECTS/COMPLICATIONS
- Hemorrhage and shock
- Infection
- Atelectasis
- Pneumonia

## HOME CARE
- Give both the patient and the caregiver *verbal* and *written* instructions. Provide them with the name and telephone number of a physician or nurse to call if questions arise.
- *General information*
  —Review the purpose and explain the type of procedure performed: partial or total nephrectomy.
  —If the nephrectomy is total, prepare the patient for dialysis (see p. 242).
- *Wound/incision care*
  —Instruct the patient on caring for the incision and changing the dressing.
     Wash hands.
     Inspect the incision for signs of infection.
     Cleanse the area with Betadine.
     If there is no evidence of drainage, leave the site open to the air. Otherwise, cover the incision with sterile gauze squares held in place with tape.
     If Steri-Strips were used, do not remove them; allow them to drop off.
  —Teach the patient how to care for the nephrostomy tube, if present.
- *Special instructions*
  —Inform the patient that showering and bathing may be resumed as recommended by the physician.
  —Explain how to measure urine output as indicated.

- *Warning signs*
  —Review the signs and symptoms that should be reported to a physician or nurse.
    Infection: incision red, warm to touch, painful, with increased or purulent drainage
    Urinary tract infection: fever, chills, hematuria, flank pain, sudden increase in urinary output
- *Activity*
  —Discuss the need to exercise to tolerance and to plan frequent rest periods. Explain that fatigue is common.
  —Encourage the patient to discuss allowances and limitations with respect to occupation, recreation, and activities.
  —Tell the patient to avoid heavy lifting (>10 pounds) for at least 6 weeks.
  —Advise the patient to avoid contact sports (e.g., wrestling, football) that could endanger the remaining kidney.
- *Diet*
  —Inform the patient that a regular diet can be followed unless there are restrictions related to the underlying reason for nephrectomy.
  —Encourage the patient to drink 8-10 glasses of fluids per day unless restrictions of the underlying disease apply.

**FOLLOW-UP CARE**

- Stress the importance of regular follow-up visits. Make sure the patient has the necessary names and telephone numbers.

# Neurogenic Bladder

—Neurogenic bladder: dysfunctional bladder caused by interruption of normal bladder innervation as a result of lesions or injuries. Types of neurogenic bladder dysfunction include reduced bladder capacity, no control of urination, and decreased perception of bladder fullness.

**CONTRIBUTING FACTORS**

- Spinal cord injury or tumor
- Stroke

- Brain tumor
- Parkinson's disease
- Multiple sclerosis
- Alzheimer's disease
- Aging
- Diabetes mellitus and resultant peripheral innervation
- Chronic alcoholism
- Systemic lupus erythematosus
- Heavy metal toxicity (e.g., mercury)
- Vascular disease
- Herpes zoster

## SIGNS/SYMPTOMS

- Urinary frequency, dribbling
- Voiding in small amounts
- Overflow incontinence
- Reduced bladder capacity
- Loss of reflex to urinate
- Loss of sensation of bladder fullness
- Inability to empty the bladder completely (residual urine)

## COMPLICATIONS

- Urinary tract infection
- Dysreflexia (associated with spinal cord injuries)
- Urinary tract stones
- Total incontinence
- Septic shock

## DIAGNOSTIC TESTS

- Describe each procedure, its purpose, and the normal feelings or sensations that are likely, as well as any preprocedural and postprocedural care (see Urinary Incontinence, p. 657).

## TREATMENT

*Medical*
- Therapy
  —Hydration: to prevent infection and stone formation
  —Bladder training: Credé's method, Kegel exercises
  —Urinary catheterization: intermittent or continuous
- Drugs
  —For underlying cause

*Surgical*
- Implantation of artificial urinary sphincter
- Implantation of neuroprosthetics (bladder pacemaker)
- Continent vesicostomy: surgical closure of the urethra at the bladder junction and an artificial opening made to the outside; a special valve is in place to allow the client to self-catheterize (see Urostomy, p. 650)

## HOME CARE

- Give both the patient and the caregiver *verbal* and *written* instructions. Provide them with the name and telephone number of a physician or nurse to call if questions arise.
- *General information*
  —Explain the factors contributing to the disorder.
- *Warning signs*
  —Review the signs, symptoms, and problems that should be reported to a physician or nurse.
    Urinary tract infection: fever, chills, flank pain
    Kidney stones: acute colicky pain in the flank or lower abdomen
    Problems with the indwelling catheter (see Indwelling Catheter, p. 406)
    Mechanical malfunction
  —Review the signs and symptoms of autonomic dysreflexia, explaining that it may be life threatening if not corrected and that it is usually caused by a distended bladder, fecal impaction, a full rectum, or sexual stimulation.
    Headache
    Decrease ($<60$) or increase ($>100$) in heart rate
    High blood pressure ($>140/90$ mm Hg)
    Blurred vision
    "Gooseflesh" and pallor below the level of the spinal injury
    Cold sweat of the head and neck
    Metallic taste in the mouth
    Nasal congestion
    Paresthesia (numbness, tingling, prickling, increased sensitivity)
- *Special instructions*
  —Discuss and demonstrate bladder training programs (see Urinary Incontinence, p. 657).
  —Advise the patient on how and where to obtain supplies.

—Explain how to avoid autonomic dysreflexia by setting up a schedule for emptying the bladder (or rectum) and maintaining free flow of urine through the tubing.

—Explain how to recognize the signs of bladder distention by visually inspecting the bladder area, feeling the bladder, and tapping the bladder area. The bladder area will be swollen and feel like a full balloon. Tapping it with the fingertips will produce a kettle drum sound and may cause dribbling.

—Demonstrate Credé's method to assist in emptying of the bladder. Tell the patient to place the outside part of the hand against the abdomen right below the umbilicus and bear down as if having a bowel movement until urination starts. The patient may have to do this several times before urination begins. When urination starts, the motion should be continued every 30 seconds until urine flow stops.

—Review the techique for intermittent or indwelling catheterization (see Indwelling Catheter, p. 406).

—Explain the option of an external condom catheter for men (see Urinary Incontinence, p. 657).

—Review the instructions for the care of implanted mechanical devices and explain the signs and symptoms of malfunction or infection.

> Wound infection or erosion at the bulb site: redness, tenderness, warmth, purulent drainage
>
> Problems with the artificial sphincter: urinary tract infection, urinary retention or incontinence, pain, swelling, fever, blood in urine
>
> Pacemaker malfunction: bladder does not empty

- *Medications*

—Explain the purpose, dosage, schedule, and route of administration of any prescribed drugs, as well as side effects to report to a physician or nurse.

- *Activity*

—Encourage the patient to verbalize concerns about changes in life-style imposed by the disorder. Encourage questions about allowances and limitations with respect to occupation, recreation, and sports.

- *Diet*

—Explain that a regular diet or one prescribed by the physician for the underlying disease should be followed.

—Advise the patient to reduce calcium intake and increase fluids to prevent the formation of renal calculi.

## FOLLOW-UP CARE

- Stress the importance of regular follow-up visits. Make sure that the patient has the necessary phone numbers.
- Assist the patient to obtain a Medic-Alert bracelet and identification card listing diagnosis, medications, and treatment.

## REFERRALS

- Provide information on home health referrals as indicated.
- Assist the patient to obtain psychologic support.

---

# Orchiectomy

—**Orchiectomy: surgical removal of one (unilateral) or both (bilateral) testes.**

## INDICATIONS

- Prostate cancer
- Testicular cancer
- Trauma

## PREPROCEDURAL TEACHING

- Review the physician's explanation of the procedure and the reason for it. Discuss the need for informed consent for surgery and anesthesia. Encourage the patient to ask questions and to discuss fears or anxieties about loss of sexual function and manhood.
- Explain that fertility may be affected and provide the patient with information on sperm banking.

### Review of Preprocedural Care

- Explain that the patient is usually admitted on the day of surgery and stays overnight after the procedure.
- Review preprocedural diagnostic tests.
  - —Alpha-fetoprotein and human chorionic gonadotropin for tumor markers
  - —Pregnancy test for certain types and stages of tumors
  - —Intravenous pyelogram and urogram

—Radionuclide imaging

—Lymphangiogram: injection of contrast dye into the lymph vessels to determine blockage

- Inform the patient that he will be asked to shower and shampoo with bactericidal soap (Safeguard, Dial, Hibiclens) the night before or morning of the procedure.
- Explain the need for NPO status from the night before the procedure.
- Discuss the possibility that the pubic hair will be shaved.

**Review of Postprocedural Care**

- Explain that analgesics and antiemetics will be administered as needed.
- Stress the importance of turning, coughing and deep breathing, and getting out of bed and moving about.
- Demonstrate use of the incentive spirometer.
- Explain that a scrotal support will be used to relieve pain and scrotal swelling; the scrotum will be elevated on a towel roll and an ice pack may be applied. Tell the patient that the pain usually lasts 24-48 hours.
- Advise the patient to avoid sitting for long periods, since this increases scrotal swelling.

**SIDE EFFECTS/COMPLICATIONS**

- Persistent pain
- Swelling
- Hemorrhage
- Wound infection
- Infertility

**HOME CARE**

- Give both the patient and the caregiver *verbal* and *written* instructions. Provide them with the name and telephone number of a physician or nurse to call if questions arise.
- Prepare the patient for chemotherapy (see p. 178) or radiation therapy (see p. 559), if ordered.
- *General information*
  —Review the procedure that was performed: unilateral (diseased testis removed, scrotum left intact) or bilateral orchiectomy. Discuss the underlying reason for the procedure (see Testicular Cancer, p. 622, or Prostate Cancer, p. 541).
  —For unilateral orchiectomy, explain that the scrotum is left in-

tact so reconstructive surgery (placement of a gel-filled testicular implant) can be done later; that sexual function resumes once the incision is healed; that monthly testicular self-examination of the remaining testis is important; and that one healthy testis can compensate for loss of function of the other so male characteristics are not affected.

—For bilateral orchiectomy, explain that the procedure is usually done for testicular cancer; that it renders the male sterile and will cause impotence if the nerves or vasculature is damaged; and that synthetic hormones may be given to replace male hormones. Provide information on impotence (see Erectile Dysfunction, p. 294).

- *Wound/incision care*
  —Demonstrate care of the surgical wound and dressing changes as needed. Explain that the dressing can be placed over the incision and held by the scrotal support.

- *Warning signs*
  —Review the signs and symptoms that should be reported to a physician or nurse.

  Difficulty urinating or inability to urinate

  Severe or persistent pain

  Wound infection: redness, warmth, tenderness, purulent drainage, fever, chills

  Nausea and vomiting

  Appearance of a mass in the opposite testicle, inguinal area, or neck

- *Medications*
  —Explain the purpose, dosage, schedule, and route of administration of any prescribed drugs, as well as side effects to report to a physician or nurse.

- *Activity*
  —Encourage the patient to discuss allowances and limitations with respect to occupation, recreation, and activities.

  —Instruct the patient to plan frequent rest periods, gradually increasing activity as tolerated. Tell him that normal activity can usually resume within 1 week.

  —Advise the patient to avoid stair climbing and sitting for long (over 2-hour) periods.

  —Suggest that the patient avoid lifting more than 10 pounds, working or exercising strenuously, or playing contact sports for the period of time specified by the physician.

- *Diet*
  —Inform the patient that he may follow a regular diet unless the physician has prescribed a special one.

## FOLLOW-UP CARE

- Stress the importance of regular follow-up visits. Make sure the patient has the necessary names and telephone numbers.

## PSYCHOSOCIAL CARE

- Encourage the patient to verbalize his feelings about changes in body image, sense of loss of manhood, fear of losing sexual function, and feminization.

## REFERRALS

- Provide information about reproduction and fertility as needed, and refer the patient to medical or community-based counseling.

# Osteomalacia

—Osteomalacia: a metabolic disease characterized by loss of mineralization of bones, resulting in softening, brittleness, and deformity. Similar to rickets in children, osteomalacia occurs when vitamin D deficiency leads to reduced absorption of phosphorus and calcium. Weight-bearing bones such as those in the spine, pelvis, and lower extremities are mostly affected and are prone to fractures. The elderly and women are at highest risk.

## CONTRIBUTING FACTORS

- Inadequate dietary intake of vitamin D
- Calcium deficiency
- Lack of sun exposure
- Intestinal malabsorption of vitamin D
  —Liver disease
  —Hypoparathyroidism
  —Small intestinal disease
- Chronic renal failure
- Chronic anticonvulsant therapy

**SIGNS/SYMPTOMS**
- Abnormal bowing and bending of long bones and vertebral column
- Bone pain and limb tenderness
- Muscle weakness and cramps
- Decreased joint range of motion
- Generalized weakness, malaise, fatigue

**COMPLICATIONS**
- Degenerative joint disease
- Bone deformities
- Bone fractures

**DIAGNOSTIC TESTS**
- Describe each procedure, its purpose, and the normal feelings or sensations that are likely, as well as any preprocedural and postprocedural care.
    —Blood tests: serum calcium, serum alkaline phosphatase, vitamin D, sedimentation rate
    —X-rays: to identify calcification of bones, fractures
    —Bone biopsy: to show excessive uncalcified bone

**TREATMENT**
*Medical*
- Therapy
    —Adjunctive therapy
    —Diet therapy: high calcium, high phosphorus
    —Physical therapy
- Drugs
    —Vitamin D replacement
    —Calcium supplements
    —Analgesics
*Surgical*
- Fracture repair as indicated

**HOME CARE**
- Give both the patient and the caregiver *verbal* and *written* instructions. Provide them with the name and telephone number of a physician or nurse to call if questions arise.

- *General information*
  —Discuss the disorder, explaining the role that vitamin D plays in calcium and phosphorus absorption, which is required for bone calcification.
  —Review the sources of vitamin D: diet, vitamin supplements, exposure to ultraviolet light. Explain that sunlight is a good source of vitamin D formation.
- *Warning signs*
  —Review the signs and symptoms that should be reported to a physician or nurse.
    Increase in or sudden appearance of bone or joint pain
- *Special instructions*
  —Discuss ways to prevent injury through maintenance of a safe environment: side rails; nonskid surfaces; clean, dry floors; adequate lighting.
- *Medications*
  —Explain the purpose, dosage, schedule, and route of administration of any prescribed drugs, as well as side effects to report to the physician or nurse.
  —Advise the patient to watch for and report any signs of vitamin D toxicity: headache, nausea, diarrhea, renal calculi.
- *Activity*
  —Encourage the patient to discuss allowances and limitations with respect to occupation, recreation, and activities.
  —Advise the patient on the use of ambulatory assistance devices such as a cane or crutches to lessen strain and load on weak bones and joints. Assist the patient to obtain the equipment.
  —Encourage and instruct the patient in range-of-motion and muscle-strengthening exercises to help maintain muscle strength and joint mobility.
  —Discuss the exercise regimen for retaining calcium in bones: isometric and resistive.
  —Advise the patient to be careful when doing activities that could lead to strain, severe stress, and fractures (e.g., rising from a chair, deep bending, exercising).
  —Discuss the need to avoid activities that can cause injury (e.g., bowling and horseback riding, which can cause vertebral decompression).
- *Diet*
  —Discuss the importance of increasing dietary calcium and vitamin D through such foods as dairy products, egg yolks, tuna,

O

liver oil, and salmon. Refer the patient to a dietitian for assistance with meal planning.

**FOLLOW-UP CARE**

- Stress the importance of regular follow-up visits. Make sure the patient has the necessary names and telephone numbers.

# Osteomyelitis

—Osteomyelitis: an acute or chronic infection of the bone caused by a bacterial, fungal, or viral organism. The most commonly involved organisms are *Staphylococcus aureus, Escherichia coli, Klebsiella, Pseudomonas,* and proteins. Chronic osteomyelitis is a bone infection that persists for years, flaring up intermittently after minor trauma to the area or when systemic resistance is low. Primary osteomyelitis is a direct invasion of bone as a result of compound fractures, penetrating wounds, bone marrow aspiration, or surgery. Secondary osteomyelitis (acute hematogenic osteomyelitis) is an infection of the bone via the patient's blood or adjacent soft tissues; it may be related, for example, to pressure sores, intravenous drug abuse, joints involved with septic arthritis, or radiation therapy.

**CONTRIBUTING FACTORS/RISK FACTORS**

- Undernourishment
- Old age
- Diabetes mellitus
- Chronic obstructive pulmonary disease
- Sickle cell disease
- Malignancies
- Peripheral vascular disease

**SIGNS/SYMPTOMS**

- Acute osteomyelitis
  —Abrupt onset of localized pain
  —Fever, chills
  —Redness, heat, swelling, infected bone
  —Malaise

—Limited motion
—Restlessness
—Irritability
• Chronic osteomyelitis
—Persistent purulent drainage from old pocket

## COMPLICATIONS

• Chronic osteomyelitis
• Amputation
• Abscess formation
• Pathologic fracture
• Joint contractures

## DIAGNOSTIC TESTS

• Describe each procedure, its purpose, and the normal feelings or sensations that are likely, as well as any preprocedural and postprocedural care.
—Blood tests
White blood cell count: elevated
Erythrocyte sedimentation rate: elevated
Blood cultures: to identify causative organism
—Bone biopsy: to obtain material for culture and sensitivity studies
—X-rays: to reveal destructive process
—Computed tomography: to detect bone changes and spread of infection to surrounding tissues
—Magnetic resonance imaging: to determine extent of acute or chronic infection

## TREATMENT

*Medical*
• Therapy
—Bed rest
—Compresses: warm, moist, or alternate warm and cold
—Hyperbaric oxygen chamber
• Drugs
—Intravenous antibiotics: therapy prescribed for 4-6 weeks
—Topical antibiotics
—Analgesics, antipyretics
*Surgical*
• Surgical decompression of infected bone: holes are drilled into the bone to localize sites of exudate; the overlying infected bone

is removed; the cavity is loosely packed for drainage purposes and to keep wound open
- External fixation devices: to stabilize bones and prevent fractures
- Saucerization (sequestrectomy): removal of necrotic bone and scar tissue to provide a healthy surface for regeneration of bone
- Bone grafting
- Microsurgical free muscle transfer: to cover the wound and eliminate dead space
- Amputation of limb: for life-threatening or persistent infections

## HOME CARE

- Give both the patient and the caregiver *verbal* and *written* instructions. Provide them with the name and telephone number of a physician or nurse to call if questions arise.
- *General information*
  —Discuss the disease process, causes and contributing factors, and the potential for chronic infection. Stress the importance of continuing prescribed antibiotic therapy.
- *Wound/incision care*
  —Explain and demonstrate wound care using aseptic technique for dressing changes. Discuss proper disposal of contaminated dressings and removal of soiled linens. Stress the importance of maintaining wound isolation.
- *Warning signs*
  —Review the signs and symptoms of infection that should be reported to a physician or nurse.
  > Fever
  > Chills
  > Increased pain
  > Malaise
  > Recurring drainage from wound
- *Special instructions*
  —Review care of the external fixator device if indicated (see p. 304).
  —Teach the patient how to use and care for the Hickman catheter (see p. 163) or other intravenous access device for home antibiotic therapy. Provide referrals for home care.
- *Medications*
  —Explain the purpose, dosage, schedule, and route of administration of any prescribed drugs, as well as side effects to report to the physician or nurse.

—Advise the patient to watch for and report any side effects of antibiotics: nausea, vomiting, diarrhea, abdominal pain.
* *Activity*
  —Explain the need for rest to conserve energy and promote healing.
  —Teach the patient range-of-motion exercises and encourage their use to maintain muscle strength and joint mobility.
  —Explain the importance of immobilizing the affected part to decrease the spread of purulent material.
  —Instruct the patient in the use of ambulatory aids (crutches, cane, wheelchair, or walker, as indicated) when he or she is allowed out of bed. Assist the patient to obtain the equipment.
* *Diet*
  —Encourage the patient to follow a nutritionally sound diet high in protein and vitamins C and D to enhance and promote healing.

**FOLLOW-UP CARE**
* Stress the importance of regular follow-up visits. Make sure the patient has the necessary names and telephone numbers.

**O**

# Osteoporosis

—Osteoporosis: an overall reduction in bone mass or density that occurs because bone resorption (breaking down of bone for other body uses) is greater than bone formation. Osteoporosis causes bone to become brittle and susceptible to fractures. Bones store calcium for other body functions; the body takes the calcium out for use through resorption. With age the process of resorption normally occurs faster than bone formation, calcium absorption becomes impaired, and vitamin D formation decreases from lack of estrogen. These changes result in a gradual decrease in bone mass or density.

**RISK FACTORS**
* Women
  —After menopause because of decreased estrogen production and inactivity

—Petite, white, or Asian because of small amount of bone mass
—Nulliparity
- Others
  —In young people after severe injury because of prolonged inactivity or immobility
  —History of rheumatoid arthritis, liver disease, certain cancers, overactive thyroid
  —Sedentary life-style, lack of exercise and weight-bearing activities
  —Smoking or alcohol abuse: interferes with calcium absorption
  —Long-term use of drugs (e.g., corticosteroids, antacids, heparin, phenytoin, isoniazid): suppresses the activity of bone-building cells
  —High caffeine intake: decreases absorption of calcium
  —Family history
  —Inadequate calcium intake

## SIGNS/SYMPTOMS

- Fractures
  —Dorsal and lumbar vertebral bodies
  —Neck and intertrochanteric regions of femur (hip fracture)
  —Distal radius
  —Vertebral compression fractures leading to:
    Loss of height
    Kyphosis (back hump)
    Back discomfort
    Constipation

## COMPLICATIONS

- Fractures of vertebrae, hip, wrist
- Respiratory compromise caused by severe kyphosis

## DIAGNOSTIC TESTS

- Describe each procedure, its purpose, and the normal feelings or sensations that are likely, as well as any preprocedural and postprocedural care.
  —Blood tests
    Serum alkaline phosphatase: decreased
    Serum hydroxyproline: increased
  —X-ray examination: to document osteoporotic fractures, spinal curvature

—Radiogrammetry, photodensitometry, single- and dual-photon absorptiometry: to measure skeletal density and detect loss of bone mass

—Computed tomography: to measure vertebral (spinal) bone density; to detect herniated or fractured vertebral disks

## TREATMENT

*Medical*

- Therapy
  —Application of back corset or neck support to prevent stress fractures
  —Moderate weight-bearing exercises to hold calcium in bone
  —High-calcium, high-protein diet
  —Nutritional supplements: calcium carbonate and vitamin D
- Drugs
  —Estrogen replacement therapy for postmenopausal women
  —Analgesics
  —Antiresorptive agents to prevent further loss of bone mass

*Surgical*

- Repair of fractures (e.g., hip, wrist)
- Laminectomy to relieve pressure on the spinal nerves or cord if vertebrae are involved (fractures, ruptured disk)

## HOME CARE

- Give both the patient and the caregiver *verbal* and *written* instructions. Provide them with the name and telephone number of a physician or nurse to call if questions arise.
- *General information*
  —Explain and discuss the disease process and the causes and contributing factors.
- *Warning signs*
  —Review the signs and symptoms of pathologic fractures that should be reported to a physician or nurse.

  Deformity
  Pain
  Edema
  Ecchymosis
  Limb shortening
  False motion, decreased range of motion
  Loss of bladder or bowel control
  Paralysis

- *Special instructions*
  —Discuss the importance of establishing home safety measures to prevent falls and injuries: placing a handrail in the bathtub, installing nightlights, and avoiding the use of throw rugs.
  —Advise the patient to use ambulatory assist devices such as a cane or walker as indicated to relieve stress on the back and joints; this will help the patient maintain balance and reduce the risk of falling.
- *Medications*
  —Explain the purpose, dosage, schedule, and route of administration of any prescribed drugs, as well as side effects to report to the physician or nurse.
  —Discuss the use of calcium supplements. Explain that calcium should be taken 2 hours before or after other medications because it can reduce absorption of other drugs. Inform the patient that increased calcium can result in kidney stone formation. This can be prevented by increasing daily fluid intake and not taking calcium supplements with iron, since iron absorption would be impaired.
- *Activity*
  —Explain the importance of weight-bearing exercises to increase bone mass. Encourage such activities as walking, tennis, and dancing to activate bone formation, improve circulation, and enhance calcium absorption.
  —Advise the patient to be careful when doing any activity (e.g., getting up from a chair or bending deeply), since falling or straining can cause severe stress and lead to fractures.
- *Diet*
  —Encourage the patient to eat foods high in calcium, including cheese, milk, dark green leafy vegetables, eggs, peanuts, sesame seeds, and oysters.
  —Instruct the patient in planning menus that provide a sufficient daily intake of foods high in or fortified with calcium and vitamin D, such as eggs, halibut, herring, dairy products, liver, salmon, and sardines.
  —Tell the patient to limit intake of alcohol and caffeine.

## FOLLOW-UP CARE

- Stress the importance of regular follow-up visits. Make sure the patient has the necessary names and telephone numbers.

# Ovarian Cancer

—Ovarian cancer: a rapidly growing tumor that is seldom diagnosed in the early stages because of the lack of signs or symptoms. More than 60% of women with ovarian cancer have advanced disease at the time of diagnosis. The most common type of ovarian cancer is serous cystadenocarcinoma; others are mucinous, endometrioid, or clear cell. Most ovarian cancer arises in the epithelium. Between 5% and 10% of tumors have their primary source in another body organ, usually the breast. Dissemination occurs through implantation of cells into the surface of the pelvic peritoneum, sigmoid colon, cecum, or terminal ileum and omentum, as well as via submesothelial lymphatics.

## RISK FACTORS

- Uninterrupted ovulation
- Age over 50 (postmenopausal)
- Nulliparity, celibacy, infertility
- Long history of menstrual irregularity
- Higher socioeconomic status
- High-fat diet
- Exposure to industrial chemicals such as asbestos and talc

Others being studied are age at menopause, history of rubella and mumps, family history of ovarian cancer, family size, and ovarian malfunctions.

## SIGNS/SYMPTOMS

- Ascites, abdominal or pelvic pain or fullness
- Weight loss
- Gastrointestinal complaints: dyspnea, indigestion
- Urinary complaints: frequency, urgency
- Menstrual irregularities: abnormal uterine bleeding

## DIAGNOSTIC TESTS

- Describe each procedure, its purpose, and the normal feelings or sensations that are likely, as well as any preprocedural and postprocedural care.
  - —Pelvic examination with bimanual manipulation: to palpate the ovaries for size and shape

—Laparoscopy with biopsy: to detect ovarian abnormality and the presence of malignant cells
—Lymphangiography: to detect the involvement of retroperitoneal nodes
—Cancer antigen 125 (CA-125): tumor marker elevated in the presence of ovarian cancer

## TREATMENT

*Medical*
* Therapy
  —Radiation therapy
      Intracavity
      External beam
  —Single-agent chemotherapy
      Chlorambucil
      Melphalan
      Doxorubicin
      Cyclophosphamide
      5-Fluorouracil
      Methotrexate
      Vinblastine
      Bleomycin
      Cisplatin
      Nitrogen mustard
      Thiotepa
      Tetracycline
  —Combination chemotherapy (including cisplatin)

*Surgical*
* Simple salpingo-oophorectomy
* Total abdominal hysterectomy with bilateral salpingo-oophorectomy and partial or complete omentectomy

## HOME CARE

* Give both the patient and the caregiver *verbal* and *written* instructions. Provide them with the name and telephone number of a physician or nurse to call if questions arise. Use visual aids in instruction.
* *General information*
  —Review the physician's explanation of the disease process. Explain that prescribed treatment will be based on the stage of cancer and age of the patient.

—Provide information about the prescribed treatment: hysterectomy (see p. 400), chemotherapy (see p. 178), or radiation therapy (see p. 559).
- *Warning signs*
  —Review the signs and symptoms that should be reported to a physician or nurse.

    Infection: redness, drainage, fever, pain

    Bleeding

    Urinary obstruction: distention, decreased output

    Bowel obstruction: distention, abdominal discomfort, flatulence, nausea, loss of appetite

    Pleural effusion: shortness of breath, fever
- *Special instructions*
  —Teach the patient methods of managing abdominal discomfort and other gastrointestinal complaints: medications; heat; small, frequent meals.
  —Discuss pain management techniques: relaxation, imagery, biofeedback.
- *Medications*
  —Explain the purpose, dosage, schedule, and route of administration of any prescribed drugs, as well as side effects to report to the physician or nurse.
- *Activity*
  —Encourage the patient to exercise as tolerated. Explain that walking is especially helpful in relieving abdominal discomfort.
- *Diet*
  —Stress the importance of adequate intake of fluids and food and obtaining sufficient calories. Suggest dietary supplements as needed.

## FOLLOW-UP CARE

- Stress the importance of follow-up medical and gynecologic examinations as ordered. Make sure the patient has the necessary names and telephone numbers.
- Advise women with young daughters to have them begin annual gynecologic examinations at onset of sexual activity or age 18.

## REFERRALS

- Assist the patient to obtain referral services for sexual psychologic counseling and support groups as needed.

# Oxygen Therapy

—Oxygen therapy: provision of oxygen to the tissue so that normal metabolism can occur; used to relieve hypoxemia and prevent hypoxia. Oxygen may be delivered as a liquid, by means of an oxygen concentrator, or from a cylinder.

## COMPLICATIONS

- Atelectasis
- Oxygen toxicity: sore throat, cough, nausea, anxiety, numbness, muscular twitching, chest pain with deep inspiration

## HOME CARE

- Give both the patient and the caregiver *verbal* and *written* instructions. Provide them with the name and telephone number of a physician or nurse to call if questions arise.
- *General information*
  —Explain the purpose of oxygen therapy.
- *Warning signs*
  —Review the signs and symptoms that should be reported to a physician or nurse.
    Irregular, shallow, or slow breathing; difficulty in breathing
    Restlessness or anxiety
    Tiredness, drowsiness, trouble waking up
    Persistent headache
    Slurred speech
    Confusion, difficulty in concentrating
    Bluish fingernails or lips
- *Special instructions*
  —Work with the social service or home health agency to find equipment and a supplier near the patient's home. Include the patient and caregiver in decision making.
  —Assist the patient to obtain a home health referral for follow-up at home.
  —Teach the patient the oxygen concentration delivery that was ordered. Explain the importance of maintaining the appropriate flow rate, since high flow rates in patients with chronic obstructive pulmonary disease can suppress the respiratory drive.

—Teach the patient how to remove and reposition the oxygen equipment to permit wiping off and drying the face, nose blowing, and eating.

—For a patient who requires humidity and aerosol therapy, provide instructions.

—Explain that humidification and adequate hydration are important because oxygen dries the mucous membranes.

—Demonstrate the use of equipment and how to fill humidifiers and nebulizers.

—Demonstrate the administration of medication via hand-held nebulizers.

—Show the patient how to care for the skin and mucous membranes, since with prolonged wear, oxygen devices can cause skin irritation and breakdown, which can provide an additional route for microorganisms.

—Demonstrate the use, care, and cleaning of equipment.

—Teach the patient how to use the oxygen source, oxygen delivery device, and humidification source.

—Demonstrate how to check water in the humidifier and nebulizer every 8 hours to maintain an adequate level and how to refill as needed.

—Explain the importance of maintaining the temperature of humidifiers between 95° and 97.8° F.

—Ensure that the humidifier is placed on a table at least 2 feet from walls and furniture, with the steam directed into the room.

—Provide instruction on oxygen management when traveling around town with oxygen: Plan ahead before travel. Call the oxygen supply company and ask what equipment is needed and how long to allot for travel between refills. Allow for a 20%-25% safety margin of oxygen supply to cover unexpected delays. Use a watch with an alarm function to remind you that the oxygen tank is running low. Practice operating the oxygen equipment before travel.

—Inform the patient that liquid oxygen is available in a small, lightweight container similar in size to a thermos bottle; advise that it be reserved for trips outside the home, since it is expensive to use continuously.

—Discuss oxygen management when traveling by automobile. Demonstrate how to secure the oxygen unit with a seatbelt and shoulder harness.

Instruct the patient or caregiver to keep the oxygen container upright at all times to avoid rapid release of oxygen. Slight tipping of liquid oxygen tanks during loading and unloading is not dangerous.

Advise the patient to store extra tanks in the trunk of the car, since tanks are too large to stand upright.

Instruct the patient to keep the car window partly open while using oxygen.

Tell camper or motor home owners to contact the oxygen supply company for installation of a liquid oxygen reservoir.

—If the patient is planning to travel by local public transportation, advise contacting the city's transportation department to check restrictions on oxygen equipment on local transportation systems.

—Stress the importance of not smoking or allowing others to smoke near the patient because of the possibility of combustion, fire, or explosion.

—Explain the necessity of checking all electrical equipment used in the same room with oxygen administration for frayed cords or potential for sparking to avoid combustion and fire or explosion.

—Tell the patient not to place carpet, clothing, or furniture over the tubing, since a leak could result.

—Demonstrate the use of an all-purpose fire extinguisher and instruct the patient to keep one near the equipment.

—Advise the patient to notify the local fire department of the presence of oxygen in the house and to request free safety inspections, if available.

• *Medications*

—Explain the purpose, dosage, schedule, and route of administration of any prescribed drugs, as well as side effects to report to a physician or nurse.

• *Activity*

—Encourage walking and other activities as tolerated. Advise the patient to use a portable oxygen source because continuous oxygen therapy can limit mobility.

## FOLLOW-UP CARE

• Stress the importance of regular follow-up visits. Make sure the patient has the necessary names and telephone numbers.

# Pacemaker Care

—**Pacemaker care: use and maintenance of an electronic device that stimulates the myocardium to control or maintain the heart rate. The pacemaker can be a temporary or permanent mode of treatment. The battery-powered pulse generator and lead system senses heart function and stimulates the myocardium to contract.**

## INDICATIONS

- Sinus node dysfunction
- Conduction blocks
- Bradyarrhythmias
- Tachyarrhythmias

## PREPROCEDURAL TEACHING

- Review the physician's explanation of implantation of the pacemaker and the reason for it; encourage the patient to ask questions and to discuss any fears or anxieties. Explain the need for informed consent.

### Review of Preprocedural Care

- Instruct the patient not to eat or drink for 6-8 hours before the procedure.
- Explain that the procedure will be done under local anesthesia and sedation and will last 1-3 hours.
- Explain that the patient's head will be positioned to one side and draped.
- Inform the patient that some pressure may be felt during the procedure.
- Explain that the lead(s) will be threaded into the right atrium through the subclavian vein via fluoroscopy.
- Tell the patient that an incision will be made under the collarbone.
- Explain that the patient will be continuously monitored during and after the procedure.

### Review of Postprocedural Care

- Tell that patient that bed rest will be maintained for the first 4-6 hours to prevent lead dislodgment.

- Explain that stiffness and soreness will be felt at the insertion site.
- Inform the patient that the arm on the side of the incision may be immobilized in a sling.
- Explain that postoperative electrocardiographic monitoring will continue for 24 hours.

## SIDE EFFECTS/COMPLICATIONS

- Pacemaker dysfunction
- Catheter dislodgment
- Stokes-Adams syndrome
- Cardiac dysrhythmias
- Infection
- Bleeding
- Perforation
- Cardiac tamponade

## HOME CARE

- Give both the patient and the caregiver *verbal* and *written* instructions. Provide them with the name and telephone number of a physician or nurse to call if questions arise.
- *General information*
  —Explain the underlying rhythm disorder, type of pacemaker (temporary or permanent), and care.
- *Warning signs*
  —Review the signs and symptoms that should be reported to a physician or nurse.

    Pacemaker dysfunction: syncope, pallor, fatigue, shortness of breath, palpitations or irregular pulse, pulse out of range of programmed settings, chest pain

    Catheter dislodgment: hiccups, twitching of chest and abdominal muscles

    Stokes-Adams syndrome: vertigo, syncope, convulsions, coma

    Fever, redness, warmth, pain, swelling, discoloration, bleeding, or drainage at incision site
- *Special instructions*
  —Teach the patient how to measure a pulse radially; explain that it should be done each day at rest.
  —Instruct the patient to inform all dentists and physicians of the pacemaker before any procedures.
  —Instruct the patient to inform airport security personnel of the pacemaker before passing through the metal detector.

Reassure the female patient that pregnancy is not contraindicated. Instruct her to inform her physician that she is planning a pregnancy so that the pacemaker can be adjusted to rate changes associated with pregnancy.

—Discuss electrical safety.

Tell the patient to avoid working with radar or electrical equipment such as diathermy or electrocautery devices, arc welding, electrical smelting furnaces, large electrical generators, CB radios with high-power linear amplifiers, radio or television transmitters while they are operating, and magnetic resonance imaging devices.

Instruct the patient to ground home appliances.

Stress the importance of using caution around strong magnetic fields, such as microwave ovens and blow dryers.

Instruct the patient to move away from any fields that interfere with pacemaker function; the pacemaker will resume normal programmed function.

Provide the patient and caregiver with written information on the pacemaker model, date of insertion, location of generator, and pacer programming.

Explain that the expected life of a pacemaker battery is 5-10 years, depending on the type of battery.

Explain that the part of the pacemaker system that may need changing is the generator.

**P**

• *Medications*

—Explain the purpose, dosage, schedule, and route of administration of any prescribed drugs, as well as side effects to report to a physician or nurse.

—Stress the importance of avoiding use of over-the-counter medications without consulting a physician.

• *Activity*

—Encourage the patient to discuss allowances and limitations with respect to occupation, recreation, and activities.

—Explain activity limitations as directed by the physician. Advise the patient to avoid heavy lifting (>10 pounds) and vigorous arm or shoulder activity. Explain that sexual activity may be resumed as tolerated.

—Demonstrate range-of-motion exercises for the affected shoulder, and tell the patient to begin them after the first 24 hours.

—Tell the patient not to drive for the first 4 weeks.

—Stress the importance of avoiding contact sports.

—Instruct the patient to avoid traveling for 3 months after pace-maker insertion.

—Advise the patient not to wear restrictive clothing over the pacemaker site.

—Tell the patient to avoid direct contact with or blows to the pacemaker site.

**FOLLOW-UP CARE**

• Stress the importance of regular follow-up visits, including the pacemaker clinic. Make sure the patient has the necessary names and telephone numbers. If telephone monitoring is available, discuss this option with the patient.

• Instruct the patient to schedule an appointment soon before the expiration date of the battery.

• Assist the patient to obtain a Medic-Alert bracelet and an iden-tification card listing the type of pacemaker, set rate, date of implantation, and name of physician.

**PSYCHOSOCIAL CARE**

• Encourage the patient to verbalize fears and concerns about the underlying rhythm disorder, need for a pacemaker, changes in life-style, and pacemaker management.

---

# Paget's Disease
## (Osteitis Deformans)

---

**—Paget's disease: a chronic inflammatory disease that results in thickening, softening, and eventual bowing of bones. Paget's disease is characterized by an initial phase of excessive bone re-sorption (breaking down of bone for other body uses), followed by excessive abnormal bone formation. The diseased bone is structurally weak and fragile, causing painful deformities, and is prone to fractures. Paget's disease usually affects the femur, tibia, lower spine, pelvis, and skull. It occurs worldwide but is extremely rare in Asia, the Middle East, Africa, and Scandina-via. In the United States it affects 3% of people over 40 years of age (mostly men). The cause of the disease is unknown.**

## SIGNS/SYMPTOMS

- Bone pain: mild to severe, aggravated by weight bearing or pressure, worse at night
- Increased warmth over involved sites
- Backache
- Skeletal deformities: kyphosis, barrel-shaped chest, bowing of the tibia or femur
- Easily bendable bones
- Pathologic fractures
- Cranial nerve compression: visual deficits, hearing loss, headaches, dysphagia
- Skull enlarged, soft, thick

## COMPLICATIONS

- Pathologic fractures
- Renal calculi
- Heart failure
- Hearing loss
- Visual changes
- Sarcoma

## DIAGNOSTIC TESTS

- Describe each procedure, its purpose, and the normal feelings or sensations that are likely, as well as any preprocedural and postprocedural care.
    —Standard x-rays: to document typical lesions of the disease, pathologic fractures, deformed bone structure
    —Blood tests: to detect elevated alkaline phosphatase, indicating new bone growth
    —Bone biopsy: to confirm the diagnosis
    —Bone scans: to identify active bone lesions
    —Magnetic resonance imaging: to detect areas of bone breakdown and bone growth

## TREATMENT

*Medical*
- Therapy
    —Orthotics (e.g., external splints, casts): to maintain reduction and help straighten bone
- Drugs
    —Hormones: to retard bone formation
    —Calcitonin

—Etidronate

—Cytotoxic antibiotic (mithramycin): to produce remission of symptoms

—Analgesics: to control pain

—Nonsteroidal antiinflammatory drugs: to control pain

*Surgical*

• Repair of pathologic fractures by closed or open reduction

## HOME CARE

• Give both the patient and the caregiver *verbal* and *written* instructions. Provide them with the name and telephone number of a physician or nurse to call if questions arise.

• *General information*

—Explain the disease process and prescribed treatment.

• *Warning signs*

—Review the signs and symptoms that should be reported to a physician or nurse.

  Cranial and spinal involvement: decreased hearing, headache, paresthesias (numbness, tingling), paralysis, visual defects (pupil inequality), changes in speech patterns, difficulty in swallowing

  Kidney stones: dysuria, hematuria

—Discuss the high risk of pathologic fracture, and explain that signs or symptoms should be reported immediately to a physician.

  Sudden increase in pain

  Hearing or sensing a bone crack

  Experiencing the inability to bear weight or use bone normally

• *Special instructions*

—Teach the patient to self-inject calcitonin. Permit time for practice, and stress the need to rotate injection sites.

• *Medications*

—Explain the purpose, dosage, schedule, and route of administration of any prescribed drugs, as well as side effects to report to the physician or nurse.

—Tell the patient to avoid over-the-counter products such as antacids and vitamins without checking with a physician.

—Instruct the patient taking etidronate to schedule medication doses 2 hours before or after meals. Advise not taking the medication with milk or foods high in calcium, since they impair absorption.

- *Activity*
  —Encourage the patient to maintain activity levels as tolerated. Encourage range-of-motion exercises of the unaffected joints to maintain joint mobility.
  —Advise the patient to avoid excessive activity but also to avoid immobility.
  —Instruct the patient in the use of ambulatory assist devices and aids (crutches, cane, walker).
  —Discuss home safety measures to prevent falls: removal of throw rugs, electrical cords, and other obstacles.
  —Advise the patient to move cautiously, avoiding sudden jerking movements, to lessen the probability of fracture.
- *Diet*
  —Instruct the patient to increase intake of foods containing vitamin D (milk, certain seafoods), calcium dairy products, and dark green vegetables.
  —Encourage fluid intake of 6-8 glasses a day to minimize renal calculus formation.

**FOLLOW-UP CARE**
- Stress the importance of follow-up visits. Make sure the patient has the necessary names and telephone numbers.

P

# Pain Management

—Pain management: dealing with the state in which a person experiences and reports severe discomfort or an uncomfortable sensation. Pain can be influenced by a variety of physiologic, psychologic, and sociologic factors. *Tolerance* is the ability to endure pain intensity. *Threshold* is the amount or degree of discomfort the patient can tolerate before terming the sensation painful. *Acute pain* is intense, has an end point, warns of actual or potential tissue damage, and resolves when healing occurs. *Chronic pain* lasts longer than 6 months and may be continuous or intermittent. Chronic pain does not serve as a warning of tissue damage.

**HOME CARE**

- Give both the patient and the caregiver *verbal* and *written* instructions. Provide them with the name and telephone number of a physician or nurse to call if questions arise.
- *General information*
  —Explain the relationship of pain to the disease process. Assist the patient to understand the source of pain.
- *Special instructions*
  —Assist the patient to identify factors or actions that trigger pain, such as activity, movements, and temperature extremes.
  —Discuss past effective and ineffective pain relief measures. Explore the past effect of pain relief measures on the patient, such as sleepiness, lethargy, and decreased energy or sexual activity.
  —Assist the patient to localize and describe the intensity of pain using a scale (e.g., 0-10, with 0 meaning absence of pain and 10 being intense pain).
  —Discuss interventions other than taking medications for intractable pain.
    Anesthetic procedures such as nerve blocks, trigger point injections, and use of nitrous oxide
    Neuroablative procedures such as cordotomy
    Physiatric supportive measures such as using a prosthesis, physical therapy, and occupational therapy
  —Discuss alternative strategies patients can use to relieve pain without taking prescribed drugs, and explain that these techniques may also augment the effect of pain medication (see Appendix E).
    Sensory interventions: massage such as back and foot massage: to relax muscular tension and increase local circulation; range-of-motion exercises (passive, assistive, or active): to relax muscles, improve circulation, and prevent pain related to stiffness and immobility; cold application: used initially to decrease tissue injury response (swelling) and decrease pain; heat application: used after cold to aid in clearance of tissue toxins and mobilize fluids; transcutaneous electrical nerve stimulation (TENS): pocket-size battery-operated device used to send mild continuous electrical impulses through the skin by means of electrodes placed on the body (see discussion below)
    Emotional interventions to increase pain threshold by controlling or reducing anxiety, fatigue, or depression): *prevention or control of anxiety:* to reduce muscle tension

and increase pain tolerance through relaxation exercises and slow, controlled breathing; *promotion of self-control:* to reduce feelings of helplessness and lack of control that contribute to anxiety and pain; *pacing of activities*

Cognitive interventions: *distraction:* focus on something unrelated to pain (e.g., conversing, watching television or videos, listening to music); humor; *guided imagery:* use of images to alter a physical or emotional state, promote relaxation, and decrease pain sensation

—Discuss the need to identify body positions of comfort; encourage attention to proper posture and body alignment. Advise the patient to immobilize or rest the affected area.

—Tell the patient to relieve pressure areas by turning or using pressure reduction devices such as an air-fluidized support system.

— Discuss the use of TENS. Explain that the mild electrical current blocks or modifies pain messages before they reach the brain and replaces them with a buzzing or tingling sensation. Inform the patient that TENS may stimulate the body's production of endorphin, a natural pain reliever. Instruct the patient in the use and home care of the TENS unit.

Apply a thin coat of gel over each entire electrode.

Place the electrodes securely on the skin with tape.

Place the electrodes close to the site of pain.

Turn the intensity knob until a slight tingling or buzzing sensation is felt on the skin. Increase the intensity if the pain is still felt or decrease the intensity if the tingling sensation causes discomfort.

Turn the TENS unit off before removing it.

Wipe the electrodes with an alcohol and water mixture after removing them from the skin.

Do not allow the unit to get wet. If it does get wet, allow it to dry thoroughly before using it again.

Replace the electrodes if the adhesive surface separates from the backing or if they no longer adhere firmly to the skin.

Replace the battery pack or recharge as needed. If there is no tingling sensation when the intensity is turned up, the batteries are weakening.

Use hypoallergenic tape to secure the electrodes to prevent redness or rash, cleanse the skin well after removing the electrodes, and apply lotion to the placement sites.

- *Medications*
  - —Explain the purpose, dosage, schedule, and route of administration of any prescribed drugs, as well as side effects to report to a physician or nurse.
  - —Give the patient general guidelines for the use of pain medications.

    Explain that a variety of pain relief measures may be necessary for some types of pain.

    Instruct the patient to use pain relief measures before pain becomes severe. Determine the patient's ability or willingness to participate actively in use of pain relief measures, and suggest pain relief measures the patient believes will be helpful.

    Rely on patient behavior that indicates pain severity rather than relying on known physical stimuli.

    Encourage the patient to try a pain relief measure at least twice before abandoning it as ineffective. Instruct the patient to keep an open mind as to what may relieve pain.

    Urge the patient to keep trying to relieve the pain and not to become discouraged.
  - —Discuss the use of nonnarcotic analgesics.

    Inform the patient that nonnarcotic analgesics include acetaminophen, aspirin, and nonsteroidal antiinflammatory drugs such as ibuprofen, indomethacin, and naproxen.

    Explain that these medications are generally well tolerated but have the potential to cause gastrointestinal ulceration, renal toxic effects, and inhibition of platelet aggregation.

    Tell the patient that if the nonnarcotic does not have a therapeutic effect initially, the dosage should be increased before another type of drug is tried.
  - —Discuss the use of narcotics, which are indicated for severe postoperative pain or intractable pain such as that associated with cancer.

    Inform the patient that narcotics include morphine, hydromorphone, and methadone and that these may be administered by intravenous drip, intrathecally, or epidurally to enhance the analgesic effect.

    Explain that fixed dosage schedules with adequate doses for pain relief provide more constant blood levels and predictable pain relief. Suggest that additional doses may be needed for breakthrough pain.

Discuss the side effects of narcotic analgesics: constipation, vomiting, and respiratory and central nervous system depression.

Review the use of narcotic agonists and antagonists: nalbuphine (Nubain), butorphanol (Stadol), pentazocine (Talwin), and buprenorphine (Buprenex).

—Explain the use of analgesic potentiators.

Inform the patient that these include phenothiazine derivatives such as promethazine (Phenergan), prochlorperazine (Compazine), and chlorpromazine (Thorazine); hydroxyzine (Vistaril); diazepam (Valium); lorazepam (Ativan); and diphenhydramine (Benadryl).

—Discuss the use of stimulants.

Inform the patient that these include cocaine, methylphenidate (Ritalin), dextroamphetamine, and caffeine.

—Discuss other types of drugs used in pain control, including tricyclic antidepressants such as amitriptyline (Elavil), imipramine (Tofranil), and doxepine (Sinequan), as well as butyrophenones such as droperidol (Inapsine) and haloperidol (Haldol).

—Discuss and demonstrate the use of equipment for administering pain relief medications.

External and implantable pumps for intravenous, epidural, and intrathecal administration of narcotic analgesics

Patient-controlled analgesia (PCA), particularly for the management of acute pain such as postoperative pain

Continuous subcutaneous infusion with an ambulatory infusion pump

Transcutaneous electrical nerve stimulation (TENS)

# Pancreatic Cancer

—**Pancreatic cancer: a highly malignant tumor that is insidious in onset and, because there are no early signs, is frequently diagnosed late in the course. Pancreatic tumors are usually adenocarcinomas arising in the head of the pancreas.**

## RISK FACTORS (KNOWN AND SUSPECTED)

- Medical history of diabetes or pancreatitis
- Cigarette smoking
- Dietary fat
- Alcoholism
- Organic chemicals such as coke, coal gas, beta-naphthylamine, and benzidine

## SIGNS/SYMPTOMS

- Weight loss, often gradual and progressive
- Pain: midepigastric, steady, dull, usually worse at night, more common in the left upper quadrant when the tumor is in the body or tail of the pancreas; lower abdominal pain in a small number of patients
- Back pain: aggravated by lying flat and relieved by sitting up and bending forward or lying curled in a fetal position
- Jaundice with itching of arms, legs, and abdomen; worse in evening and at night
- Weight loss
- Constipation, bloating, flatulence
- Depression

## COMPLICATIONS

- Thrombophlebitis
- Diabetes mellitus
- Bleeding tendencies
- Ascites

## DIAGNOSTIC TESTS

- Describe each procedure, its purpose, and the normal feelings or sensations that are likely, as well as any preprocedural and postprocedural care.
  - —Computed tomography, ultrasound: to determine the size and location of the lesion
  - —Fine-needle aspiration biopsy: to identify the type of tumor
  - —Endoscopic retrograde cholangiopancreatography: to determine more precisely the size and location of the tumor
  - —Angiography: to determine vascular involvement of the tumor
  - —Laparoscopy: to detect metastatic abdominal lesions
  - —Cancer antigen 19-9, carcinoembryonic antigen: nonspecific tumor markers elevated in the presence of pancreatic cancer

**TREATMENT**

*Medical*
- Therapy
  —Radiation therapy
  - High-dose external beam
  - Interstitial seed of iodine-125 or iridium-192
  - Brachytherapy
  - Intraoperative radiation therapy
- Drugs
  —5-Fluorouracil alone or with radiation therapy
  —Nitrosoureas, mitomycin-C, doxorubicin

*Surgical*
- Pancreatoduodenectomy (Whipple procedure)
- Total pancreatectomy
- Palliation: anastomosis of jejunum to distended common bile duct to relieve jaundice and itching

**HOME CARE**

- Give both the patient and the caregiver *verbal* and *written* instructions. Provide them with the name and telephone number of a physician or nurse to call if questions arise.
- *General information*
  —Review the physician's explanation of the disease process and prescribed treatment.
- *Warning signs*
  —Review the signs and symptoms that should be reported to a physician or nurse.
  - Weight loss, dehydration
  - Anorexia, constipation, bloating, flatulence, or other signs and symptoms of gastrointestinal distress
  - Pain uncontrolled by prescribed medication
- *Special instructions*
  —Teach the patient to use frequent baths, lotions, and ointments to soothe skin and lessen itching.
  —Teach the patient alternative methods of pain management to supplement or enhance pain medications (see Pain Management, p. 501).
- *Medications*
  —Explain the purpose, dosage, schedule, and route of administration of any prescribed drugs, as well as side effects to report to the physician or nurse.

—Teach the self-administration of insulin if diabetes develops (see Diabetes Mellitus, p. 236).

—Encourage the patient to use pain medications to maintain an acceptable level of comfort.

• *Diet*

—Stress the importance of adequate intake of fluids and food. Encourage small, frequent meals and the use of nutritional supplements.

## FOLLOW-UP CARE

• Stress the importance of follow-up visits. Make sure the patient has the necessary names and telephone numbers.

## PSYCHOSOCIAL CARE

• Encourage expressions of fear and feelings about death. Assist the patient and family to seek counseling.

• Encourage independence as much as possible.

## REFERRALS

• Assist the patient to obtain referral services, including home health and hospice care.

# Pancreatitis

—Pancreatitis: inflammation of the pancreas. Acute pancreatitis has a sudden onset, usually following a large meal or large intake of alcohol. The acute form is a type of autodigestion of the pancreas by its own enzymes, progressing to a necrotic form. Chronic pancreatitis is progressive functional damage to the pancreas.

## CONTRIBUTING FACTORS

• Excessive use of alcohol
• Gallbladder disease
• Cancer
• Physical trauma to abdomen
• Duodenal ulcer

- Mumps
- Drug toxicity: oral contraceptives, glucocorticoids, sulfon-amides, chlorothiazides, azathioprine

## SIGNS/SYMPTOMS

- Acute
  —Constant, severe epigastric pain
  —Pain radiating to back or left shoulder, somewhat relieved by sitting
  —Nausea and vomiting
  —Extreme malaise
  —Decreased urine output
  —Jaundice with gallbladder involvement
  —Fever, chills
  —Rapid pulse, low blood pressure
  —Discoloration of the flank or abdomen
  —Agitation, confusion related to electrolyte imbalance
- Chronic
  —Constant, dull epigastric pain
  —Sharp pain with radiation to the back
  —Pain relieved by sitting forward
  —Pain increased by eating or lying flat
  —Greasy, foul-smelling stools
  —Weight loss
  —Nausea and vomiting
  —Malnutrition
  —Fat-soluble vitamin deficiencies
  —Symptoms of diabetes mellitus

## COMPLICATIONS

- Acute
  —Acute respiratory distress syndrome
  —Electrolyte imbalance, cardiac dysrhythmias
  —Circulatory or renal failure
  —Shock, hemorrhage
  —Disseminated intravascular coagulation
- Both acute and chronic
  —Jaundice
  —Paralytic ileus
  —Hyperglycemia
  —Infection and abscesses

—Wound infection
—Surgical fistulas

## DIAGNOSTIC TESTS

• Describe each procedure, its purpose, and the normal feelings or sensations that are likely, as well as any preprocedural and postprocedural care.
—Stool for fat analysis
—X-ray of abdomen
—Ultrasound of abdomen
—Computed tomography of abdomen
—Upper gastrointestinal series
—Cholangiography
—Acute
  Urine studies: urinalysis, amylase
  Blood studies: complete blood count, blood urea nitrogen, glucose, calcium, albumin
  Pancreatic enzymes, amylase, lipase
—Chronic
  Urinalysis
  Blood studies: complete blood count, glucose, alkaline phosphatase, amylase, bilirubin
  Endoscopic retrograde cholangiopancreatography

## TREATMENT

*Medical*
• Therapy
—Acute pancreatitis
  Intravenous hydration
  NPO and nasogastric tube
  Bed rest
  Peritoneal lavage
  Nutritional support (total or partial parenteral nutrition, jejunostomy feeding)
• Drugs
—Acute pancreatitis
  Analgesics
  Antacids
  Antibiotics
  Anticholinergics
  Histamine $H_2$ blocker

—Chronic pancreatitis
    Analgesics, digestants (pancreatic enzyme supplements)
    Antacids
    Histamine $H_2$ blocker

*Surgical*

- Acute pancreatitis
    —Surgical drainage of pseudocysts
    —Surgical drainage of pancreatic abscesses
    —Surgery for gallbladder duct obstruction
- Chronic pancreatitis
    —Secondary treatment for pain complications (cysts, abscesses)
    —Surgery involving the pancreas or small intestine
    —Islet cell (for insulin) preservation
    —Autotransplantation of islet cell preparations
    —Autotransplantation of pancreas segments
    —Closed-loop insulin infusion system

## HOME CARE

- Give both the patient and the caregiver *verbal* and *written* instructions. Provide them with the name and telephone number of a physician or nurse to call if questions arise.
- *General information*
    —Explain the disease process, underlying cause, and contributing factors. Stress the importance of initiating measures to prevent further attacks.
    —Describe prescribed treatment. Explain that surgery is generally not indicated for pancreatic pseudocysts in abscess form.
- *Warning signs*
    —Review the signs and symptoms that should be reported to a physician or nurse.
        Severe epigastric pain relieved by sitting
        Nausea and vomiting
        Greasy, foul-smelling or clay-colored stools
        Weight loss
        Dark urine
        Pseudocyst: epigastric pain radiating to the back
- *Special instructions*
    —Discuss skin care, including the use of nonalcoholic lotions or creams to treat itchy, dry skin.
    —Discuss nonmedication measures for coping with pain, such as relaxation techniques and guided imagery.

- *Medications*
  —Explain the purpose, dosage, schedule, and route of administration of any prescribed drugs, as well as side effects to report to the physician or nurse.
  —Teach the patient how and when to take prescribed enzyme therapy. Instruct the patient to take enzymes with meals or snacks.
  —Teach the self-administration of insulin if diabetes develops (see Diabetes Mellitus, p. 236).
- *Diet*
  —Inform the patient that a high-carbohydrate, low-protein, low-fat diet or one prescribed by the physician should be followed.
  —Stress the importance of avoiding alcohol, caffeinated beverages (coffee, tea, soda), and spicy or irritating, gas-producing foods.

**FOLLOW-UP CARE**

- Stress the importance of follow-up visits. Make sure the patient has the necessary names and telephone numbers.

**REFERRALS**

- Obtain counseling and refer the patient to a community-based alcohol treatment program as needed.

# Parkinson's Disease
## (Paralysis Agitans)

—Parkinson's disease: a syndrome characterized by progressive muscle rigidity, bradykinesia (slowing of the ability to initiate voluntary movements), and involuntary tremors. Parkinson's disease often develops after age 60, and deterioration progresses for an average of 10 years, with death usually resulting from aspiration pneumonia or some other infection. Parkinson's disease involves degeneration of dopamine-producing cells in the brain, which leads to degeneration of neurons in the basal ganglia. Once cell loss reaches 80%, symptoms appear. There is no definable cause.

**CONTRIBUTING FACTORS**

- Drug exposure (e.g., neuroleptic drugs or reserpine)
- Carbon monoxide poisoning
- Manganese poisoning
- Tumors or infarcts involving the midbrain

**SIGNS/SYMPTOMS**

- Initial symptoms
  —Weakness, tendency to tremble (usually in one hand)
  —Slowness or awkwardness of affected limb
  —Some loss of facial expression
  —Deliberate quality of speech
  —Tendency to posture arm flexed at elbow
  —May progress to other side of body after 1-2 years
- Autonomic dysfunction
  —Skin: oily, perspiration, seborrhea
  —Intermittent, profuse diaphoresis
  —Gastric retention
  —Urgency or hesitation in urination
  —Urinary retention
  —Orthostatic hypotension
  —Dysphasia
- Equilibrium
  —Festination (leaning of trunk farther with each step)
  —Propulsion (forward stepping with leaning of trunk)
  —Retropulsion (backward stepping with leaning of trunk)
  —Lateropulsion (sidewise stepping with leaning of trunk)
- Face
  —Masklike facies (blank facial expression)
  —Decreased eye blinking
- Gradual dementia
  —Initial
      Forgetfulness
      Minor confusional episodes
      Depression
  —Later
      Irritability, nervousness
      Mood swings
      Paranoia and visual hallucinations
      Frank delirium
      Social isolation

- Hands
  —Fingers extended with metacarpophalangeal joints flexed approximately 30 degrees
  —Handwriting
  —Letters becoming progressively smaller (micrographia)
  —Tremulous writing
- Nutrition
  —Impaired deglutition
  —Drooling, excessive salivation
  —Weight loss
  —Failure of cricopharyngeal muscles to relax; choking
  —Constipation
- Posture and rigidity
  —Shuffling gait without arm swing
  —Akinesia (most evident in spinal musculature)
  —Stooped body posture
  —Impaired mobility; self-care deficits
- Speech
  —Involuntary repetition of sentences
  —Decreased amplitude
  —Soft, rapid monotone
- Tremors
  —Lips, jaw, tongue, facial muscles, axial muscles, limb muscles
  —Fingers: pill-rolling movement
  —Head: to-and-fro tremor
  —Usually resting tremors (most apparent when affected area is at rest): paralysis agitans
  —Exaggerated by stress and anxiety

## COMPLICATIONS

- Dementia
- Tardive dyskinesia (in drug-induced parkinsonism)
- Debilitation
- Sundowning

## DIAGNOSTIC TESTS

- Describe each procedure, its purpose, and the normal feelings or sensations that are likely, as well as any preprocedural and postprocedural care.
  —Serum examination: mild microcytic anemia
  —Chest x-ray: slight scoliosis

—Computed tomography, skull x-ray: normal results, or computed tomography may show cerebral atrophy when there is history of chronic dementia

—Electroencephalogram: normal results or slowing and disorganization

—Cineradiographic study of swallowing: abnormal pattern

—Gastrointestinal studies: hypomotility; delayed emptying of stomach, varying degrees of large bowel distention (frank megacolon in patients with severe constipation)

## TREATMENT

*Medical*

- Therapy
  —Treatment is done on an outpatient basis except for complications or elective surgery. The patient's physical limitations may require many adjustments in the home for activities of daily living.
- Drugs
  —Antiparkinson agents
  —Antidepressants
  —Antihistamines
  —Antioxidants (may be beneficial, but there is insufficient evidence to confirm)
  —Vitamin E in a low dose; 400 IU daily may be suggested

*Surgical*

- Stereotactic thalamotomy: to control tremors and rigidity by producing a small lesion in the ventrolateral nucleus of the thalamus

## HOME CARE

- Give both the patient and the caregiver *verbal* and *written* instructions. Provide them with the name and telephone number of a physician or nurse to call if questions arise.
- *General information*
  —Discuss the causes, symptoms, and treatment modalities for Parkinson's disease and explain procedures as they occur.
- *Medications*
  —Explain the purpose, dosage, schedule, and route of administration of any prescribed drugs, as well as side effects to report to the physician or nurse.
  —Explain that the patient must take medications with food to reduce gastric irritation and nausea.

- Activity
  - —Encourage the patient to discuss allowances and limitations with respect to occupation, recreation, and activities.
  - —Urge the patient to maintain activity to whatever degree is possible.
  - —Advise the patient to use a cane as necessary for walking.
  - —Instruct the patient in safety measures to prevent injury.
  - —Explain the need for speech therapy.
  - —Stress the importance of frequent skin care and oral hygiene.
  - —Teach the patient about the importance of bladder and bowel programs.
  - —Explain that following a daily exercise program can slow progression of the disease.
  - —Advise the patient about the importance of diversional activities.
  - —Emphasize the need for independence; tell caregivers to avoid overprotection and to permit the patient to perform self-care, including feeding, dressing, and walking.
- *Diet*
  - —Encourage the patient to follow a high-residue, high-bulk, high-roughage diet to promote gastrointestinal motility.
  - —Advise the use of natural laxatives such as prune juice to maintain regular bowel evacuation.
  - —Instruct the patient to control protein intake to minimize blocking of L-dopa.
  - —Encourage a fluid intake of 2000 ml per day, unless contraindicated, to maintain voiding.
  - —Suggest acidifying urine with orange or cranberry juice to minimize the potential for infection.
  - —Inform the patient of the need for a high-calorie, soft diet, and instruct the patient to take small bites and eat slowly.
  - —Discuss strategies to help with meals: cut food for the patient, place all utensils within easy reach, use a blender for thicker foods, use braces or splints to help with tremor, use a straw and bib to help with drooling.

## FOLLOW-UP CARE

- Stress the importance of continued outpatient care: physician visits, physical therapy, and home nursing care. Make sure the patient has the necessary names and telephone numbers.

## PSYCHOSOCIAL CARE

- Explain to the family the need to encourage social participation.
- Explain that although physically disabled, the patient is intellectually normal.
- Stress the importance of verbalization about loss of self-esteem, sexuality, and body functions.
- Advise the patient of the importance of expressing feelings.

## REFERRALS

- Ensure that the patient has the following addresses and phone numbers to obtain printed information: Parkinson's Disease Foundation, 710 W. 168th St., New York, NY 10032, phone (800) 344-8872; or United Parkinson's Foundation, 1501 N.W. 9th Ave., Miami, FL 33136, phone (800) 327-4545.

# Percutaneous Transluminal Coronary Angioplasty

—Percutaneous transluminal coronary angioplasty: nonsurgical, invasive procedure in which a balloon-tipped catheter is introduced, usually through an artery in the groin. Under fluoroscopy, the catheter is moved to specific areas of the coronary arteries of the heart that are narrowed by atherosclerotic plaque. The balloon is inflated to flatten the plaque and allow more blood and oxygen to reach the tissues.

## INDICATIONS

- Occluded or nearly occluded coronary arteries

## PREPROCEDURAL TEACHING

- Review the physician's explanation of the procedure and the reason for it; encourage the patient to ask questions and to discuss any fears or anxieties.

### Review of Preprocedural Care

- See Cardiac Catheterization (p. 144).

**Review of Postprocedural Care**

- Explain that the introductory catheter sheath remains in place after the procedure and the patient will spend 10-36 hours in the coronary care unit (CCU) for continuous monitoring.
- Stress the importance of flat bed rest. Explain that the head may be raised 15 degrees for meals only and only while the sheath is in place.
- Emphasize the need to keep the catheterized leg straight. Tell the patient that a light restraint may be applied as a reminder.
- Explain that frequent checks of vital signs, the groin, leg pulses, color, and temperature will be done.
- Inform the patient that a urine catheter or condom catheter may be in place overnight.
- Explain that intravenous hydration will continue overnight.
- Discuss removal of the sheath. Explain that it will occur 6-12 hours after the procedure; that pressure will be applied to the groin for 20-30 minutes manually or by special C clamp until there is no evidence of bleeding, with a 5-pound sandbag for 6-8 hours afterward; that flat bed rest will be maintained for 6-8 hours afterward, with bed rest overnight; and that vital signs, including pedal pulses and groin check, will be monitored frequently.
- Explain that the patient is usually moved out of the CCU after the sheath is removed and the condition is stabilized.
- Inform the patient that he or she will probably be allowed out of bed the next morning and may walk around. If heparin is being administered intravenously, the patient may get out of bed, take a few steps, and sit in the chair. The urine catheter is removed.

## COMPLICATIONS

- Failure to dilate coronary arteries
- Bleeding (groin)
- Rupture or dissection of coronary artery(ies)
- Heart attack
- Cardiac arrest
- Clot formation (leg or coronary arteries)
- Renal hypersensitivity to contrast dye (decreased urine)
- Abrupt reclosure of the coronary artery

## HOME CARE

- Give both the patient and the caregiver *verbal* and *written* instructions. Provide them with the name and telephone number of a physician or nurse to call if questions arise.

- *General information*
  —Review the explanation of the procedure and findings.
- *Warning signs*
  —Review the signs and symptoms that should be reported to a physician or nurse.

    Infection: redness; swelling; warm to touch; purulent drainage

    Active bleeding of the groin or an enlarging hematoma of the area: discoloration, firmness, tenderness

    Numbness or tingling of the affected extremity

    Angina unrelieved or shortness of breath

    Irregular pulse, lightheadedness, dizziness

    Constipation

- *Special instructions*
  —Explain that a Band-Aid over the puncture site may be changed and may not be needed after a day or two.
  —Inform the patient that if bleeding does occur at the groin site, pressure should be applied immediately, the patient should lie flat, and the physician should be called at once.
- *Medications*
  —Explain the purpose, dosage, schedule, and route of administration of any prescribed drugs, as well as side effects to report to a physician or nurse.
- *Activity*
  —Encourage the patient to discuss allowances and limitations with respect to occupation, recreation, or activities.
  —Discuss the need to avoid heavy lifting (>10 pounds), heavy exercise, straining with bowel movements, and sexual relations for about a week after the procedure or as advised by the physician.
  —Tell the patient that showering or bathing is permitted but that very hot water should not be used.
- *Diet*
  —Emphasize the need to limit or avoid alcohol as advised by the physician.

## FOLLOW-UP CARE

- Stress the importance of regular follow-up visits. Make sure the patient has the necessary names and telephone numbers.

# Pericardiocentesis

—**Pericardiocentesis: withdrawal of blood or fluid from the pericardial sac via percutaneous needle puncture.**

## INDICATIONS

- Relief of cardiac compression and withdrawal of pericardial fluid for analysis secondary to pericarditis or pericardial effusion

## PREPROCEDURAL TEACHING

- Review the physician's explanation of the procedure and the reason for it; encourage the patient to ask questions and to discuss any fears or anxieties. Explain the need for informed consent.

### Review of Preprocedural Care

- Instruct the patient not to eat or drink 4-6 hours before the procedure.
- Explain that the procedure will be performed under local anesthesia and sedation will be given.
- Inform the patient that the skin will be cleansed from the left costal margin to the xiphoid process.
- Explain that the patient will be positioned with the head of the bed elevated 20-30 degrees.
- Tell the patient that laboratory tests and a 12-lead electrocardiogram will be completed before the procedure.
- Explain that vital signs will be monitored throughout the procedure, including pulsus paradoxus and pulse pressure.
- Inform the patient that emergency treatment and medications will be readily available.
- Explain that oxygen will be administered by mask or cannula.

### Review of Postprocedural Care

- Inform the patient that signs and symptoms of complications or recurrence of cardiac tamponade or effusion will be monitored.
- Explain that bed rest will be ordered.
- Tell the patient that heart sounds and blood pressure will be monitored.

## SIDE EFFECTS/COMPLICATIONS

- Puncture of coronary artery, ventricle, or lung
- Dysrhythmias, including ventricular fibrillation
- Laceration of the lung
- Pneumothorax
- Air embolism
- Cardiac tamponade
- Myocardial injury

## HOME CARE

- Give both the patient and the caregiver *verbal* and *written* in-structions. Provide them with the name and telephone number of a physician or nurse to call if questions arise.
- *General information*
  —Review any explanation of the procedure and specific follow-up care.
- *Warning signs*
  —Review the signs and symptoms that should be reported to a physician or nurse.
  
  Dyspnea
  Palpitations
  Chest pain
  Lightheadedness
  Fever

## FOLLOW-UP CARE

- Stress the importance of regular follow-up visits for care of the specific disease process. Make sure the patient has the necessary names and telephone numbers.

# Pericarditis

—Pericarditis: **inflammatory process of the outer lining of the heart, which leads to the formation of a serous fluid and fibrous adhesion. The thickening and scarring of the lining can restrict the movement of the heart muscles. The condition may be acute or chronic.**

## CAUSES/CONTRIBUTING FACTORS/RISK FACTORS

- Infection: bacterial, viral, fungal
- Myocardial infarction
- Trauma from surgery
- Tuberculosis
- Tumors
- Drugs
- Radiation
- Autoimmune diseases
- Idiopathic factors

## SIGNS/SYMPTOMS

- Sudden sharp chest pain radiating to the shoulder, back, and arm
- Pain that worsens when lying down or with inspiration and is relieved by leaning forward
- Fever and chills
- Nausea
- Shortness of breath
- Anxiety
- Fatigue

## COMPLICATIONS

- Pericardial effusion
- Cardiac tamponade
- Chronic constriction of myocardium

## DIAGNOSTIC TESTS

- Describe each procedure, its purpose, and the normal feelings or sensations that are likely, as well as any preprocedural and postprocedural care.
    —Blood tests: white blood cell count, blood urea nitrogen, erythrocyte sedimentation rate, cardiac enzymes
    —12-Lead electrocardiogram: to identify diffuse ST elevation
    —Chest x-ray: to detect enlarged cardiac silhouette
    —Echocardiogram: to detect accumulation of fluid around the heart

## TREATMENT

*Medical*
- Therapy
    —Pericardiocentesis: needle aspiration of excess fluid from pericardial sac

- Drugs
  —Nonsteroidal antiinflammatory drugs
  —Steroids
  —Analgesics
  —Antibiotics

*Surgical*
- Pericardial window: open pericardial drainage
- Pericardiectomy: surgical removal of visceral and parietal pericardium

## HOME CARE

- Give both the patient and the caregiver *verbal* and *written* instructions. Provide them with the name and telephone number of a physician or nurse to call if questions arise.
- *General information*
  —Discuss the development of pericarditis, causes and contributing factors, care, and treatment.
- *Warning signs*
  —Review the signs and symptoms that should be reported to a physician or nurse.
  
  Recurrence of symptoms
  
  Chest pain
  
  Fever
  
  Signs and symptoms of cold and flu
- *Special instructions*
  —Instruct the patient to avoid people with colds or flu and to get medical attention at once if an infection, cold, or flu is suspected.
  —Advise the patient that sitting up and leaning forward on a table may ease chest discomfort.
  —Inform the patient that a feeling of wellness does not necessarily mean that inflammation is completely resolved.
- *Medications*
  —Explain the purpose, dosage, schedule, and route of administration of any prescribed drugs, as well as side effects to report to the physician or nurse.
  —Stress the importance of not stopping medications without notifying the physician.
- *Activity*
  —Explain the need to increase activity gradually, avoid activities that require large amounts of energy, and take frequent rest periods during the day.

- *Diet*
  —Advise the patient to follow the prescribed diet.

**FOLLOW-UP CARE**
- Stress the importance of follow-up visits. Make sure the patient has the necessary names and telephone numbers.

# Pernicious Anemia
## (Hyperchromic Macrocytic Anemia)

—Pernicious anemia: an anemia caused by decreased absorption of vitamin $B_{12}$. Deficiency of an intrinsic factor essential for absorption of vitamin $B_{12}$ causes production of red blood cells with increasingly fragile cell membranes, which leads to widespread destruction of the cells and results in low hemoglobin levels. Deficiency of vitamin $B_{12}$ causes gastric, intestinal, and neurologic abnormalities.

**CAUSES/CONTRIBUTING FACTORS/RISK FACTORS**
- Primary
  —Genetic predisposition
  —Immunologically related diseases (thyroiditis, myxedema, Graves' disease)
- Secondary
  —Surgical removal of a portion of the stomach, limiting the amount of productive mucosa

**SIGNS/SYMPTOMS**
- Classic trilogy of signs: weakness; beefy red, sore tongue; numbness and tingling in the extremities
- Gastrointestinal
  —Nausea and vomiting
  —Anorexia
  —Weight loss
  —Flatulence

- —Diarrhea
- —Constipation
- —Pallor
- —Jaundice
- Neurologic
  - —Lack of coordination
  - —Impaired fine finger movement
  - —Lightheadedness
  - —Headache
  - —Altered vision (blurred, double vision)
  - —Ringing in the ears
  - —Irritability
  - —Depression
  - —Poor memory
  - —Impaired judgment
  - —Paresthesias of hands and feet

## COMPLICATIONS

- Paralysis
- Psychotic behavior: paranoia, hallucinations, delusions
- Loss of bowel and bladder control
- Fatal if left untreated
- Cardiomegaly, congestive heart failure
- Gastritis
- Infections: pulmonary, urinary
- Peptic ulcer disease (4-5 times greater in this population)

## DIAGNOSTIC TESTS

- Describe each procedure, its purpose, and the normal feelings or sensations that are likely, as well as any preprocedural and postprocedural care.
  - —Schilling test: definitive for diagnosis of pernicious anemia
  - —Bone marrow biopsy: increased megaloblasts
  - —Gastric analysis: elevated pH, no free hydrochloric acid
  - —Therapeutic trial with parenteral vitamin $B_{12}$: increased reticulocyte count in 4-5 days following injection
  - —Laboratory tests
    Red blood cells: <3 million
    Mean corpuscular volume, mean corpuscular hemoglobin concentration: elevated

White blood cell count, mean corpuscular hemoglobin: decreased

Bilirubin: unconjugated forms elevated

Serum vitamin $B_{12}$: decreased

Serum folate: decreased

Hemoglobin: decreased

## TREATMENT

*Medical*

- Therapy
  - —Blood transfusions
  - —Diet high in vitamin $B_{12}$
- Drugs
  - —$B_{12}$ replacement therapy
  - —Folic acid (Folvite)
  - —Iron replacement
  - —Ferrous sulfate (Feosol); ferrous gluconate (Fergon)
  - —Digestants: hydrochloric acid
  - —Antifungal, analgesic mouth rinse

## HOME CARE

- Give both the patient and the caregiver *verbal* and *written* instructions. Provide them with the name and telephone number of a physician or nurse to call if questions arise.
- *General information*
  - —Explain and discuss pernicious anemia, its causes, and contributing factors.
  - —Review symptoms of the disease. Explain that most symptoms will recede with treatment.
- *Warning signs*
  - —Review the signs and symptoms that should be reported to a physician or nurse.

    Pulmonary infection: fever, cough, production of sputum

    Urinary tract infection: frequency, urgency, burning with urination, foul-smelling urine

    Neurologic disturbances: increasing weakness, lack of coordination, irritability, confusion

- *Special instructions*
  —Explain that the weakened condition may predispose the patient to infection. Stress the importance of avoiding large crowds and individuals who have or are suspected of having infections.
  —Discuss oral care if the mucous membranes and tongue are red, swollen, and painful.
  > Rinse the mouth every 2 hours while awake with dilute mouthwash or normal saline.
  > Use a soft-bristled toothbrush or sponge cleaners as indicated. Use water-soluble jelly on the lips.
  > Medicate with topical analgesics as ordered for severe discomfort.
  —Discuss safety measures.
  > Advise a patient who has sensory deficits to avoid exposure of the extremities to extreme heat and cold.
  > Encourage the use of assistive devices for ambulation (walker, cane) as indicated.
  > Encourage the use of nonslipping, well-fitting shoes.
  > Instruct the patient to remove hazards such as loose rugs and furniture that blocks walkways.
- *Medications*
  —Explain the purpose, dosage, schedule, and route of administration of any prescribed drugs, as well as side effects to report to the physician or nurse.
  —Explain the importance of taking vitamin $B_{12}$ on a lifelong basis.
  —Instruct the patient to avoid taking over-the-counter medications without first consulting the physician or nurse.
  —Teach the patient or caregiver the proper injection technique for administering vitamin $B_{12}$, or arrange for monthly clinic visits for injection.
  —For injections administered by the patient or caregiver, provide information about obtaining vitamin $B_{12}$, needles, syringes, and alcohol sponges. Teach the proper method for disposing of needles and syringes.
- *Activity*
  —Encourage the patient to discuss allowances and limitations with respect to occupation, recreation, and activities.
  —Encourage the patient to pace activities, allow for frequent rest periods, and avoid overexertion.

—Encourage the patient to participate in regular exercise as tolerated to prevent complications from motor deficits.
- *Diet*
  —Encourage a diet that is high in vitamin $B_{12}$ (eggs, fish, meat, milk).
  —Encourage the patient to take 2500 ml of fluid daily (unless contraindicated) and to avoid hot liquids.
  —Teach the patient to eat small, frequent meals and between-meal snacks to enhance appetite.
  —Discuss the need to avoid foods that may irritate the gastrointestinal tract (spicy, flatus-forming, and caffeine).
  —Encourage the patient to weigh daily at the same time of day and in the same clothing and to record and report steady or rapid weight losses to the physician.

## FOLLOW-UP CARE

- Stress the importance of follow-up medical and laboratory evaluations. Make sure the patient has the necessary names and telephone numbers.

# Pheochromocytoma
## (Chromaffin Tumor)

—**Pheochromocytoma: a chromaffin cell tumor of the sympathetic nervous system that produces excessive amounts of epinephrine and norepinephrine. Pheochromocytoma is characterized by paroxysmal or sustained hypertension, increased metabolism, and hyperglycemia and occurs most commonly in women between the ages of 30 and 40. Although this disorder is potentially fatal, the prognosis is generally good with treatment. Most tumors are benign.**

## CAUSES/PRECIPITATING FACTORS

- Adrenal chromaffin cell tumor in adrenal medulla or sympathetic ganglia

- Extraadrenal chromaffin cell tumor in abdomen, thorax, urinary bladder, or neck
- Inherited as an autosomal dominant trait
- Postural drainage
- Exercise
- Laughing
- Smoking
- Urination
- Change in body or environmental temperature
- Vasovagal stimulus
- Anything that puts pressure on the tumor (e.g., pregnancy)

**SIGNS/SYMPTOMS**

- Persistent or paroxysmal hypertension
- Headache
- Palpitations
- Visual blurring
- Nausea and vomiting
- Weight loss
- Severe diaphoresis
- Feelings of impending doom
- Precordial or abdominal pain
- Tachypnea
- Pallor or flushing
- Tremors

**COMPLICATIONS**

- Cerebrovascular accident
- Retinopathy
- Heart disease
- Dysrhythmia
- Kidney failure

**DIAGNOSTIC TESTS**

- Describe each procedure, its purpose, and the normal feelings or sensations that are likely, as well as any preprocedural and postprocedural care.
  —Computed tomography or magnetic resonance imaging: to identify adrenal gland lesions
  —Computed tomography, x-ray, or abdominal aortography: to identify extraadrenal lesions

—Laboratory tests

Total plasma catecholamine: 10-50 times higher than normal

24-Hour urinalysis: increased secretion of catecholamines and metabolites

## TREATMENT

*Medical*

- Drugs
  - —Alpha-adrenergic blocking agents

    Phentolamine (Regitine)

    Phenoxybenzamine (Dibenzyline)
  - —Beta-adrenergic blocking agents

    Propranolol (Inderal)
  - —Tyrosine inhibitors

    Alpha-methylparatyrosine
  - —Glucorticoids, mineralocorticoids: for surgical patients
  - —Analgesics: for headache, postsurgical pain

*Surgical*

- Removal of pheochromocytoma

## HOME CARE

- Give both the patient and the caregiver *verbal* and *written* instructions. Provide them with the name and telephone number of a physician or nurse to call if questions arise.
- *General information*
  - —Discuss pheochromotytoma and its causes and precipitating factors. Explain that surgery is the preferred treatment.
  - —Provide the patient with information about adrenalectomy if performed (see p. 13).
- *Warning signs*
  - —Review the signs and symptoms of an acute attack that should be reported to a physician or nurse.

    Headache

    Nausea

    Dizziness

    Palpitations

    Dyspnea

    Diaphoresis
- *Special instructions*
  - —Demonstrate to the patient and caregiver how to measure and record blood pressure at home. Permit time for practice. Advise the patient on where to obtain equipment.

—Instruct the patient to weigh daily at the same time, on the same scale, and wearing the same clothing.

—Review precipitating events and discuss how to avoid them.

—Teach stress reduction techniques: meditation, breathing exercises, imagery.

—Instruct surgical patients to monitor for infection (respiratory or urinary tract): fever; cough; foul-smelling sputum; burning, frequency, or urgency with urination; foul-smelling urine.

—Instruct the patient to inspect the surgical site daily for signs of infection: drainage, separation of suture line, redness, swelling.

- *Medications*

  —Explain the purpose, dosage, schedule, and route of administration of any prescribed drugs, as well as side effects to report to the physician or nurse.

  —Instruct the patient to avoid taking over-the-counter medications without first consulting the physician or nurse.

- *Activity*

  —Encourage the patient to discuss allowances and limitations with respect to occupation, recreation, and activities.

- *Diet*

  —Advise the patient to avoid tyramine-containing foods (e.g., aged cheese, wine).

  —Encourage the patient to eat small, frequent meals.

**FOLLOW-UP CARE**

- Stress the importance of follow-up medical and laboratory evaluations. Make sure the patient has the necessary names and telephone numbers.

- Discuss the need to wear a Medic-Alert bracelet and carry an identification card at all times.

# Photodynamic Therapy
## (Laser Therapy)

—Photodynamic therapy: treatment involving injecting a patient with an intravenous photosensitizing agent such as dihematoporphyrin ether (DHE), waiting 48-72 hours for the drug to concentrate in malignant cells, and then exposing the cancerous area to laser light delivered through a scope such as a cystoscope or bronchoscope.

## INDICATIONS

- Possible cure for early stages of skin and bladder cancers
- Palliation of advanced lung, esophageal, and pelvic cancers
- Alleviation of symptoms caused by obstructive primary or secondary cancer
- Tumor debulking with relief of bleeding, infection, pain, and symptoms of obstruction

## PREPROCEDURAL TEACHING

- Review the physician's explanation of the procedure and the reason for it; encourage the patient to ask questions and to discuss any fears or anxieties.

### Review of Preprocedural Care

- Assure the patient that the procedure is painless.

### Review of Postprocedural Care

- Teach the patient to stay out of sunlight for up to 6 weeks after treatment because of tissue photosensitivity.
- If the procedure is used to treat bladder cancer, inform the patient that severe urinary frequency and urgency may be experienced and bladder capacity decreased; that bladder capacity usually returns to normal within 3 months; and that oral analgesics, antispasmodics, and prophylactic antibiotics may be prescribed.

# Pleural Effusion

—Pleural effusion: accumulation of fluid (blood, pus, chyle, serous fluid) in the pleural space between visceral and parietal pleura (lining of the lung). Types of effusion include exudate, which is an often dark yellow or amber fluid resulting from a disease of the pleural surface or an obstruction in the lymphatic system, and transudate, which is fluid produced when the flow of protein-free fluid is disturbed.

## CAUSES/CONTRIBUTING FACTORS

- Exudate
  - —Neoplastic diseases
  - —Viral infections
  - —Tuberculosis
  - —Empyema pneumonia
  - —Chest trauma
  - —Pancreatitis
  - —Rheumatic fever
  - —Collagen-vascular disease
  - —Uremia
  - —Pulmonary embolism
  - —Subphrenic abscess
- Transudate
  - —Peritoneal dialysis
  - —Pericarditis
  - —Cirrhosis
  - —Congestive heart failure
  - —Myxedema
  - —Sarcoidosis
  - —Hypoproteinemia
  - —Nephrotic syndrome
  - —Atelectasis

## SIGNS/SYMPTOMS

- Shortness of breath
- Respiratory difficulty
- Localized chest pain
- Asymmetric chest expansion
- Elevated temperature
- Fatigue
- Cough

## COMPLICATIONS

- Pneumothorax
- Atelectasis
- Empyema

**DIAGNOSTIC TESTS**

- Describe each procedure, its purpose, and the normal feelings or sensations that are likely, as well as any preprocedural and postprocedural care.
  —Chest x-ray
  —Thoracentesis
  —Pleural biopsy

**TREATMENT**

*Medical*

- Therapy
  —Bed rest
  —Chest tube insertion
  —Thoracentesis
- Drugs
  —Antibiotics
  —Antipyretics
  —Pain management medications
  —Nitrogen mustard instillation or tetracycline via chest tube

**HOME CARE**

- Give both the patient and the caregiver *verbal* and *written* instructions. Provide them with the name and telephone number of a physician or nurse to call if questions arise.
- *General information*
  —Explain the underlying cause and contributing factors.
- *Warning signs*
  —Review the signs and symptoms that should be reported to a physician or nurse.
    Difficulty in breathing
    Chest pain
    Elevated temperature
    Persistent cough
    Symptoms of cold or flu
- *Special instructions*
  —Discuss measures to prevent respiratory infections: avoiding persons with infections, especially upper respiratory infections; obtaining influenza vaccinations as ordered.
  —Instruct and demonstrate coughing and deep breathing to maintain lung aeration, and encourage the patient to perform them.
  —Demonstrate the use of the incentive spirometer.

- *Medications*
  —Explain the purpose, dosage, schedule, and route of administration of any prescribed drugs, as well as side effects to report to the physician or nurse.
  —Instruct the patient to avoid taking over-the-counter medications without first consulting the physician or nurse.
- *Activity*
  —Advise the patient of the importance of exercising to tolerance, avoiding fatigue, and planning rest periods.

**FOLLOW-UP CARE**

- Stress the importance of follow-up visits. Make sure the patient has the necessary names and telephone numbers.
- Emphasize the importance of not smoking and of avoiding secondhand smoke.

# Pneumonia and Pneumonitis

—**Pneumonia: an inflammatory process of the respiratory bronchioles and alveolar spaces caused by infection. Bacterial pneumonia is usually caused by** *Streptococcus, Staphylococcus,* **or** *Haemophilus.* **The infection can start from an upper respiratory infection such as "strep" throat or from inhaling fluid or other foreign substances into the lungs.** *Viral pneumonia* **is commonly caused by influenza A. It is transmitted by respiratory droplets.** *Mycoplasma* **pneumonia, which is most common in school-age children and young adults, spreads among family members. Transmission is believed to be by infected respiratory secretions. Aspiration pneumonia syndrome occurs as a result of aspiration when the patient is in an altered state of consciousness (e.g., seizure, use of drugs or alcohol, anesthesia, acute infection, or shock).**

—**Pneumonitis: noninfectious bronchial and alveolar inflammation.**

**SIGNS/SYMPTOMS**

- Chills and fever (102°-106° F [38.8°-41.1° C])

- Difficult and painful respirations
- Pleuritic pain
- Shortness of breath and grunting
- Tachypnea
- Diaphoresis
- Loss of appetite or upset stomach
- Generalized fatigue that is worse than you would expect from a cold
- Cough that produces greenish yellow sputum progressing to pink or rusty
- Restlessness
- Cyanosis
- Disorientation or confusion and low-grade fever in elderly
- Anxiety

**COMPLICATIONS**

- Atelectasis
- Empyema
- Acute respiratory distress syndrome
- Superinfection pericarditis
- Lung abscess

**DIAGNOSTIC TESTS**

- Describe each procedure, its purpose, and the normal feelings or sensations that are likely, as well as any preprocedural and postprocedural care.
    - Chest x-ray: to evaluate the pulmonary system; to detect patchy or diffuse infiltrates
    - Sputum examination for Gram stain and culture and sensitivity tests: to identify microorganisms present so that appropriate antiinfective agents can be prescribed
    - White blood cell count: increased ($>11,000/\mu l$) in the presence of bacterial pneumonia; normal or low in viral or *Mycoplasma* pneumonia
    - Blood culture and sensitivity: to determine the presence of bacteremia and aid in identification of the causative organism
    - Serologic studies: to diagnose viral pneumonia; relative rise in antibody titer suggests viral infection
    - Arterial blood gases
    - Bronchoscopy

**TREATMENT**

*Medical*

- Therapy
  —Fluid management
  —Parenteral therapy
  —Oxygen therapy
  —Chest physiotherapy
  —Artificial airway or mechanical ventilation support
- Drugs
  —Antipyretics
  —Antibiotics

**HOME CARE**

- Give both the patient and the caregiver *verbal* and *written* instructions. Provide them with the name and telephone number of a physician or nurse to call if questions arise.
- *General information*
  —Explain the underlying cause and contributing factors.
- *Warning signs*
  —Review the signs and symptoms that should be reported to a physician or nurse.
    Elevated temperature
    Diaphoresis
    Difficulty in breathing
    Persistent cough
    Cold or flu
- *Special instructions*
  —Explain the importance of avoiding transmission of disease: turn head away when coughing, cover mouth with tissue, use tissue only once, dispose of tissue in waste container, and wash hands after handling soiled tissues and before and after using the bathroom.
  —Explain the need to avoid recurrence of disease: avoid persons with infections, especially upper respiratory infections.
  —Administer the influenza vaccine as ordered.
  —Demonstrate and explain the importance of postural drainage and deep breathing exercises. Tell the patient to continue deep breathing exercises four times a day for 6-8 weeks.
  —Explain the need to use a vaporizer or humidifier at home. Advise the patient on obtaining the equipment from a drugstore or pharmacy.

- *Medications*
  —Explain the purpose, dosage, schedule, and route of administration of any prescribed drugs, as well as side effects to report to the physician or nurse.
    Antibiotics
    Antipyretics
    Analgesics: for chest pain
    Cough suppressants: for nonproductive cough
  —Instruct the patient to avoid taking over-the-counter medications without first consulting the physician or nurse.
- *Activity*
  —Explain the importance of a gradual convalescence.
  —Explain the need to limit exercise and activity to tolerance, to avoid fatigue, and to plan two or three rest periods during the day.
  —Explain the need for 7-8 hours of sleep every night.
- *Diet*
  —Explain the importance of maintaining a diet as tolerated.
  —Advise the patient to drink at least 6-8 glasses of fluids (up to 300 ml) daily unless contraindicated.

**FOLLOW-UP CARE**
- Stress the importance of follow-up visits. Make sure the patient has the necessary names and telephone numbers.

---

# Polycystic Kidney Disease

—**Polycystic kidney disease: hereditary kidney disease characterized by multiple fluid-filled cysts that enlarge and eventually compress and replace the functioning kidney tissue. In the adult form the onset is insidious, symptoms appear between 30 and 50 years of age, and the disease progresses slowly to renal failure.**

**SIGNS/SYMPTOMS**
- Early
  —Hypertension
  —Increased urine output
  —Urinary tract infection

- Late
  —Abdominal pain and distention
  —Lumbar pain
  —Widening abdominal girth
  —Palpable kidneys
  —Hematuria
  —Proteinuria
  —Decreased urine output

## COMPLICATIONS

- Ruptured cysts causing infection and bleeding
- Severe hypertension
- Abscesses
- Ureteral obstruction from clots
- Renal failure

## DIAGNOSTIC TESTS

- Describe each procedure, its purpose, and the normal feelings or sensations that are likely, as well as any preprocedural and postprocedural care.
  —Blood studies: electrolytes, protein, blood urea nitrogen, creatinine
  —Urine studies: urinalysis, culture and sensitivity, 24-hour urine for creatinine clearance
  —X-ray of kidney, ureter, bladder
  —Intravenous pyelogram, urogram
  —Renal computed tomography

## TREATMENT

*Medical*

- Therapy
  —Bed rest if bleeding
  —Dietary restrictions on sodium, potassium, protein
  —Dialysis for end-stage renal disease
- Drugs
  —Antihypertensives
  —Diuretics
  —Antibiotics

*Surgery*

- Intervention if cysts break and cause abscesses (see Abdominal Surgery, p. 3)

- Intervention if bleeding too heavily (see Abdominal Surgery)
- Nephrectomy
- Kidney transplant

## HOME CARE

- Give both the patient and the caregiver *verbal* and *written* instructions. Provide them with the name and telephone number of a physician or nurse to call if questions arise.
- *General information*
  —Explain the disease process and outcome.
- *Warning signs*
  —Review the signs and symptoms that should be reported to a physician or nurse.

    Sudden change in urine: color, blood, decreased amount, odor

    Sudden onset of flank pain

    Fever, chills

    Urinary tract infection: fever; chills; painful urination; low back or flank pain; cloudy, foul-smelling urine (ammonia or fishy smell); or blood in urine

- *Special instructions*
  —Instruct the patient in prevention of urinary tract infections: increased fluid intake (amount will depend on stage of disease), regular emptying of bladder, good perineal area care after urination and defecation, and thorough handwashing before and after toileting.
  —Instruct the patient to take, monitor, and record blood pressure and provide parameters to report.
  —Instruct the patient to weigh daily at the same time, using the same scale, and wearing the same clothing.
- *Medications*
  —Explain the purpose, dosage, schedule, and route of administration of any prescribed drugs, as well as side effects to report to the physician or nurse.
- *Activity*
  —Advise the patient to identify and avoid activities that may precipitate pain.
  —Encourage the patient to discuss allowances and limitations with respect to occupation, recreation, and activities.
  —Tell the patient to exercise to tolerance but to avoid contact sports (e.g., football, soccer, basketball).

—As the disease advances, encourage the patient to take frequent rest periods and avoid fatigue.
* *Diet*
  —Explain that the diet depends on the stage of the disease and includes restrictions on sodium, potassium, and protein. Fluids are encouraged at first and then restricted if kidney function decreases.

**FOLLOW-UP CARE**

* Stress the importance of follow-up visits. Make sure the patient has the necessary names and telephone numbers.

# Prostate Cancer

—Prostate cancer: cancer of the prostate gland, the most common site of cancer in men. Prostate cancer is rare in men under 50 years of age. The incidence and mortality are increasing, especially among African-Americans. Most prostate cancers are adenocarcinomas, which grow slowly, spread via the lymphatics through the pelvic region and into the pelvic bones, and spread via the blood to the lungs, liver, kidneys, and bones (vertebrae, pelvis, femur, and ribs). The rest are ductal (transitional cell and squamous cell carcinoma, endometrioid cancer, or sarcoma). Acinar dysplasia/prostatic intraepithelial neoplasia is a premalignant lesion.

**CAUSES/CONTRIBUTING FACTORS**

* Influence of endogenous hormones, especially dihydrotestosterone
* Genetic influences
* Dietary fat
* Exposure to certain viruses, pathogens, or industrial chemicals
* Urbanization

**SIGNS/SYMPTOMS**

* Early
  —Weak urinary stream
  —Frequency

—Dysuria
—Difficulty starting and stopping urination
- Pain in lower back, pelvis, or upper thighs
- Bilateral obstruction with renal insufficiency
- Late
  —Hematuria
  —Bone pain, urinary frequency, decreased stream, dribbling

## DIAGNOSTIC TESTS

- Describe each procedure, its purpose, and the normal feelings or sensations that are likely, as well as any preprocedural and postprocedural care.
  —Digital rectal examination: to palpate the prostate gland and detect abnormalities
  —Needle biopsy via perineal or transrectal route: to detect malignant cells
  —Transrectal ultrasonography: to determine the presence and characteristics of the lesion
  —Computed tomography and magnetic resonance imaging: to determine the size and extent of the lesion
  —Lymphangiography: to determine the extent of paraaortic and pelvic node involvement
  —Prostate-specific antigen: tumor marker that is elevated in the presence of prostate cancer

## TREATMENT

*Medical*
- Therapy
  —Radiation therapy
    External beam
    Interstitial implant
    General preprocedural and postprocedural care (see Radiation Therapy, p. 559)
- Drugs
  —Single-agent chemotherapy
    Cyclophosphamide
    5-Fluorouracil
    Doxorubicin
    Methotrexate
    Cisplatin
    Mitomycin-C
    Dacarbazine

—Hormone therapy
    Diethylstilbestrol
    Premarin
    Estradiol
    Stilphostrol
    Estramustine phosphate
—Medical adrenalectomy
    Aminoglutethimide
    Ketoconazole
    Spironolactone
    Glucocorticoids
—Antiandrogens
    Cyproterone acetate
    Flutamide
    Megestrol acetate
—Gonadotropin-releasing hormone agonists
    Leuprolide
    Zoladex
    Buserelin

*Surgery*

- Transurethral resection
- Radical prostatectomy
- Bilateral orchiectomy
- General preprocedural and postprocedural care (see Prostatectomy, p. 544)

## HOME CARE

- Give both the patient and the caregiver *verbal* and *written* instructions. Provide them with the name and telephone number of a physician or nurse to call if questions arise.
- *General information*
  —Review the physician's explanation of the disease, possible causes or contributing factors, type and stage of tumor, and prescribed treatment.
  —Discuss actual and potential sexual dysfunction associated with the prescribed therapy. Encourage questions (see Testicular Cancer, p. 622).
- *Warning signs*
  —Review the signs and symptoms that should be reported to a physician or nurse.
      Decreased output
      Edema

Hypertension

Weight gain

- *Special instructions*
  —Discuss methods of pain management (see Pain Management, p. 501).
- *Medications*
  —Explain the purpose, dosage, schedule, and route of administration of any prescribed drugs, as well as side effects to report to the physician or nurse.
- *Activity*
  —Stress the importance of adequate fluid intake, exercise, and rest.

## FOLLOW-UP CARE

- Stress the importance of follow-up visits, including an annual digital rectal examination if the prostate was not removed. Make sure the patient has the necessary names and telephone numbers.

## PSYCHOSOCIAL CARE

- Encourage the verbalization of feelings regarding body image, self-esteem, and sexuality.

## REFERRALS

- Assist the patient to obtain referral services, access to support groups, and sexual counseling services.

# Prostatectomy

—**Prostatectomy: removal of part or all of the prostate gland to relieve obstruction of urinary flow.** *Transurethral resection of the prostate* **(TURP) is removal of part of the hypertrophied prostate by means of a cystoscope or rectoscope inserted through the urethra. A spinal or light general anesthetic is used, and the hospital day is 3 or more days.** *Laser ablation prostatectomy* **is the passage of a laser scope through the urethra to ablate part of the prostate. The patient is under gen-**

eral or spinal anesthesia. The surgery is performed on the day of admission and the patient usually stays overnight. *Open prostatectomy* is surgical removal of part of the prostate through an incision in the lower abdomen or perineum because of an enlarged prostate or such complications as recurrent bladder stones, bladder diverticula, immobile hip joints, or localized cancer. *Radical prostatectomy* is removal of the entire prostate, including the covering capsule and ducts within, through a surgical incision in the lower abdomen. Removal is based on diagnosis of cancer, including the capsule.

## INDICATIONS

- Benign prostatic hypertrophy
- Prostate cancer

## PREPROCEDURAL TEACHING

- Review the physician's explanation of the procedure and the reason for it; encourage the patient to ask questions and to discuss any fears or anxieties. Explain the need for informed consent for surgery, anesthesia, and blood transfusions.

### Review of Preprocedural Care

- Inform that patient that routine blood and urine studies, a chest x-ray, and an electrocardiogram will be performed.
- Explain that bowel preparation with an enema will be needed the night before.
- Instruct the patient to shower and shampoo with bactericidal soap (e.g., Dial, Safeguard, Hibiclens) the night before.
- Discuss the need for NPO status from midnight the night before.
- Mention the possibility that the pubic hair will be shaved before the operation.
- Explain that some procedures can affect sexual function.
  - —TURP or open prostatectomy: semen may go into the bladder rather than out during ejaculation (retrograde ejaculation); does not cause impotence; affects fertility
  - —Radical prostatectomy: depends on extent of surgery and whether nerves are spared; may or may not affect ejaculatory function
  - —Laser ablation prostatectomy: ejaculatory function often preserved, although diminished in volume

## Review of Postprocedural Care

- For general postoperative care, see Abdominal Surgery (p. 3).
- Explain that the urine will be blood colored (bright red), then turn a darker tea color, and then lighten within about 1 week. Tell the patient that the urine may become pink-tinged with excessive walking or sitting.
- Explain that stress incontinence or dribbling after urinary catheter removal may occur and that pelvic (Kegel) exercises may improve the condition.
- Explain the possibility of frequent dressing changes with the flat Penrose drain.
- Tell the patient that sitting for long periods (over 2 hours) may stimulate bleeding during the first week.
- Discuss care after TURP.
  - Explain that the patient will be remain in the hospital for 3 or more days.
  - Inform the patient that drainage tubes will be in place after surgery: a three-way urinary catheter in the urethra for continuous bladder irrigation.
  - Tell the patient that traction of the urinary catheter will be in place for a time after surgery.
  - Discuss the use of elastic stockings or alternating pressure stockings while the patient is in bed.
  - Stress the importance of deep breathing and coughing.
- Discuss care after laser ablation prostatectomy.
  - Tell the patient that surgery will be on the day of admission and an overnight stay will be required.
  - Explain that a urinary catheter usually stays in place about 5 days.
- Discuss care after open and radical prostatectomy.
  - Tell the patient that surgery will be performed on the day of admission and a 3- to 5-day stay will be needed.
  - Explain the drainage tubes that may be used: urinary catheter for 7-10 days or more; suprapubic catheter; flat Penrose drainage tube under the tissue near the incision; Jackson-Pratt (self-suction) drain near the incision.

## COMPLICATIONS

- TUR syndrome (TURP)
- Shock

- Blood clots in legs or elsewhere
- Stress incontinence
- Dribbling
- Retrograde ejaculation
- Impotence
- Pain
- Infection: fever, chills, redness, tenderness at incision site
- Paralytic ileus
- Constipation

## HOME CARE

- Give both the patient and the caregiver *verbal* and *written* instructions. Provide them with the name and telephone number of a physician or nurse to call if questions arise.
- *General information*
  —Explain the type of procedure and the reason for it. Discuss the drainage catheters and tubes that will be left in place.
- *Warning signs*
  —Review the signs and symptoms that should be reported to a physician or nurse.
    Obstructed urinary catheter: feeling of fullness in bladder, feeling of need to urinate, spasms of bladder, leakage of urine around catheter, decreased or no urine in bag for 4 hours
    Infection: fever, chills, redness, swelling, purulent drainage from the operative area
    Urinary tract infection (see Urolithiasis, p. 666)
    Epididymitis, especially after TURP (see Epididymitis, p. 286)
    Persistent pain in operative area
    Gross blood or clots from catheter
    Constipation
- *Special instructions*
  —Advise the patient on how and where to obtain supplies.
  —Explain and demonstrate care of the urinary catheter (see Indwelling Catheter, p. 406).
  —Instruct the patient to avoid sexual activity until permitted by the physician (different with each procedure). Remind the patient that retrograde ejaculation may occur after TURP.
  —Teach Kegel exercises to tighten the perineum and encour-

age return of sphincter control after removal of the urethral catheter (see Urinary Incontinence, p. 657).

—Tell the patient to shower daily. Suggest the use of sitz baths to ease perineal discomfort.

—Discuss the need to avoid use of rectal suppositories or enemas unless ordered by the physician.

• *Medications*

—Explain the purpose, dosage, schedule, and route of administration of any prescribed drugs, as well as side effects to report to a physician or nurse.

—Advise the patient to avoiding using over-the-counter medications without discussing them with the physician.

• *Activity*

—Encourage the patient to discuss allowances and limitations with respect to occupation, recreation, or activities.

—Instruct the patient to allow for frequent rest periods, gradually increasing activity as allowed and tolerated.

—Advise the patient to avoid long car rides (over 2 hours) or rides over bumpy roads.

• *Diet*

—Inform the patient that a regular diet or one prescribed by the physician for the underlying condition should be followed.

—Caution the patient to avoid alcohol for 1 month.

—Advise avoiding caffeine (coffee, tea, cola) as directed.

—Encourage a high-fiber diet to prevent constipation and facilitate bowel movements. Explain that straining can cause bleeding.

—Encourage intake of water or juices (cranberry, prune, plum), 6-10 glasses a day, to induce frequent urination.

## FOLLOW-UP CARE

• Stress the importance of regular follow-up visits. Make sure the patient has the necessary names and telephone numbers.

## PSYCHOSOCIAL CARE

• Assist the patient, family, and caregiver to obtain emotional and fertility counseling if needed.

## REFERRALS

• Assist the patient to obtain home health care if needed.

# Pulmonary Embolism

—Pulmonary embolism: an obstruction of a pulmonary blood vessel by an embolus. An embolus is a clot made up of blood, fat, air, or amniotic fluid. The emboli cause decreased perfusion of the lung, resulting in decreased oxygenation (hypoxemia). Damage to the lung depends on the number of clots and the extent of obstruction to pulmonary circulation. The most common source of pulmonary embolism is venous thrombosis of the leg, thigh, or pelvis.

## CONTRIBUTING FACTORS

- Venostasis (e.g., prolonged bed rest, obesity, advanced age, pregnancy, postpartum period)
- Fractures, injury of pelvis
- Increased blood coagulability (e.g., use of oral contraceptives high in estrogen [>100 μg per pill])
- Systemic disease: chronic lung disease, congestive heart failure, atrial fibrillation, thromboembolism, thrombophlebitis or vascular surgery, diabetes mellitus

## SIGNS/SYMPTOMS

- Shortness of breath
- Complaints of pain when breathing
- Restlessness
- Apprehension
- Diaphoresis
- Cyanosis, pallor
- Tachypnea
- Tachycardia
- Bloody sputum (rare)
- Cough

## COMPLICATIONS

- Extended or recurrent pulmonary embolism
- Pulmonary infarction
- Atelectasis
- Pulmonary hypertension

- Right ventricular failure
- Decreased cardiac output
- Shock
- Cardiopulmonary arrest

## DIAGNOSTIC TESTS

- Describe each procedure, its purpose, and the normal feelings or sensations that are likely, as well as any preprocedural and postprocedural care.
  - —Chest x-ray: to evaluate the pulmonary and cardiac systems
  - —Lung (ventilation/perfusion) scan: to identify defects in blood perfusion of the lung
  - —Pulmonary angiogram: definitive study for pulmonary embolism
  - —Electrocardiogram: to differentiate between pulmonary embolism and myocardial infarction
  - —Arterial blood gases: to determine acid-base balance and need for oxygen
  - —Serum assays: elevated lactate dehydrogenase, bilirubin, fibrin split products, and fibrin degradation

## TREATMENT

*Medical*
- Therapy
  - —Bed rest
  - —Oxygen therapy
  - —Cardiac monitor
- Drugs
  - —Anticoagulants: heparin, coumadin
  - —Thrombolytics: streptokinase, urokinase; to speed the process of clot lysis

*Surgical*
- Insertion of umbrella filter for multiple emboli

## HOME CARE

- Give both the patient and the caregiver *verbal* and *written* instructions. Provide them with the name and telephone number of a physician or nurse to call if questions arise.
- *General information*
  - —Explain the disorder, underlying causes, and contributing factors.

—Provide information on prevention for patients at risk for pulmonary embolism.

—Stress the importance of not smoking or using tobacco products. Explain to the patient that nicotine causes constriction and damage to intimal cells.

• *Warning signs*

—Review the signs and symptoms that should be reported to a physician or nurse.

   Sudden, sharp chest pain

   Bloody sputum

   Elevated temperature

• *Medications*

—Explain the purpose, dosage, schedule, and route of administration of anticoagulants, as well as side effects to report to the physician or nurse (see Anticoagulation Therapy, p. 42).

—Tell the patient to avoid medications that enhance the response to coumadin (e.g., aspirin, nonsteroidal antiinflammatory drugs [ibuprofen], cimetidine, trimethaphan). Drugs that decrease the response to coumadin include antacids, diuretics, oral contraceptives, and barbiturates.

—Explain the need to check for bleeding in urine, stools, and sputum if the patient is sent home with a prescription for anticoagulants.

• *Activity*

—Discuss the importance of exercising to tolerance with planned rest periods. Tell the patient to perform regular exercise such as walking.

—Teach strategies to prevent venous pooling: avoid sitting or standing for long periods, elevate legs while sitting, and do not cross legs. Demonstrate proper application of antiembolic stockings if ordered.

## FOLLOW-UP CARE

• Stress the importance of follow-up visits. Make sure the patient has the necessary names and telephone numbers.

• Provide information and referral to smoking cessation programs as indicated. Provide literature prepared by the American Heart Association.

# Pulmonary Hypertension

—Pulmonary hypertension: increased pulmonary artery pressure resulting from progressive disease of the pulmonary vessels or lung tissue. Pulmonary hypertension occurs as a primary disease or secondary to existing cardiac or pulmonary disease. In primary hypertension the small pulmonary arteries become narrow as a result of thickening of the intimal lining of the lung. Primary hypertension affects primarily women between 20 and 40 years of age.

## CAUSES/CONTRIBUTING FACTORS
- Primary pulmonary hypertension
  —Unknown
- Secondary pulmonary hypertension
  —Congenital heart disease that causes left-to-right shunting
  —Acquired heart disease that results in left ventricular failure (e.g., rheumatic valvular heart disease)
  —Chronic hypoxia related to chronic obstructive pulmonary disease
  —Pulmonary embolus
  —Pulmonary stenosis

## SIGNS/SYMPTOMS
- Increasing dyspnea on exertion and at rest
- Tachypnea
- Chest pain
- Dizziness
- Syncope
- Apprehension, fear
- Cyanosis (secondary hypertension)

## COMPLICATIONS
- Right-sided heart failure
- Sudden death

## DIAGNOSTIC TESTS

- Describe each procedure, its purpose, and the normal feelings or sensations that are likely, as well as any preprocedural and postprocedural care.
  —Chest x-ray: to detect enlargement of the pulmonary artery and right atrium and ventricle
  —Electrocardiograam: to detect arrhythmias
  —Echocardiogram: to evaluate the structure and function of the heart
  —Arterial blood gases: to determine acid-base balance and need for oxygen
  —Cardiac catheterization: invasive procedure to visualize the heart and major blood vessels

## TREATMENT

*Medical*
- Therapy
  —Oxygen therapy
  —Hemodynamic monitoring
  —Cardiac monitoring
  —Isovolumetric phlebotomy (secondary hypertension)
- Drugs
  —Primary hypertension: vasodilators, diuretics, calcium channel blockers

*Surgical*
- Lung transplantation

## HOME CARE

- Give both the patient and the caregiver *verbal* and *written* instructions. Provide them with the name and telephone number of a physician or nurse to call if questions arise.
- *General information*
  —Explain the disorder, underlying causes, and contributing factors.
- *Warning signs*
  —Review the signs and symptoms that should be reported to a physician or nurse.
    Decreased activity tolerance
    Changes in color
    Consistency of sputum
    Increased cough

Swelling of legs, ankles, or abdomen

Erythrocytosis: headache, muscle aches, blurred vision, increased fatigue, hemoptysis, epistaxis

- *Special instructions*
  —For patients with secondary hypetension, explain that a compensatory polycythemia (erythrocytosis) occurs as a result of shunting (arteriovenous mixing) and that a hematocrit greater than 45% may be within normal limits for the patient. Provide individual hematocrit parameters.
  —Provide the patient with information regarding oxygen therapy (see p. 492) if ordered and assist the patient to obtain equipment from medical supply houses.
  —Demonstrate and provide information on adaptive breathing techniques.
  —Explain the value of relaxation techniques, such as music therapy, deep breathing, meditation, and biofeedback.
  —Stress the importance of not smoking or using tobacco products. Explain that smoking increases the workload of the heart by causing vasoconstriction.

- *Medications*
  —Explain the purpose, dosage, schedule, and route of administration of any prescribed drugs, as well as side effects to report to the physician or nurse.
  —Tell the patient to avoid taking aspirin or iron; advise checking labels of all over-the-counter medications.

- *Activity*
  —Discuss the importance of exercising to tolerance, avoiding fatigue, and planning rest periods. Confer with the physician about the type of exercise.
  —Tell the patient to avoid activities involving sudden strenuous movement, push-pull exercise, or heavy lifting.
  —Advise the patient to avoid exertion on hot, humid, or smoggy days.
  —Explain that activities involving isotonic exercises (walking, bicycling, swimming) are permissible as long as the patient is aware of actions to take during episodes of fatigue or dyspnea (e.g., stop the activity and take a rest).
  —Teach energy-saving procedures: sitting while shaving, combing hair, dressing, cooking, and taking a shower.
  —Stress the importance of avoiding dehydration by drinking fluids on hot days and avoiding strenuous activity.

**FOLLOW-UP CARE**

- Stress the importance of follow-up visits. Make sure the patient has the necessary names and telephone numbers.
- Provide information and referral to smoking cessation programs as indicated.

# Pulse Taking

—**Pulse taking: measurement of the pulse, the regular contraction and expansion of an artery as the wave of blood passes through the blood vessel. Common sites for taking arterial pulses are the wrist (radial), neck (carotid), forehead (temporal), back of knee (popliteal), and inside of elbow (antecubitus). The most common sites for patients to take their own pulse are the wrist and neck.**

**HOME CARE**

- Give both the patient and the caregiver *verbal* and *written* instructions. Provide them with the name and telephone number of a physician or nurse to call if questions arise.
- Explain what the pulse is, why the patient needs to take his or her pulse, and what to do if the pulse is too fast, too slow, or irregular.
- Explain that a number of factors can affect the pulse rate: exercise; stress; stimulants such as tobacco, caffeine, recreational or illicit drugs, and alcohol; cold or allergy medication; and imbalances of electrolytes such as sodium and potassium.
- Instruct the patient in taking the pulse, and permit time for return demonstration and practice.
    —Use two fingers, the pointer and middle fingers (the thumb is not suitable because it contains a pulse).
    —Place the two fingers *lightly* at the point of throbbing and pulsation.
        Radial pulse (on the inside of the wrist): start at the outside of the wrist; slide the two fingers slightly inward until the pulse is felt.

Carotid pulse (to the right or left of the throat area): start at the center of the throat just under the chin; slide the two fingers to the right or left about 1 inch until a pulsation is felt.

- Instruct the patient to count the pulses for 30 seconds and multiply by 2. Explain that this is the pulse rate per minute.
- Instruct the patient to record the pulse rate and indicate what he or she was doing or eating if the rate is slower, faster, or irregular compared with his or her normal rate. See Appendix G for a sample pulse-taking diary.

# Pyelonephritis

—Pyelonephritis: **inflammatory disease process from acute and chronic effects caused by bacterial infection of the lower urinary tract. The incidence is greater in females because they have a shorter urethra and lack the antibacterial secretions of the prostate that men have.**

## CONTRIBUTING FACTORS

- Lower urinary tract infection
- Urologic procedures involving a catheter or instrument
- Urethral obstruction caused by stone, clots, stricture, or tumor
- Congenital weakness of the bladder and ureter junction (allows reflux of urine)
- Neurogenic bladder
- Glomerulonephritis
- Polycystic kidney disease
- Diabetes mellitus
- Analgesic abuse (e.g., Tylenol)
- Benign prostatic hypertrophy
- History of unexplained fevers or bed-wetting
- Pregnancy

## SIGNS/SYMPTOMS

- Urinary frequency, urgency, burning
- Decreased urine output
- Cloudy, foul-smelling urine (ammonia like or fishy)

- Blood in urine
- Flank pain and tenderness
- High fever
- Shaking chills
- Malaise, fatigue, weakness
- Loss of appetite
- Nausea and vomiting

## COMPLICATIONS

- Generalized bacterial infection (septic shock)
- Scarring of the kidney tissue
- Kidney abscess
- Kidney stones
- Necrosis of kidney tissue

## DIAGNOSTIC TESTS

- Describe each procedure, its purpose, and the normal feelings or sensations that are likely, as well as any preprocedural and postprocedural care.
  - —Urinalysis, culture and sensitivity
  - —X-ray of kidneys, ureter, and bladder (KUB)
  - —Intravenous pyelogram and urogram
  - —Blood culture and sensitivity for persistently high temperature

## TREATMENT

*Medical*
- Therapy
  - —Hydration intravenously or orally to achieve urine output of at least 2000 ml per day
- Drugs
  - —Antibiotics
  - —Antipyretics
  - —Analgesics

*Surgical*
- Intervention only if obstruction present (see Urolithiasis, p. 666, and Nephrectomy, p. 469).

## HOME CARE

- Give both the patient and the caregiver *verbal* and *written* instructions. Provide them with the name and telephone number of a physician or nurse to call if questions arise.

- *General information*
  —Explain the disease process, underlying causes, and contributing factors.
- *Warning signs*
  —Review the signs and symptoms that should be reported to a physician or nurse.
    Recurrence of symptoms
- *Special instructions*
  —Discuss methods of preventing recurrent urinary tract infection: empty bladder regularly, avoid prolonged bladder distention, wash hands before and after toileting.
  —For a female patient, advise her to keep the perineal area clean and dry, wipe front to back after toileting, avoid the use of feminine hygiene sprays, urinate before and after sexual intercourse to prevent (re)infection, report vaginal discharge and follow through with treatment, wear cotton underpants and avoid nylon underpants, and wear loose, nonrestrictive clothing.
  —Teach the patient the method of obtaining midstream urine for culture and sensitivity.
  —Teach the self-monitoring urine test for bacteria.
- *Medications*
  —Explain the purpose, dosage, schedule, and route of administration of any prescribed drugs, as well as side effects to report to the physician or nurse.
  —Stress the importance of completing the antibiotic course even if feeling better.
- *Activity*
  —Encourage the patient to discuss allowances and limitations with respect to occupation, recreation, and activities.
- *Diet*
  —Tell the patient to follow a regular diet or the one prescribed by the physician.
  —Stress the importance of drinking 10-15 glasses of clear fluids (water or cranberry, plum, or prune juice) per day.
  —Tell the patient to avoid caffeinated beverages (coffee, tea, cola) and alcohol, especially during a urinary tract infection episode.

## FOLLOW-UP CARE

- Stress the importance of follow-up medical and laboratory evaluations. Make sure the patient has the necessary names and telephone numbers.

# Radiation Therapy

—**Radiation therapy: the major treatment modality in cancer care. Radiation therapy involves the use of gamma rays to disturb proliferation of cells by decreasing the rate of mitosis or impairing DNA synthesis, thereby reducing tumor mass. Radiation is used at all phases of the cancer trajectory: curative, adjuvant, and palliative.**

## TYPES OF RADIATION DELIVERY SYSTEMS

- External beam/teletherapy: the patient lies on a table at a distance from the source and is exposed to a prescribed dose of radiation on a daily basis. The radiation field usually includes the tumor and draining lymphatics.
- Implant therapy/brachytherapy (close therapy): sealed sources implanted directly into the tumor or cavity surrounding the tumor. The sources used (cesium, iridium) are nonpenetrating and deposit most of the dose in a small area. The goal is to deliver a high dose to a small volume of tissue. The patient is radioactive for the time the source is in place (usually 3-5 days). Precautions (time, distance, shielding) are necessary.
- Radiopharmaceutical/isotope therapy: use of unsealed sources such as liquids to treat cancers. The most commonly used is iodine-131 for thyroid cancer; the half-life is 8 days.
- Interstitial thermoradiotherapy: combination of heat with radiation. The dose can be delivered locally, regionally, or systemically (whole body) by electromagnetic, radiofrequency, or ultrasound techniques.
- Intraoperative radiation therapy: provides direct visualization and treatment of tumors to control local recurrences.
- Combination of chemotherapy and radiation therapy: to treat residual disease after surgery.
- Radiosensitizers: nonhypoxic or hypoxic agents used to increase lethal effects of radiation.

## SIDE EFFECTS/COMPLICATIONS

- Acute (during treatment to 6 months), subacute (after 6 months), or chronic (with variable time to expression). Side effects are seen sooner in the skin, mucous membranes, and hair follicles and later in the vascular system and muscles. Early side effects are believed to be reparable; late effects are more often permanent.

- General effects: fatigue, anorexia
- Transient erythema: as early as first treatment; dry or wet desquamation in second or third week (see box on p. 562)
- Pulmonary effects: increased cough that is productive or nonproductive; dyspnea; pneumonitis (dyspnea, cough, fever, night sweats); late effect is fibrosis, usually asymptomatic
- Gastrointestinal effects: vomiting, anorexia, diarrhea, gastric distention
- Toxic effects: depend on site of irradiation, volume of tissue irradiated, total dosage delivered, time frame

## DIAGNOSTIC TESTS

- Describe each procedure, its purpose, and the normal feelings or sensations that are likely, as well as any preprocedural and postprocedural care.
  —Complete blood cell count
  —Electrolytes
  —Urinalysis

## TREATMENT

*Medical*

- Drugs
  —Antiemetics
  —Antibiotics
  —Antidiarrheals
  —Blood products

## HOME CARE

- Give both the patient and the caregiver *verbal* and *written* instructions. Provide them with the name and telephone number of a physician or nurse to call if questions arise.
- *General information*
  —Reinforce the physician's explanation of therapy: the type to be delivered, frequency and length of treatment (weeks), and expected side effects versus toxic effects.
  —Explain that high-dose radiation therapy causes sterility.
  —For women undergoing radiation therapy for endometrial cancer, explain that vaginal shrinkage may occur.

- *Warning signs*
  —Review the signs and symptoms that should be reported to a physician or nurse.

  > Skin reactions: redness, itching, swelling, dry or moist desquamation (see the box on p. 562), pain
  >
  > Mucositis
  >
  > Nausea, vomiting
  >
  > Diarrhea
  >
  > Tachycardia
  >
  > Dyspnea
  >
  > For women undergoing radiation therapy for endometrial cancer: vaginal or rectal bleeding, foul-smelling discharge, abdominal pain, hematuria

- *Special instructions*
  —Discuss the need to prevent infection by avoiding large crowds and persons with upper respiratory tract infections.
  —Instruct the patient in skin care, including maintenance of dye markings and the need to avoid use of soap and other ointments, sunbathing, and heat applications (see box on p. 562).
  —Teach the patient the importance of oral hygiene if receiving oral, head, or neck radiation therapy (see Cancer Care, p. 138).

- *Activity*
  —Teach the patient how to manage fatigue and maintain mobility, for example, planning activities before and after treatment based on energy level.
  —Encourage the patient to continue working and other activities of daily living as tolerated, including regular exercise.

- *Diet*
  —Teach the patient the importance of a regular diet with small, frequent feedings as necessary.
  —Advise the patient to avoid eating several hours before and after treatment to prevent nausea.
  —Encourage fluid intake of up to 3000 ml per day.

**FOLLOW-UP CARE**

- Stress the importance of keeping all scheduled treatment, laboratory, and medical follow-up appointments. Make sure the patient has the necessary names and telephone numbers.

**REFERRALS**

- Refer the patient to support groups and other community resources as needed.

## SKIN CARE DURING EXTERNAL BEAM THERAPY

External beam radiation therapy can cause mild to severe skin reactions, based on how much radiation is given and how often, how much skin area is treated, and the type of radiation used. Usually in the first 2 weeks of treatment, the skin over the area being treated with radiation turns pink or red, becomes sensitive to sunlight, loses hair, or develops a rash. With more treatments, a condition called dry desquamation may develop; the skin may peel and become painful and weepy. Patients most likely will notice a skin reaction 10 days to 2 weeks after treatment has been completed. Hair loss from the treated scalp begins about 10 days after the first treatment.

***Prevention of skin reactions***

To prevent skin reactions or make them less severe, instruct the patient to do the following.

- Clean skin with warm, not hot, water.
- After washing, rinse with tepid water and pat dry with a soft towel.
- Do not soak in a tub. Do not remove the treatment field markings during bathing. Avoid soap as much as possible. If soap is needed for adequate cleansing, use Aveeno, Dove, or some other mild, unscented soap that will not dry the skin.
- Do not use heating pads, hot packs, or ice on the area being treated.
- Do not use perfumed or powdered products on the treated skin. Do not use ointments or menthol rubs.
- Shave with an electric razor.
- Protect the skin from heat, cold, and sunlight by using a sunscreen with a sun protection factor of 15 or higher. Shield the face and neck with a scarf or wide-brimmed hat.
- Wear loose-fitting clothing. Tight clothes and belts rub and irritate already sensitive skin.

## SKIN CARE DURING EXTERNAL BEAM THERAPY—cont'd

### *Prevention of skin reactions—cont'd*
- Do not put adhesive bandages, such as Band-Aids, on treated skin.
- Use a light dusting of cornstarch to prevent itching and to remove moisture in neck creases and armpits and beneath the breasts.

### *Treatment of skin reactions*
For dry desquamation, use pure aloe vera gel, vitamin A and D ointments, Lubriderm, or other water-soluble, nonirritating substances.

For moist desquamation, apply cool compresses moistened with water or normal saline. Special ointments may be prescribed. Moisture vapor–permeable film or other sterile dressings, such as Op-Site or Tegaderm, may be applied to the area to protect it while it heals. Moist desquamation usually heals 1-2 weeks after treatment ends.

For pain in the treated area, an over-the-counter analgesic such as aspirin, acetaminophen (e.g., Tylenol), or ibuprofen (e.g., Motrin, Advil) may be used. After the skin heals, it may still be sensitive to heat, cold, and sunlight. Some chemotherapy drugs cause "radiation recall," which is a return of the previous skin reaction, usually seen as redness in the treated area.

For hair loss, discuss with the patient that this is likely to occur during treatment. Instruct the patient to select scarves, hats, wigs, or hairpieces before treatment. Have the stylist match the real hair style to the wig so that the difference is less obvious when the patient begins to wear the wig. Hair loss is usually temporary but depends on the amount of radiation received, gender, age, and whether the patient also receives cancer chemotherapy.

Discuss the signs and symptoms to report to the physician or nurse: rash; dry, itchy, flaky areas; peeling and weeping; pain.

**R**

# Renal Failure

—Renal failure: inability to meet normal demands of kidney function. Acute renal failure is the sudden and rapid deterioration of kidney function resulting from obstruction, decreased blood flow, or renal disease. Acute renal failure is usually reversible but has high morbidity and mortality if not treated. Chronic renal failure is the slow, progressive loss of kidney function, leading to end-stage renal disease. It is an irreversible process, requiring dialysis or kidney transplantation.

## CAUSES/CONTRIBUTING FACTORS

- Acute renal failure
  —Nephrotoxic exposure: drugs, chemicals, metals, contrast dyes
  —Infection
  —Shock: hemorrhagic, septic, cardiogenic, hypovolemic
  —Trauma: burns
- Congestive heart failure
  —Renal thrombus, stenosis, obstructions (calculi)
  —Chronic renal failure
  —Diabetes mellitus
  —Glomerulonephritis
  —Chronic pyelonephritis
  —Polycystic kidneys
  —Small kidneys
  —Tuberculosis
  —Tumors
  —Recent surgery (cardiac or vascular)
  —Several organ failure
  —Advanced age

## SIGNS/SYMPTOMS

- Acute renal failure
  —Decrease (<400 ml/24 hr) or absence of urine output
  —Lethargy, confusion, irritability, headache
  —Nausea, vomiting, constipation, diarrhea
  —Shortness of breath on exertion or when flat

- Chronic renal failure
  —General malaise and fatigue, sleepiness, apathy, confusion
  —Loss of appetite, metallic taste, nausea, vomiting
  —Skin: itching; dry, discolored skin; easy bruising; sallow color; thin, brittle nails and hair
  —Decreased urine output, anuria
  —Peripheral neuropathy: burning, pain of soles of feet or "restless legs"
  —Cardiovascular: anemia, hypertension, shortness of breath, peripheral edema
  —Amenorrhea in women, impotence in men

## COMPLICATIONS

- Acute renal failure
  —Pericarditis
  —Fluid and electrolyte imbalance
  —Infection and sepsis
  —Chronic renal failure
- Chronic renal failure
  —Cardiovascular: dysrhythmias, pericarditis, congestive heart failure, accelerated atherosclerosis
  —Pulmonary edema
  —Musculoskeletal: calcium deposits in blood vessels or joints, bone disease and disturbed vitamin D metabolism
  —Peripheral neuropathy
  —Metabolic encephalopathy
  —Peptic ulcer disease
  —Fluid-electrolyte imbalance

## DIAGNOSTIC TESTS

- Describe each procedure, its purpose, and the normal feelings or sensations that are likely, as well as any preprocedural and postprocedural care.
  —Blood tests: blood urea nitrogen, creatinine, electrolytes, uric acid
  —Urine tests: urinalysis, osmolality, electrolytes, creatinine clearance, uric acid
  —X-ray of kidneys, ureter, bladder (KUB)
  —Renal computed tomography
  —Intravenous pyelogram
  —Renal biopsy

**TREATMENT**

*Medical*

- Therapy
  —Treatment of underlying cause
  —Fluid and electrolyte management
  —Dialysis
  —Diet high in carbohydrates, low in protein and potassium
- Drugs
  —Antihypertensives
  —Anabolic steroids
  —Vitamins, iron, minerals, antacids

*Surgical*

- Single or bilateral nephrectomy
- Kidney transplant

**HOME CARE**

- Give both the patient and the caregiver *verbal* and *written* instructions. Provide them with the name and telephone number of a physician or nurse to call if questions arise.
- *General information*
  —Explain the underlying cause or contributing factors of the condition. Explain the type of renal failure and disease process.
  —Explain and prepare the patient for dialysis as ordered (see p. 242).
- *Warning signs*
  —Review the signs and symptoms that should be reported to a physician or nurse.
    Urine output decreased (<1 cup per 8 hours) or absent
    Elevated blood pressure (>140/90 mm Hg)
    Rapid weight gain (>2 pounds in 24 hours)
    Swelling (edema) of feet, ankles, abdomen
    Excessive muscle weakness
    Palpitations or irregular pulse
    Shortness of breath on exertion or flat
    General malaise and fatigue, increased sleepiness, drowsiness
    Loss of appetite, loss of weight
    Burning feet or "restless legs," paresthesias
    Muscle cramps (especially legs), twitching
    Excessive bruising or easy bruising

- *Special instructions*
  —Discuss skin care and grooming: keep nails short and clean; bathe daily but avoid long hot baths or showers; avoid vigorous towel rubbing; use lanolin, nonalcohol, superfatted soaps and emollient lotions for itchy skin; use mild shampoo with conditioners; avoid scratching the skin to prevent skin breaks and infection.
  —Instruct the patient in oral hygiene: brush the teeth using a soft-bristled toothbrush; use mouthwash after each meal for breath control; eat hard or sour candy for breath control and dry mouth.
  —Discuss the need for perineal care after toileting.
  —Instruct the patient in and demonstrate techniques for taking and recording blood pressure, temperature, and pulse (rest 5 minutes before taking). Provide a timetable and parameters to report. Allow time for practice using home blood pressure equipment.
  —Explain the need to weigh daily at the same time and wearing the same clothes, after urination, and before eating. Instruct the patient to keep a log of weight.
- *Medications*
  —Explain the purpose, dosage, schedule, and route of administration of any prescribed drugs, as well as side effects to report to the physician or nurse.
  —Advise patients taking diuretics to take them in the morning to avoid having to get up in the night.
- *Activity*
  —Discuss the need to pace activities as tolerated.
  —Instruct the patient in the use of ambulatory aids as needed (walker, cane, wheelchair).
  —Discuss energy-conserving techniques and the use of home assist devices such as a shower chair or bath bars as needed.
  —Tell the patient to schedule rest periods between activities.
  —Encourage the patient to discuss allowances and limitations with respect to occupation, recreation, and activities.
- *Diet*
  —Review the prescribed diet with the patient.
  —Discuss the need to restrict sodium, potassium, phosphate, and protein. Explain that salt intake can be reduced by not eating "fast" or convenience-type foods, avoiding use of table salt, not cooking with salt, reading all labels, and rinsing canned vegetables before cooking and eating.

**R**

—Advise the patient to eat a high-calorie, high-carbohydrate diet.

—Encourage a diet high in fiber to prevent constipation.

—Instruct a patient who is nauseated to take antiemetics half an hour before eating and to eat smaller, more frequent meals.

—Review prescribed fluid restrictions. Explain that levels are usually based on the previous day's urine output plus 500-800 ml over intake. Encourage the patient to spread fluid intake over the day, particularly during mealtimes and when active. Suggest using ice chips to control thirst.

## FOLLOW-UP CARE

• Stress the importance of follow-up medical and laboratory evaluations. Make sure the patient has the necessary names and telephone numbers.

• Encourage and assist the patient to obtain a Medic-Alert bracelet and identification card.

## PSYCHOSOCIAL CARE

• Encourage the patient and caregiver to verbalize fears and feelings about the disease process.

• Encourage independence and participation in planning care. Refer the patient to counseling to help the patient and caregiver cope with the disease and its outcomes.

## REFERRALS

• Provide referrals for home health, hospital, and community resources.

# Renal Transplant

—**Renal transplant: implantation of a kidney from a living relative or a cadaver donor into a recipient to restore renal function. Implantation of the donor organ is preceded by nephrectomy of the diseased kidney.**

## INDICATIONS

- End-stage renal disease

## PREPROCEDURAL TEACHING

- Review the physician's explanation of the procedure and the reason for it; encourage the patient to ask questions and to discuss any fears or anxieties. Explain the need for informed consent for surgery, anesthesia, and blood transfusions.

### Review of Preprocedural Care

- Explain that when a suitable donor is found, the patient will be called in for the transplantation.
- Review the comprehensive workup and evaluation for a patient awaiting transplant.
  - Blood studies for blood typing and tissue typing for compatibility, as well as electrolytes, creatinine, and blood urea nitrogen
  - Cystometrogram to evaluate bladder capacity and urination reflex
  - Voiding cystourethrography to evaluate bladder filling and emptying
  - Urine studies of creatinine and blood urea nitrogen
  - Transplant coordinator workup
  - Social worker and psychiatry workup
- Discuss the peroperative procedures once the donor is identified.
  - Hemodialysis (depending on time of last run)
  - Urinalysis to evaluate for infection
  - Blood studies for electrolytes, creatinine, blood urea nitrogen
  - Electrocardiogram, chest x-ray
- Explain that the patient will be NPO from the time of notification (if a cadaver kidney) or from the night before (if donor is a living relative).
- Discuss the need for a small cleansing enema.
- Inform the patient of the need to shower with bactericidal soap (e.g., Hibiclens, Safeguard, Dial).
- Discuss the probability that the abdomen and pubic area will be shaved.
- Review the regimen of oral immunosuppressants.
- Inform the patient that the surgery lasts 3-4 hours or more and the patient will be under general anesthesia.

**Review of Postprocedural Care**

- For general postprocedural care, see Abdominal Surgery (p. 3).
- Explain that the patient is usually in the intensive care unit for the night after the surgery.
- Explain that the patient may be returned to surgery for removal of the transplanted kidney if hyperacute rejection occurs.
- Describe the drainage tubes that may be used: urethral catheter for 2-3 days or more (urine will be blood tinged for several days), Jackson-Pratt bulb (self-suction) drain near the incision line.
- Inform the patient that analgesics will be available for pain. Stress the importance of explaining the type and severity of pain.
- Explain that dialysis may be needed until the kidney starts working (2-30 or more days with cadaver kidney). A kidney from a living related donor usually starts working immediately.

**COMPLICATIONS**

- Rejection of transplanted kidney
- Wound infection
- Urinary tract infection
- Pulmonary problems
- Hemorrhage, shock
- Paralytic ileus
- Renal artery stenosis, thrombosis, or aneurysm
- Side effects of immunosuppressants
- Gastrointestinal bleeding
- Diabetes
- Glaucoma
- Cushing's syndrome

**HOME CARE**

- Give both the patient and the caregiver *verbal* and *written* instructions. Provide them with the name and telephone number of a physician or nurse to call if questions arise.
- *General information*
  —Review renal transplantation, reinforcing the importance of lifelong immunosuppressant treatment.
  —Review the signs of rejection, explaining that it may occur at any time, even years later.
- *Wound/incision care*
  —Demonstrate wound care and dressing change (see Nephrectomy, p. 469). Assist the patient to obtain necessary supplies.

- *Warning signs*
  —Review the signs and symptoms that should be reported to a physician or nurse.

    Infection: redness, tenderness, pain, swelling, warm to touch, purulent drainage

    Rejection: decreased or absent urine output; large amounts of dilute urine; hematuria; flulike symptoms (elevated temperature [>100° F], malaise, nausea, vomiting, diarrhea); reddening, swelling, and tenderness of the transplant area; sudden weight gain (>3 pounds a day); increased blood pressure; increased pulse (>100)

    Urinary tract infection

    Sudden onset of acute pain in operative area

    Inability to take medications

- *Special instructions*
  —Stress the importance of avoiding exposure to crowds and persons with known or suspected infections for at least 3 months after surgery.
  —Explain the importance of recording daily weight (weighing at the same time, with the same clothing, after urination, and before eating). Instruct the patient to report a gain of 2 or more pounds a day or 4 or more pounds a week.
  —Explain and demonstrate how to measure and record intake and output for the first 3 weeks.
  —Explain the importance of taking and recording temperature, pulse, and blood pressure (same arm, same time, 5-minute rest period before measurement) twice daily. Help the patient obtain equipment for home use.
  —Inform the patient that strong or direct sunlight should be avoided because immunosuppressants increase susceptibility to skin cancer (especially lymphoma). They also decrease susceptibility to cancer of the cervix, vulva, and perineum and Kaposi's sarcoma.

- *Medications*
  —Explain the purpose, dosage, schedule, and route of administration of any prescribed drugs, as well as side effects to report to a physician or nurse.
  —Provide detailed instructions on immunosuppressant therapy and side effects.
  —Tell the patient to avoid over-the-counter medications unless approved by the physician.
  —Stress the importance of not missing doses of medications.

- *Activity*
  —Encourage the patient to discuss allowances and limitations with respect to occupation, recreation, or activities.
  —Tell the patient to begin exercise slowly and increase level gradually, taking frequent rest breaks.
  —Advise the patient to avoid heavy lifting (>10 pounds) and contact sports such as football, soccer, and basketball.
  —Discuss the need to avoid driving for 2 weeks.
  —Instruct the patient to avoid positions that place pressure on the transplant site (lap seat belt on long car trip).
  —Explain the need to refrain from sexual activity for at least 6 weeks or until advised by the physician. Emphasize that women should avoid pregnancy until approved by a physician. Provide contraceptive information.
- *Diet*
  —Tell the patient to follow a regular diet or one prescribed by the physician.
  —Advise the patient of the tendency to overeat because steroids stimulate the appetite.
  —Explain the need for a low-potassium diet if the patient is taking cyclosporine.
  —Tell the patient not to drink alcohol until allowed by the physician.

**FOLLOW-UP CARE**
- Stress the importance of regular follow-up medical and laboratory visits. Make sure the patient has the necessary names and telephone numbers. Remind the patient to take the log of weight and vital signs to each medical appointment.
- Explain the importance of notifying the physician of dentist appointments, having eye examinations every 6 months for glaucoma and cataracts, and having annual pelvic examinations (for females).
- Encourage and assist the patient to obtain a Medic-Alert bracelet and identification card listing the diagnosis, medication, and other information.

**REFERRALS**
- Assist the patient, family, or caregiver to obtain emotional support and family planning counseling as needed.

# Replacement of Knee or Shoulder

—Total knee replacement: replacement of the knee joint with a prosthesis to provide stability and motion. The femoral condylar cartilage and the tibial condylar surfaces are replaced with the prosthesis.

—Total shoulder replacement: placement of a prosthesis into the humeral shaft after removal of the head of the humerus.

## INDICATIONS

• Degenerative disease: rheumatoid arthritis, osteoarthritis

## PREPROCEDURAL TEACHING

• Review the physician's explanation of the procedure and the reason for it; encourage the patient to ask questions and to discuss any fears or anxieties. Explain the need for informed consent for surgery and anesthesia.

### Review of Preprocedural Care

• Review properative studies: x-rays, serologic and urologic studies to show the presence of infection, anemia, and electrolyte status.
• Explain that the patient will be NPO from midnight of the night before.
• Inform the patient of the need to shower with bactericidal soap (e.g., Hibiclens, Safeguard, Dial).
• Discuss the probability that the operative site will be shaved.
• Explain that ice may be applied before surgery to lessen edema (knee replacement).

### Review of Postprocedural Care

• Explain that the patient will be in the hospital for 4-5 days.
• Inform the patient that bed rest will be required for 24-48 hours. After knee replacement, the operative leg will be elevated on a pillow.
• Discuss the drainage tubes (Hemovac) that may be used, and explain that wound drainage will be moderate, decreasing in amount.

- Tell the patient that a regular diet will be resumed in 2-3 days.
- Discuss the frequency of checks for vital signs, peripheral pulse, and neurovascular status.
- Explain that after shoulder replacement a sling and swathe may be used for joint immobilization or a shoulder spica or airplane splint may be used with the arm elevated on a pillow.
- Review postoperative exercises: range of motion for unaffected joints; isometric exercises; quadriceps setting, gluteal contractions, and flexion-extension exercises (for knee replacement); exercises of fingers, wrist, and elbow (for shoulder replacement).
- Introduce the use of the continuous passive motion (CPM) device (after knee replacement). Explain that the operative extremity is positioned in a sling in the device and the leg is moved through preset limits of range of motion.
- Review activity levels. After knee replacement, ambulation without weight bearing is permitted in 3-5 days and weight bearing in 10-14 days. After shoulder replacement, ambulation as tolerated with a shoulder immobilizer is permitted after 48 hours.

**COMPLICATIONS**

- Hemorrhage/hematoma formation
- Infection
- Thrombophlebitis
- Fat embolus
- Compartment syndrome (after knee replacement)
- Atelectasis
- Pneumonia
- Displacement of prosthesis

**HOME CARE**

- Give both the patient and the caregiver *verbal* and *written* instructions. Provide them with the name and telephone number of a physician or nurse to call if questions arise.
- *General information*
  —Review the type of procedure performed and any specific limitations.
- *Warning signs*
  —Review the signs and symptoms that should be reported to a physician or nurse.
     Increased pain in knee or shoulder area
     Redness, swelling, redness in calf of one leg
     Fever

Shortness of breath or chest pain

Decreased ability to move shoulder, arm, or knee

- *Special instructions*
  —Instruct the patient in the proper use of ambulatory aids: walker, crutches, and cane (for knee replacement).
- *Medications*
  —Explain the purpose, dosage, schedule, and route of administration of any prescribed drugs, as well as side effects to report to a physician or nurse.

    Antibiotics

    Analgesics

    Anticoagulants

  —Stress the importance of having prothrombin time checked and observing for bleeding if the patient is taking anticoagulants (see p. 42).
- *Activity*
  —Advise the patient that full movement takes 3-6 months to return after joint replacement surgery. Review strengthening and range-of-motion exercises to help strengthen muscles and regain joint mobility and flexibility.

## FOLLOW-UP CARE

- Stress the importance of regular follow-up visits with the physician and physical therapist until recovery is complete. Make sure the patient has the necessary names and telephone numbers.

R

# Restrictive Cardiomyopathy

—**Restrictive cardiomyopathy: cardiomyopathy is a heart muscle disorder resulting in impaired function of the heart's pumping action. A less common form, restrictive cardiomyopathy, occurs when the heart loses its elasticity and cannot fill completely and contract effectively. This occurs when fibroelastic tissue infiltrates the heart, resulting in a thick and stiff heart.**

## CAUSES

- Endomyocardial fibroelastosis

## SIGNS/SYMPTOMS

- Exercise intolerance
- Fatigue
- Dyspnea
- Orthopnea
- Chest pain
- Peripheral edema

## COMPLICATIONS

- Heart failure
- Sudden death
- Arrhythmias
- Systemic emboli
- Heart failure

## DIAGNOSTIC TESTS

- Inform the patient that several diagnostic procedures may be done to aid in the diagnosis of this condition. Describe each procedure, its purpose, and the normal feelings or sensations that are likely, as well as any preprocedural and postprocedural care.
  —Chest x-ray: to show the enlarged heart and increased pressure in the pulmonary arteries
  —Electrocardiogram: to determine the extent and location of muscle involvement and show low voltage and conduction disturbance
  —Echocardiogram: to detect thickness of the heart muscle or fluid in the pericardial sac and the ability or inability of the heart muscle to move
  —Radionuclide studies: to show infiltration of the heart muscle and detect its pumping ability
  —Cardiac catheterization: to identify a decrease in heart muscle, elevated pressures during the filling of the heart, and the cause of the restriction
  —Endomyocardial biopsy: to determine the cause

## TREATMENT

*Medical*

- Drugs
  —Digitalis: to strengthen and regulate the heart
  —Diuretics: to aid the kidney in eliminating salt and fluid

—Oral vasodilators: to reduce the amount of blood coming into the heart and thus reduce the heart's workload; to relax the muscles against which the heart pumps
—Anticoagulants: to prevent clots from forming

## HOME CARE

• For home care see Heart Failure (p. 352).

---

# Retinal Detachment

**—Retinal detachment: partial or complete separation of the sensory layers of retina (the inner lining of the eyeball) from the posterior retinal lining, creating a subretinal space that fills with fluid. The retina is an extension of the central nervous system that receives images and transmits them to the brain. Retinal detachment is usually unilateral and spontaneous. It occurs more often in males. A retinal tear is a jagged break in the retina. A retinal hole is a break in the retina that allows liquid vitreous to seep between retinal layers; the condition is associated with trauma and aging.**

## CONTRIBUTING FACTORS

• Myopia
• Cataract surgery
• Eye trauma
• Degenerative changes caused by aging
• Systemic diseases
  —Severe hypertension
  —Chronic glomerulonephritis
  —Diabetes
  —Retinal vein occlusion
  —Retinal tumors, inflammation

## SIGNS/SYMPTOMS

• Floating spots
• Recurrent flashes of light

- Blurred or sooty vision
- Unilateral vision loss: gradual and painless

## COMPLICATIONS
- Vision impairment
- Blindness

## DIAGNOSTIC TESTS
- Describe each procedure, its purpose, and the normal feelings or sensations that are likely, as well as any preprocedural and postprocedural care.
    —Ophthalmoscopy: to show retinal pallor; hanging retina; crescent-shaped, red-orange tear(s); bulging retina

## TREATMENT
*Surgical*
- Retinal tears and holes
    —Photocoagulation: to burn and eventually seal localized tears or breaks; used frequently in torn areas that are small or with retinal holes to prevent further detachment
    —Cryothermy: placement of a frozen metal probe on the conjunctiva near the tear, causing scleral inflammation, which leads to scar tissue formation and reattachment
    —Diathermy: application of a heated probe to the scleral surface over the site of the retinal break, causing burning that leads to an inflammatory response and eventual scarring and healing
- Retinal detachment
    —Scleral buckling: placement of a band similar to a piece of belt around the sclera at the site of detachment, drawing the sclera closer to the retina to facilitate attachment

## PREPROCEDURAL TEACHING
- Review the physician's explanation of the procedure and the reason for it; encourage the patient to ask questions and to discuss any fears or anxieties.
- Explain that retinal detachment rarely heals spontaneously and that surgical correction is necessary to seal the retina.

### Review of Preprocedural Care
- Inform the patient that complete bed rest is necessary to restrict eye movements.

- Explain that sedation is used and bilateral eye patches are applied to restrict eye movement and that the head will be positioned to promote reattachment.
- Tell the patient that mydriatics and cycloplegics are given to dilate the pupil and decrease movement of intraocular structures.
- Explain the need to cleanse the face with bactericidal soap and the possibility that the eyelashes will be cut off to minimize the chance of infection.

### Review of Postprocedural Care

- Explain the importance of avoiding activities that increase intraocular pressure: straining, coughing, sneezing, bending, vomiting.
- Tell the patient that to minimize excessive eye movement, the patient will need to avoid shaving, brushing teeth, washing face, and combing the hair.
- Explain that moderate pain can be expected in the first 24-48 hours but can be relieved with prescribed analgesics. Instruct the patient to report the presence of *sudden severe pain,* which can signal occurrence of hyphema.
- Advise the patient that eye patches will be worn for several days after eye surgery to prevent eye movement.
- Discuss the need for the patient to be placed in a specific position for several days according to the location of the detachment (e.g., may be prone) and type of surgical procedure; bed rest is maintained if there is macular involvement.
- Explain that the eyelid may be swollen after surgery and that ice packs will be applied.

### HOME CARE

- Give both the patient and the caregiver *verbal* and *written* instructions. Provide them with the name and telephone number of a physician or nurse to call if questions arise.
- *General information*
    —Explain the underlying cause or contributing factors of the condition. Discuss the purpose and type of procedure performed.
- *Warning signs*
    —Review the signs, symptoms, and complications that should be reported to a physician or nurse.
    Sudden loss of vision
    Severe pain in eyeball

Heavy shower of floaters

Flashing lights

Purulent drainage

Persistent redness

Swelling

Fever

Postsurgical complications: hyphema, retinal re-detachment, infection, thrombophlebitis

- *Special instructions*
  - —Remind the patient to lie in the recommended position following the scleral buckling procedure.
  - —Advise the patient to apply cold compresses to the eye to reduce swelling and ease discomfort.
  - —Explain the importance of wearing dark glasses to minimize photophobia and pain when eyedrops (mydriatics) are used.
  - —Instruct the patient to wear an eye shield at night for protection (for 2-4 weeks).
  - —Discuss lid hygiene: remove any drainage with a cotton ball moistened with tap water; gently sweep the cotton ball from the inner to outer aspect of the lid, using a new cotton ball with each sweeping motion.
  - —Explain that floaters may appear after surgery and can disappear in weeks or last for years.
  - —Explain the importance of avoiding rubbing, touching, and bumping of the operative eye.
- *Medications*
  - —Explain the purpose, dosage, schedule, and route of administration of any prescribed drugs, as well as side effects to report to the physician or nurse.
  - —Tell the patient to avoid using over-the-counter eyedrops or ointments without checking with the physician.
  - —Teach the patient the procedure for administering eyedrops and emphasize the importance of washing the hands thoroughly before administration.
- *Activity*
  - —Explain the importance of avoiding activities that can increase intraocular pressure: constipation (straining); sneezing; jarring head movements; heavy exercise; heavy lifting; bending; driving. Tell the patient to avoid sexual activity for 4-6 weeks or as prescribed by a physician.
  - —Inform the patient that watching television is permitted but

reading should generally be avoided for the first week or as directed by the physician.

—Discuss the need to remove hazards at home to avoid injury (e.g., remove loose rugs).

## FOLLOW-UP CARE

• Stress the importance of follow-up visits until recovery is complete. Make sure the patient has the necessary names and telephone numbers.

# Rheumatic Fever

—Rheumatic fever: a systemic inflammatory disease that develops following a beta-hemolytic streptococcal infection of the upper respiratory tract (e.g., tonsillitis, nasopharyngitis, otitis media). Rheumatic fever most commonly involves the heart, synovial joint linings, skin, and central nervous system. The mitral valve is affected in 75%-80% of cases and the aortic valve in less than 5%. Healing may be complete, or scarring may develop because of chronic inflammation.

## SIGNS/SYMPTOMS

• Fever
• Migratory joint pains (growing pains). polyarthritis
• Swelling, redness, effusion of joints
• Skin lesions: trunk, extremities
• Subcutaneous nodules: knuckles, wrists, knees
• Chorea (purposeless jerky movements)

## COMPLICATIONS

• Heart failure
• Pericarditis
• Endocarditis
• Myocarditis
• Valvular heart disease: mitral and aortic most commonly affected
• Cardiac arrhythmias

## DIAGNOSTIC TESTS

- Describe each procedure, its purpose, and the normal feelings or sensations that are likely, as well as any preprocedural and postprocedural care.
  - —White blood cell count, C-reactive protein, sedimentation rate: to determine the inflammatory process
  - —Streptomycin or antistreptolysin O titer: to detect beta-hemolytic streptococcal infection
  - —Throat cultures
  - —Electrocardiogram
  - —Chest x-ray
  - —Echocardiogram

## TREATMENT

*Medical*

- Therapy
  - —Bed rest during acute phase
- Drugs
  - —Antibiotics: penicillin, erythromycin
  - —Antipyretics, salicylates: aspirin

## HOME CARE

- Give both the patient and the caregiver *verbal* and *written* instructions. Provide them with the name and telephone number of a physician or nurse to call if questions arise.
- *General information*
  - —Explain the disease process, causes, contributing factors, care, and treatment.
- *Warning signs*
  - —Review the signs and symptoms that should be reported to a physician or nurse.
    - Recurrent streptococcal infections: sudden sore throat, throat redness, swollen lymph glands, pain on swallowing, fever, headache, nausea
    - Reaction to penicillin therapy: rash, fever, chills
- *Special instructions*
  - —Review potential sources of reinfection and discuss preventive measures.
    - Maintain good oral hygiene, with daily care and regular visits to the dentist.

Avoid persons with upper respiratory infection. Report and treat all skin boils (furuncles).

Avoid scratching and infecting skin acne.

—Explain the signs of cardiac complications and instruct the patient to watch for them: chest pain (pericarditis), shortness of breath, increasing fatigue, palpitations, swelling of ankles and feet (heart failure, valvular heart involvement).

—Explain the need for prophylactic antibiotic therapy before invasive procedures that predispose to bacteremia if there has been valve involvement, including dental or gum therapy, urologic and gynecologic procedures, childbirth.

- *Medications*

—Explain the purpose, dosage, schedule, and route of administration of any prescribed drugs, as well as side effects to report to the physician or nurse.

—Stress the importance of completing antibiotic therapy to prevent recurrence and discuss the need for lifelong prophylactic antibiotic coverage in the presence of valve involvement.

—Discuss the hypersensitivity reaction to penicillin. Warn the patient that reaction after long-term use is possible. Instruct the patient to stop penicillin therapy and call the physician immediately if a reaction occurs.

- *Activity*

—Explain the need for strict bed rest that may continue for up to 5 weeks during the acute phase. As activities are resumed, instruct the patient to avoid fatigue, plan regular rest periods, and avoid strenuous activities.

—Encourage the patient to discuss allowances and limitations with respect to occupation, recreation, and activities.

—Suggest nonstressful diversional activities during the convalescent period. For adolescents and young adults, suggest home study and tutoring programs.

## FOLLOW-UP CARE

- Stress the importance of regular follow-up visits. Make sure the patient has the necessary names and telephone numbers.
- Emphasize the importance of informing the dentist and other physicians of rheumatic fever and the possible need for prophylactic antibiotic therapy.

# Ruptured Disk
## (Herniated or Slipped Disk, Herniated Nucleus Pulposus)

—Ruptured disk: a chronic condition occurring when all or part of the nucleus pulposus, the soft, gelatinous, cushioning center of cartilage between each two vertebrae, is pushed through the disk's weakened or torn outer ring (anulus fibrosus). This results in exertion of pressure on the spinal nerves as they exit the spinal canal, causing back pain and other signs of nerve root irritation (sciatica). Ruptured disk typically occurs in adult men under 45 years of age. The lumbar and lumbosacral regions are most frequently affected (95%). Cervical disks may also rupture, usually because of degenerative changes.

### CAUSES/CONTRIBUTING FACTORS
- Severe trauma or strain
- Intervertebral joint degeneration caused by aging

### SIGNS/SYMPTOMS
- Sciatica: severe low back pain radiating to the buttocks, legs, and feet
- Sudden pain following coughing, sneezing, bending, or lifting
- Muscle spasm and tenseness
- Loss of sensation and motor control to the extremities

### COMPLICATIONS
- Paresis
- Motor weakness
- Sensory changes
- Footdrop
- Loss of bowel, bladder control

### DIAGNOSTIC TESTS
- Describe each procedure, its purpose, and the normal feelings or sensations that are likely, as well as any preprocedural and postprocedural care.

—Straight leg raising test: positive when the patient complains of posterior leg (sciatic) pain versus back pain when the leg is lifted; pain is increased with foot dorsiflexion
—Back x-rays: to document decreased disk space
—Computed tomography: to show disk rupture
—Magnetic resonance imaging: to confirm disk rupture and show compression sites on the spinal nerve
—Myelogram: to show the site of rupture
—Diskogram: to show disk degeneration and rupture

## TREATMENT

*Medical*

- Therapy
  —Skin traction with pelvic belt
  —Bed rest in position of comfort: side lying or recumbent with pillow under knees
  —Ice massage of lumbosacral area to lessen edema
  —Back support or metal back brace
  —Ultrasound diathermy with back massage
  —Exercise regimen after acute pain and inflammation have subsided; to strengthen back and abdominal muscles
- Drugs
  —Antiinflammatory (nonsteroidal) medications
  —Analgesic and antipyretic medications
  —Muscle relaxants
  —Narcotics
  —Antianxiety agents

*Surgical*

  —Percutaneous diskectomy: removal of the disk by insertion of a metal canal under fluoroscopy
  —Microdiskectomy: removal of the affected disk by microscopic surgery through a 1-inch incision
  —Nuclear diskectomy
  —Laminectomy: excision of part of the lamina and removal of the protruding disk
  —Spinal fusion: to stabilize the spine; indicated if more than one disk is involved
  —Chemonucleolysis: injection of enzyme (chymopapain) directly into the disk to dissolve prolapsed tissue

## HOME CARE

- Give both the patient and the caregiver *verbal* and *written* instructions. Provide them with the name and telephone number of a physician or nurse to call if questions arise.
- *General information*
  —Discuss the disorder and contributing factors.
- *Warning signs*
  —Review the signs and symptoms that should be reported to a physician or nurse.
      Continued presence of pain
      Paresthesia (numbness, tingling sensation in extremities)
      Muscle spasms
      Changes in bowel, bladder function
- *Special instructions*
  —Explain and instruct the patient in the use and application of the back brace, support, or belt. Discuss use of the skin traction belt. Advise and assist the patient to obtain the necessary home equipment.
- *Medications*
  —Explain the purpose, dosage, schedule, and route of administration of any prescribed drugs, as well as side effects to report to the physician or nurse.
  —Discuss nonsteroidal antiinflammatory drugs (NSAIDs), and warn the patient not to take over-the-counter analgesics or muscle relaxants with NSAIDs without checking with the physician.
- *Activity*
  —Explain the need for initial complete bed rest (up to 2 weeks) to decrease inflammatory responses and to reduce pressure in the spine, which relieves pressure on the irritated nerve root and decreases pain. Instruct the patient to assume the position of greatest comfort: semi-Fowler's or side lying with knees always flexed. Caution the patient not to lie on the stomach.
  —Advise the patient to use a urinal, bedpan, or bedside commode during the period of bed rest to avoid walking. Assist the patient to obtain the equipment.
  —Teach body mechanics and principles of lifting, moving, and carrying (see p. 87) once acute pain eases.
  —Demonstrate back exercises to strengthen muscles (see p. 89).

- *Diet*
  —Explain the importance of a high fluid intake and a diet high in fiber roughage to prevent constipation during the period of bed rest.
  —Discuss the need to maintain a weight appropriate for age, sex, and height. If the patient is overweight, explain that excess body weight aggravates the strain on the spine. Refer the patient to a dietitian for a weight control diet.

## FOLLOW-UP CARE

- Stress the importance of regular follow-up visits to the physician and physical therapist until recovery is complete. Make sure the patient has the necessary names and telephone numbers.

# Saphenous Vein Ligation and Stripping

—Saphenous vein ligation and stripping: a procedure used in the treatment of varicose veins. Such enlarged, tortuous, dilated veins usually occur in the lower extremities. As the veins dilate and venous valve function decreases, they become less functional, resulting in venous stasis and thrombus formation.

## INDICATIONS

- Varicose veins

## PREPROCEDURAL TEACHING

- Review the physician's explanation of the procedure and the reason for it; encourage the patient to ask questions and to discuss any fears or anxieties. Explain the need for informed consent.

### Review of Preprocedural Care

- Tell the patient that all hair will be removed from the surgical leg.
- Instruct the patient to take two showers with hexachlorophene within 12 hours before the procedure.
- Instruct the patient not to eat or drink after midnight before the procedure.

- Explain that all visible varicose veins that are to be stripped will be marked with dye with the patient standing.
- Inform the patient that sedation will be given the night before the procedure.

## SIDE EFFECTS/COMPLICATIONS

- Ecchymosis, bleeding
- Numbness
- Ulceration
- Infection
- Thromboembolic disease
- Scars

## HOME CARE

- Give both the patient and the caregiver *verbal* and *written* instructions. Provide them with the name and telephone number of a physician or nurse to call if questions arise.
- *General information*
  —Review any explanation about the procedure and specific follow-up care.
- *Wound/incision care*
  —Discuss and demonstrate proper care of the incision.
- *Warning signs*
  —Review the signs and symptoms that should be reported to a physician or nurse.
      Fever
      Redness, warmth, pain, edema, or purulent drainage from incision sites
- *Special instructions*
  —Instruct the patient to wear support stockings. Assist the patient to obtain appropriate supplies and proper size.
  —Advise the patient to avoid wearing constrictive clothing and knee-high stockings.
- *Medications*
  —Explain the purpose, dosage, schedule, and route of administration of any prescribed drugs, as well as side effects to report to a physician or nurse.
  —Encourage the patient to take pain medications.
- *Activity*
  —Advise the patient to take frequent rest periods during the day and elevate the legs above the heart while sitting for at least 6 weeks after the procedure.

—Tell the patient to avoid prolonged periods of sitting and standing and to change positions at frequent intervals.

—Advise not crossing the legs while sitting.

—Encourage the patient to initiate a walking program.

—Stress the importance of weight reduction, if indicated. Provide referral to community resources and weight reduction programs.

**FOLLOW-UP CARE**

- Stress the importance of regular follow-up visits. Make sure the patient has the necessary names and telephone numbers.

# Sarcoidosis

—Sarcoidosis: a multisystem granulomatous disorder of unknown etiology, characteristically producing pulmonary infiltrates, lymphadenopathy, and skin lesions. In most cases the process is benign and self-limiting without residual effects. Sarcoidosis is most common in young adults and African-Americans between 20 and 40 years of age.

**SIGNS/SYMPTOMS**

- Weight loss, anorexia
- Fever, night sweats, joint pain, fatigue
- Respiratory: clubbing of fingers, dyspnea, cough
- Palpitations
- Skin nodules: over face, neck, and extremities
- Bone cysts in hands and feet
- Nasal mucosal lesions
- Hair loss
- Blurred vision, eye pain, drainage, infection

**COMPLICATIONS**

- Pulmonary fibrosis
- Cor pulmonale

## DIAGNOSTIC TESTS

- Describe each procedure, its purpose, and the normal feelings or sensations that are likely, as well as any preprocedural and postprocedural care.
  - —Kveim skin test: positive 3-6 weeks
  - —Skin and lymph node biopsy
  - —Bronchoscopy: transbronchial biopsy, open lung biopsy, bronchoalveolar lavage
  - —Gallium-67 scan
  - —Chest x-ray
  - —Pulmonary function tests
  - —Serum tests: complete blood count, creatinine protein, erythrocyte sedimentation rate, angiotensin-converting enzyme level

## TREATMENT

*Medical*

- Therapy
  - —Chest physiotherapy
  - —Heat therapy and joint supports for arthritis
- Drugs
  - —Systemic or topical steroids
  - —Azathioprine (Imuran)
  - —Optic agents: methylcellulose eyedrops
  - —Antiarrhythmic agents
  - —Calcium-chelating medication
  - —Antiarthritic treatment: salicylates, nonsteroidal antiinflammatory drugs, corticosteroids
  - —Vitamin D supplements

## HOME CARE

- Give both the patient and the caregiver *verbal* and *written* instructions. Provide them with the name and telephone number of a physician or nurse to call if questions arise.
- *General information*
  - —Explain and discuss sarcoidosis, its causes, and contributing factors.
- *Warning signs*
  - —Review the signs, symptoms, and complications that should be reported to a physician or nurse.
    - Shortness of breath
    - Red, watery eyes

Dizziness

Chest pain

Swollen joints

Unusual fatigue

Fever

- *Special instructions*

—Teach the importance of chest physiotherapy (breathing exercises, postural drainage): as prophylaxis or treatment of chronic pulmonary disease.

—Stress the importance of avoiding large crowds and individuals who are known to have active infections.

—Instruct the patient to weigh daily to detect steady weight loss.

- *Medications*

—Explain the purpose, dosage, schedule, and route of administration of any prescribed drugs, as well as side effects to report to the physician or nurse.

Topical and systemic corticosteroids (see Steroid Therapy, p. 608)

—Teach the patient aseptic technique for administering eyedrops to avoid contamination.

Wash any drainage from the eye.

Wash hands.

Look up toward the ceiling.

Pull down the lower lid while holding the medication tip 1-2 cm from the eye.

Instill drop(s).

Wipe any excess medication from the face.

—Teach the patient aseptic technique for administering ointment.

Wash any drainage from the eye.

Wash hands.

Pull down lower lid and apply a thin stream of ointment just inside the lower lid without touching the eye or surrounding area.

Close the eyes and rotate them to distribute medication.

Replace the cap and store as directed.

- *Activity*

—Encourage the patient to discusss allowances and limitations with respect to occupation, recreation, and activities.

—Discuss energy conservation and breathing exercises.

—Encourage the patient to pace activities, allow for adequate rest periods, and avoid overexertion.

- *Diet*
  —Encourage a low-salt, low-potassium, low-calcium diet with vitamin D supplements.
  —Advise the patient to eat small, frequent meals to meet nutritional needs.

**FOLLOW-UP CARE**

- Stress the importance of follow-up medical and laboratory evaluations. Make sure the patient has the necessary names and telephone numbers.
- Discuss the need for routine chest x-rays and pulmonary function tests to monitor the disease process.
- Emphasize the importance of wearing a Medic-Alert bracelet and carrying an identification card at all times.

# Sickle Cell Anemia

—Sickle cell anemia: a chronic hemolytic disorder that occurs as the result of a genetic mutation transmitted from parent to child. Sickle cell anemia is characterized by abnormal, crescent-shaped, rigid, and elongated red blood cells. These "sickled" cells interfere with circulation because they cannot get through the microcirculation and are destroyed in the process. Sickle cell crises occur in two forms: vasoocclusive and aplastic. In vasoocclusive crisis, the more common form, the collection of misshapen red blood cells in the smaller blood vessels (e.g., peripheral, renal) results in blockage of blood flow, tissue hypoxia, and death. Sickle cell anemia is seen primarily in African-Americans. In aplastic crisis, infection results in a decreased availability of functioning red blood cells because of bone marrow aplasia, iron deficiency, or splenic destruction of red blood cells.

**CAUSES**

- Genetic hereditary disorder

## SIGNS/SYMPTOMS

- General
  —Fatigue
  —Dyspnea on exertion
  —Delayed sexual maturity
- Crisis
  —Severe pain: bone, abdomen, chest, joints, muscles
  —Jaundice
  —Pallor
  —Joint swelling
  —Fever (low-grade)
  —Lethargy
  —Leg ulcers

## COMPLICATIONS

- Stroke
- Renal failure
- Respiratory failure
- Myocardial infarction
- Hemolytic anemia

## DIAGNOSTIC TESTS

- Describe each procedure, its purpose, and the normal feelings or sensations that are likely, as well as any preprocedural and postprocedural care.
  —Stained blood smear
  —Sickle cell slide preparation of blood
  —Sickle turbidity test (HbS)
  —Hemoglobin electrophoresis (HbS)
  —Red blood cell life span

## TREATMENT

*Medical*

- Therapy
  —Rest
  —Oxygen
  —Intravenous fluids and electrolytes
- Drugs
  —Analgesics
  —Antiinfectives (low-dose penicillin)
  —Deferoxamine (chelating agent)

—Sedatives

—Iron supplements

## HOME CARE

- Give both the patient and the caregiver *verbal* and *written* instructions. Provide them with the name and telephone number of a physician or nurse to call if questions arise.
- *General information*
  —Explain and discuss sickle cell disorder, its causes, and contributing factors.
- *Warning signs*
  —Review the signs, symptoms, and complications that should be reported to a physician or nurse.

  Jaundice

  Dyspnea

  Severe joint or abdominal pain

  Headaches

  Vertigo

  Sleepiness with difficulty awakening

  Persistent fever (more than 2 days)

  Hematuria
- *Special instructions*
  —Alert the patient to avoid factors that precipitate sickle cell crisis: high altitude, drinking iced liquids, vigorous exercise.

  —Discuss the importance of avoiding persons with infections, such as upper respiratory infections. Tell the patient to seek early treatment of infection.

  —Advise the patient to discuss the need for vaccinations (e.g., *Haemophilus influenzae* B) with the physician or nurse.

  —Stress the importance of seeking early treatment for crisis. Explain that hospitalization may be necessary.

  —Teach the patient to blow the nose gently, avoid coughing, and avoid straining on elimination.

  —Teach the patient to avoid trauma and extremes of temperature and to protect extremities from injury because of impaired circulation.

  —Demonstrate how to monitor oral intake, urinary output, and urine protein level.

  —Alert the patient to the need to have family members tested for HbS. Refer carriers to genetic counseling.

  —For a female patient, explain that women have a high risk for pulmonary or renal complications. Stress the importance of planning pregnancies and provide birth control information.

- *Medications*
  —Explain the purpose, dosage, schedule, and route of administration of any prescribed drugs, as well as side effects to report to the physician or nurse.
- *Activity*
  —Encourage the patient to discuss allowances and limitations with respect to occupation, recreation, and activities.
  —Teach range-of-motion exercises and encourage regular physical activity to prevent bone mineralization.
  —Explain the need for balance between activity and rest.
- *Diet*
  —Discuss the need for a well-balanced diet.
  —Encourage the patient to eat small, frequent meals.
  —Encourage fluid intake to prevent dehydration.

## FOLLOW-UP CARE

- Stress the importance of follow-up medical and laboratory evaluations. Make sure the patient has the necessary names and telephone numbers.

## REFERRALS

- Assist the patient to obtain psychosocial counseling as needed. Refer to hospital and community support groups as indicated.
- Refer patients planning to have children to genetic counseling.

**S**

# Sigmoidoscopy

—**Sigmoidoscopy: passage of a rigid or flexible scope for direct visualization of mucosa or biopsy of lesions of the sigmoid colon, rectum, and anal canal.**

## INDICATIONS

- Changes in bowel habits
- Rectal bleeding
- Diverticulosis

- Polyps
- Ulcerative colitis
- Crohn's disease
- Irritable bowel syndrome
- Benign tumors
- Anorectal fistulas
- Weight loss
- Anemia

## PREPROCEDURAL TEACHING

- Review the physician's explanation of the procedure and the reason for it; encourage the patient to ask questions and to discuss any fears or anxieties. Discuss the need for informed consent.

### Review of Preprocedural Care

- Explain that preprocedural care varies according to the suspected diagnosis.
- Inform the patient that light meals or a clear liquid diet may be ordered for 48 hours before the procedure.
- Discuss the need to be NPO for 8 hours before the procedure.
- Explain that a bowel prep consisting of laxatives or enemas may be ordered.
- Discuss what will happen during the procedure.
  - —The patient is positioned in a knee-chest position on a tilting table or a left lateral position with the right buttock elevated.
  - —Air may be insufflated to allow better passage of the scope and better visualization.
  - —A light sedative or analgesics will be given; atropine may be given to limit gastrointestinal secretions.
- Reassure the patient that safety and privacy will be ensured.

### Review of Postprocedural Care

- Explain that the patient will remain on bed rest for 1-2 hours after the procedure to allow monitoring for signs and symptoms of complications.
- Explain that flatus will result from air inserted during the procedure and cannot be controlled, but is temporary and may be relieved with ambulation.

## COMPLICATIONS

- Bowel perforation
- Vasovagal stimulation

**HOME CARE**

• Give both the patient and the caregiver *verbal* and *written* instructions. Provide them with the name and telephone number of a physician or nurse to call if questions arise.

• *General information*

—Review any explanation about the procedure and specific follow-up care. Advise the patient that there may be slight rectal bleeding if biopsy specimens were taken.

• *Warning signs*

—Review the signs and symptoms that should be reported to a physician or nurse.

Abdominal pain and distention

Rectal bleeding

Fever

Pallor and diaphoresis

• *Activity*

—Explain that the patient should avoid vigorous activity on the day of the procedure but then may resume activities as tolerated.

• *Diet*

—Tell the patient that a regular diet or one prescribed by the physician for the underlying disease may be followed.

**FOLLOW-UP CARE**

• Stress the importance of regular follow-up visits. Make sure the patient has the necessary names and telephone numbers.

**S**

# Spinal Cord Injury

—Spinal cord injury (for chronic care following acute rehabilitation): physical injury that transects, lacerates, stretches, or compresses the spinal cord, resulting in compromised blood supply, hemorrhage, edema, or ischemia. Neurologic deficits are caused by the interruption in neuronal function and transmission of nerve impulses. The neurologic deficits depend on the lesions and the level of injury. Spinal cord injuries are classified according to type, cause, site, mechanism of injury, stability, and degree of spinal cord function loss.

## CAUSES/CONTRIBUTING FACTORS/RISK FACTORS

- Motor vehicle accidents
- Diving or other sports accidents
- Industrial accidents
- Falls
- Assaults, including gunshot wounds
- Degenerative changes or diseases of the spinal cord

## SIGNS/SYMPTOMS

- Signs and symptoms depend on degree, type, and level of injury
- Loss of muscle function below the level of injury, including respiratory muscles
- Loss of sensation: proprioception, pain, temperature, touch, and pressure below the level of injury
- Loss of spinal reflexes below the level of injury
- Pain at level of injury
- Loss of vasomotor tone
- Bladder and bowel dysfunction
- Priapism: abnormal prolonged or constant penile erection, seldom associated with sexual arousal
- Autonomic dysreflexia: bradycardia, sweating above level of injury, elevated temperature, headache, nausea, nasal congestion, paroxysmal hypertension

## COMPLICATIONS

- Contractures
- Decubiti
- Urinary calculi and urinary tract infection
- Pneumonia
- Autonomic dysreflexia
- Sexual dysfunction
- Paralytic ileus
- Respiratory failure
- Sepsis
- Spinal shock

**DIAGNOSTIC TESTS**

- Describe each procedure, its purpose, and the normal feelings or sensations that are likely, as well as any preprocedural and postprocedural care.
    - X-ray of spine: to detect fracture, deformity, or displacement of vertebrae
    - Computed tomography or magnetic resonance imaging: to detect changes in the spinal cord or vertebrae
    - Myelography: to show disruption of the spinal canal
    - Arterial blood gases: to assess effectiveness of respirations
    - Serum electrolytes
    - Complete blood count with differential

**TREATMENT**

*Medical*

- Therapy
    - Stryker or Foster frame or kinetic treatment table
    - Skeletal traction
    - Cervical collar
    - Assistive devices: splints, braces, wheelchair
    - Nerve stimulation
    - Physical therapy
    - Occupational therapy
    - Neurologic rehabilitation
    - Psychologic counseling, including sexual counseling
      Bladder and bowel retraining program
    - Nutritional counseling
    - NPO until chewing, swallowing, and gastrointestinal functioning are established
    - Feedings parenteral or enteral
    - Antiembolic stockings
    - Intermittent urinary catheterization
- Drugs
    - Corticosteroids
    - Osmotic diuretics
    - Anticoagulants
    - Analgesics
    - Antacids and $H_2$ blockers
    - Stool softeners and laxatives
    - Antianxiety agents
    - Muscle relaxants

—Antispasmodics
—Antibiotics
—Anticholinergics
—Antihypertensives

*Surgical*

- Laminectomy: to relieve compression from a hematoma; to remove bone fragments or penetrating objects
- Spinal fusion: to stabilize spine
- Cervical tongs or halo traction: to immobilize the cervical spine
- Body cast or Harrington rods: to immobilize the thoracic spine
- Tracheostomy: to provide long-term ventilatory support
- Tenotomies, myotomies, neurectomies, rhizotomy, muscle transplants: to treat spasticity

## HOME CARE (FOR CHRONIC CARE FOLLOWING LONG-TERM REHABILITATION)

- Give both the patient and the caregiver *verbal* and *written* instructions. Provide them with the name and telephone number of a physician or nurse to call if questions arise. Provide spinal cord injury instruction sheets to assist in instruction.
- *General information*
  —Explain and discuss the spinal cord injury, care, treatment, and rehabilitation needs.
- *Warning signs*
  —Review the signs, symptoms, and complications that should be reported to a physician or nurse.
    Skin breakdown or poor response to decubitus treatment
    Urinary tract infection: urinary frequency, urgency, retention, or incontinence; suprapubic distention; pain or burning with urination; malodorous urine; cloudy or bloody urine; fever; chills; flank pain
    Renal calculi: pain that may be sharp, sudden, and intense or dull and aching in the flank area; urinary frequency; voiding in small amounts; hematuria
    Upper respiratory infection: changes in respirations, color change in sputum, fever
    Respiratory distress
    Autonomic dysreflexia: bradycardia, sweating above level of injury, elevated temperature, headache, nausea, nasal congestion, paroxysmal hypertension
    Lack of bowel movement for more than 3 days or impaction

Thrombophlebitis: erythema, warmth, edema in calves or
  thighs

Sudden changes in motor or sensory function

Loose or dislodged pins or vest

- *Special instructions*
  —Discuss skin care.

    If the patient is confined to bed or wheelchair, instruct the
      patient to use a mirror to check skin for breakdown.

    Instruct the caretaker on perineal care following elimina-
      tion: wash gently with mild soap, rinse well with warm
      water, pat dry, and apply skin protector.

    Advise the removal of sharp objects, crumbs, and wrinkles
      from bed and chairs.

    Advise the patient to regulate bath water temperature and
      avoid application of extreme hot and cold temperatures
      because of loss of temperature sensation.

    Instruct the patient to change position at least every 15-30
      minutes when in wheelchair and at least every 2 hours
      when in bed. Instruct the patient to set an alarm clock to
      wake during the night to turn.

  —Discuss urinary elimination.

    Stress the importance of following the bladder retraining
      program.

    Teach the patient to observe for urinary distention every
      2-4 hours.

    Reinforce or teach methods to stimulate voiding reflex.

    Teach intermittent self-catheterization.

    Teach and demonstrate care of the indwelling urinary cath-
      eter.

  —Discuss bowel elimination.

    Stress the importance of following the bowel retraining
      program.

    Attempt to establish the previous bowel pattern with regu-
      lar, convenient times or 30 minutes after meals.

    Reinforce or teach methods to stimulate a bowel movement.

    Massage the abdomen from the right side to the left to
      stimulate the gastrointestinal tract.

    Suggest bearing down, bending forward, or applying
      manual abdominal pressure during defecation.

    Teach the patient the signs of rectal fullness: goosebumps,
      perspiration, rising of hair on arms and legs, and sense
      of fullness.

**S**

Instruct the patient to sit on the bedpan, toilet, or commode at the scheduled time for bowel movement. Encourage the patient to sit erect during defecation, if possible.

Tell the patient to avoid sitting on the bedpan, toilet, or commode for more than 20 minutes.

Teach the patient the signs of impaction: no formed stools for more than 3 days or semiliquid stools.

—Teach the patient or caregiver about preventing and managing autonomic dysreflexia, including noxious stimuli that cause autonomic dysreflexia.

—Explain the need to use anesthetic jelly liberally for urinary catheterization and insertion of suppository or enema.

—Stress the importance of following the prescribed rehabilitation program for the specific spinal cord injury.

—Assist the patient in obtaining assistive aids for self-care, mobility, support, and physical exercises.

—Assist the patient and caregiver to identify adaptations needed in the home environment: obtaining special beds with trapeze or special mattress, widening doorways, installing ramps for wheelchairs.

—Provide alternative methods of dealing with chronic pain: visualization, guided imagery, meditation, relaxation, biofeedback.

• *Medications*

—Explain the purpose, dosage, schedule, and route of administration of any prescribed drugs, as well as side effects to report to the physician or nurse.

—Stress the importance of not taking over-the-counter medications without consulting the physician.

• *Activity*

—Encourage the patient to discuss allowances and limitations with respect to occupation, recreation, and activities.

—Demonstrate range-of-motion exercises to the family or caregiver and instruct them to assist the patient with exercises.

—Advise the patient that the prone position may help relieve pressure on susceptible areas and help decrease contractures and spasms in hips and knees.

—Stress the importance of performing range-of-motion, muscle-strengthening, and stretching exercises.

—Instruct the patient to schedule rest periods with activities and exercises.

—Explain the need to plan activities to avoid fatigue.

—Discuss ways to protect the legs from injury during movement and transfers.

—Advise the patient to take warm baths and massage to help prevent spasticity.

—Instruct the patient on the use of splints or high-top shoes that are cut off at the toes to help prevent foot contractures in patients with spasticity.

—Advise the patient to avoid stimuli that trigger spasm: cold, anxiety, fatigue, emotional distress, infection, bowel or bladder distention, ulcers, pain, tight clothing, maintaining one position for too long. Advise the family and caregivers that touch should be firm, gentle, and steady.

• *Diet*

—Assist the patient to plan a high-calorie, high-protein, high-fiber diet.

—Advise the patient to avoid foods that cause an upset stomach or diarrhea.

—Provide the patient with a list of specific gas-producing foods to avoid.

—Encourage the patient to drink plenty of fluids, up to 2 liters a day, unless contraindicated.

—Encourage the patient to drink cranberry juice or take vitamin C to decrease urine pH.

—Encourage the patient to drink prune juice to help prevent constipation.

—Advise the patient to drink fluids at even intervals throughout the day.

—Instruct the patient to restrict fluid intake before bedtime.

—Advise the patient to avoid alcohol and caffeine-containing foods and beverages. Provide the patient with a list of specific caffeine-containing foods and beverages.

—Advise the patient to limit milk and dairy products to minimize the risk of renal calculi.

—Instruct the family and caregiver to assist with feedings as necessary.

## FOLLOW-UP CARE

• Stress the importance of follow-up medical and laboratory evaluations. Make sure the patient has the necessary names and telephone numbers.

- Assist the patient in obtaining a Medic-Alert bracelet and identification card listing diagnosis, medication, and treatment.

## PSYCHOSOCIAL CARE

- Assist the patient to establish realistic goals and implement alternative methods for communication and mobility.
- Encourage the patient to continue to express concerns related to injury, disability, loss of mobility, body image changes, and feelings of grief.
- Advise the family to avoid overprotectiveness.
- Encourage decision making and promote independence in the patient.
- Encourage the family to verbalize concerns related to injury, disability, and effects on their life-style.
- Offer specific suggestions of ways to achieve sexual gratification or manage common problems related to spinal cord injury and sexual activity.
- Allow the patient and partner to verbalize concerns regarding sexual activity.

## REFERRALS

- Refer the patient to a social worker for further support, counseling, and financial assistance, if appropriate.
- Refer the patient for sexual counseling.
  - —For males: sexual dysfunction, primarily inability to ejaculate
  - —For females: for contraceptive and reproductive counseling because uterine contractions of labor may cause autonomic dysreflexia in women with spinal cord injuries at T8 or above
- Assist the patient to obtain referral to home health care or custodial care services.
- Refer the patient to community resources, local support groups, and vocational rehabilitation agencies.
- Assist the patient to obtain referral to spinal cord injury organizations.
  - —Spinal Cord Injury Foundation
  - —National Spinal Cord Injury Association, 600 West Cummings Park, Suite 2000, Woburn, MA 01801, (617) 935-2722
  - —Information Center for Individuals with Disabilities, 29 Stanhope Street, P.O. Box 256, Boston, MA 02117, (617) 450-9888.

—American Paralysis Association, 500 Morris Avenue, Springfield, NJ 07081, (800) 225-0292 or in New Jersey (201) 379-2690

—Spinal Cord Injury Hotline (800) 526-3456

# Sprains and Strains

—**Sprains and strains: muscle and ligament injuries. Sprains and strains vary in severity and tissues affected, but the treatment is often the same. A sprain is a tear, usually in a muscle but sometimes in a ligament or tendon, that may be partial or complete tearing of the fibers from their attachments. A strain is a "pull" caused by an acute or chronic overstretching or overuse; it may involve a muscle but usually affects ligaments or tendons. The tearing or stretching caused by these injuries leads to bleeding into tissues, which sets up an inflammatory reaction. Both sprains and strains are classified according to severity.**

## SIGNS/SYMPTOMS

* First-degree strain: excess pull or stretch
  —Mild pain
  —Edema with some bruising (bleeding into tissues)
  —Muscle spasm
  —Tenderness
  —Slight loss of function or strength
* First-degree sprain: ligament fibers partially torn
  —Mild pain
  —Slight edema
  —Local tenderness
  —No joint instability
  —Slight change in function for a short time
* Second-degree strain: tear or disruption of some muscle fibers
  —Increased pain and edema
  —Redness
  —Bleeding
  —Change in function
  —Local heat

S

- Second-degree sprain: incomplete tear of ligament
  —Moderate edema
  —Local pain and tenderness
  —Moderate joint instability
  —Inability to carry out usual activities
- Third-degree strain: complete disruption of muscle fibers, with possible rupture of fascia
  —Severe pain
  —Muscle spasm
  —Pronounced edema
  —Marked ecchymosis with hematoma formation
  —Marked tenderness
  —Loss of function
- Third-degree sprain: full or complete tear of ligament or tendon
  —Severe pain
  —Edema: minimal to marked
  —Joint disability
  —Loss of function

## COMPLICATIONS

- Chronic joint disability
- Neurovascular dysfunction of extremity
- Posttraumatic arthritis

## DIAGNOSTIC TESTS

- Describe each procedure, its purpose, and the normal feelings or sensations that are likely, as well as any preprocedural and postprocedural care.
  —Stress radiographs: to evaluate severity of injury
  —Magnetic resonance imaging: to confirm the extent of ligamentous injury or disruption

## TREATMENT

*Medical*

- Therapy
  —"RICE"
      **R**est: let the injured area rest; how long depends on severity of injury
      **I**ce: apply ice packs to the affected area to decrease swelling and bruising

Compression: elastic or Ace bandages to wrap injured area; cast or splint for severe sprains or strains; bandage should be wrapped firmly around the injury, but not so much that blood flow is restricted

Elevation: raising the injured area above the heart to reduce swelling (foot higher than knee; hand higher than elbow)

- Drugs
  —Analgesics
  —Antiinflammatory agents

*Surgical*

- Indicated for third-degree sprains or strains
- Open reduction and repair of torn or avulsed tissues: to restore full joint function
- Ligament or tendon reattachment or removal: if severely damaged

## HOME CARE

- Give both the patient and the caregiver *verbal* and *written* instructions. Provide them with the name and telephone number of a physician or nurse to call if questions arise.
- *General information*
  —Explain the nature and extent of injury (first, second, or third degree).
- *Warning signs*
  —Review the signs and symptoms of neurovascular impairment caused by tightness of the cast or dressing. Explain that they should be reported to a physician or nurse.
    Skin color: red, blue, purple
    Skin temperature: injured tissues are cooler than surrounding tissue; warm or hot skin
    Swelling: injured area will be swollen, but skin around it should not be tight
    Sudden increase in pain
    Inability to bend fingers or toes of affected extremity
    Numbness and tingling in fingers or toes
    Decreased capillary refill: pink color takes longer than 4 seconds to return when pressure is applied to the fingernails or toenails of injured limb
- *Special instructions*
  —Instruct the patient in the use of required ambulatory aids (e.g., crutches, cane).

—Teach the patient the proper method of applying Ace bandages: from distal to proximal on the limb to aid venous constriction and venous return. Advise the patient to loosen the bandage if signs of neurovascular impairment are noted.

—Instruct the patient to apply ice packs for the first 24-72 hours or longer to lessen bleeding and edema, depending on injury.

- *Medications*

—Explain the purpose, dosage, schedule, and route of administration of any prescribed drugs, as well as side effects to report to the physician or nurse.

- *Activity*

—Depending on the severity of injury, discuss how long mobility will be impaired: 24-72 hours for first-degree sprains and strains; 10 days to 3 or more weeks for second- and third-degree injuries.

—Stress the importance of maintaining rest and immobilization of the affected limb for the prescribed time. Explain that returning to activity while there is still swelling or bleeding may cause further injury and delayed healing and recovery.

—Discuss the need to elevate the injured limb. Instruct the patient not to elevate it too high because this could reduce blood flow and thus increase swelling.

—Instruct the patient in progressive active range-of-motion and rehabilitative exercises as prescribed by the physician depending on severity of injury.

**FOLLOW-UP CARE**

- Stress the importance of follow-up medical and laboratory evaluations. Make sure the patient has the necessary names and telephone numbers.

---

# Steroid Therapy
## (Corticosteroid Therapy)

---

**—Steroid therapy: use of corticosteroids as replacement therapy for adrenal insufficiency, for inflammation suppression, for control of allergic reactions, and for reducing the risk of graft rejection in transplantation. The length of time the pa-**

tient remains on steroid therapy depends on the underlying condition for which it is prescribed; it can be lifelong or temporary. Corticosteroids are classified according to their biologic activities: glucocorticoids (carbohydrate and protein metabolism), mineralocorticoids (electrolyte and water metabolism), and androgens (anabolic and masculinizing). They are administered systemically (parenteral or oral) or topically (skin).

## CAUTIONS

- Hypertension and diabetes mellitus can be exacerbated.
- Concurrent infections can be masked.
- Therapy should be used with caution in patients who are predisposed to peptic ulceration, thrombophlebitis, adrenal suppression, and mood swings.
- Gradual withdrawal of exogenous corticosteroids is necessary to prevent adrenal insufficiency.

## COMPLICATIONS

- Steroid-induced diabetes
- Hypertension
- Osteoporosis
- Peptic ulcer
- Thromboembolism
- Hypokalemia
- Pseudotumor cerebri
- Development of Cushing's syndrome

## HOME CARE

- Give both the patient and the caregiver *verbal* and *written* instructions. Provide them with the name and telephone number of a physician or nurse to call if questions arise.
- Initiate the teaching plan as soon as it is known that the patient will be discharged with a prescription for steroid therapy.
- *General information*
  —Review the explanation of the condition that requires steroid therapy, the type of steroid therapy (systemic or topical) that is prescribed, benefits, dosage, time of administration, side effects, importance of taking the medication at the prescribed time and not skipping a dose, and what to do if a dose is missed.

- *Warning signs*
  —Review the signs and symptoms that should be reported to a physician or nurse.
    Euphoria
    Gastrointestinal pain or bleeding
    Bruising
    Thrombophlebitis
    Hypertension
    Cushingoid features: moonface, acne
    Hirsutism
    Osteoporosis
    Mood swings
- *Special instructions*
  —Tell the patient to refill medication prescriptions 1-2 weeks before the supply runs out and to store medication in a cool place, avoiding extremes of temperature.
  —Explain that normal signs of infection may be masked by steroid therapy and that the physican or nurse should be consulted at the onset of symptoms.
  —Instruct the patient to take oral steroids with milk or antacids to decrease gastric irritation.
  —Explain that the oral form of the medication comes in various dosages and that the patient must be sure to take the appropriate dose at the prescribed time.
  —Discuss the need for and process of gradually withdrawing oral medication. Instruct the patient to monitor for and report the return of symptoms during withdrawal.
  —If the medication is administered topically, discuss the dosage and appropriate administration. Caution the patient to use the medication only as prescribed.
- *Activity*
  —Encourage the patient to discuss allowances and limitations with respect to occupation, recreation, or activities.
- *Diet*
  —Instruct the patient to increase protein intake to combat osteoporosis.

## FOLLOW-UP CARE

- Stress the importance of regular follow-up visits. Make sure the patient has the necessary names and telephone numbers.

• Discuss the importance of wearing a Medic-Alert bracelet and carrying an information card giving the name and dosage of the drug.

# Stroke
## (Cerebrovascular Accident)

—**Stroke: a disruption in oxygen supply to cerebral cells, resulting in ischemia of an area of the brain and associated neurologic deficits.**

## CAUSES/CONTRIBUTING FACTORS/RISK FACTORS

• Ischemic stroke
  —Thrombosis: atherosclerosis, hypertension, hematologic disorders
  —Embolus: atrial fibrillation, extracranial clot formations, valvular heart disease
  —Systemic hypoperfusion: circulatory failure, hypovolemia, systemic hypotension, hypoxia
• Hemorrhagic stroke
  —Hypertension
  —Aneurysm
  —Vascular malformations
  —Trauma
  —Systemic hemorrhagic disorders

## SIGNS/SYMPTOMS

• Symptoms are dependent on location and size of the lesion and extent of injury; they may appear on the side of the body opposite the lesion or may occur bilaterally
• Altered level of consciousness: drowsiness, stupor, coma
• Behavioral changes: apathy, irritability, memory loss, disorientation
• Loss of sensation and reflexes: usually unilateral; may be temporary or permanent
• Flaccid or spastic muscle tone
• Unequal pupils

- Ptosis of eyelid
- Visual disturbances: blurring or loss of vision
- Drooping mouth
- Weakness or paralysis: unilateral or bilateral
- Communication dysfunction
  —Aphasia: expressive or receptive language impairment
  —Apraxia: impairment in the ability to perform purposeful acts or to manipulate objects
  —Agnosia: impairment in the ability to recognize familiar objects or persons
- Dysphagia
- Bowel and bladder incontinence
- Nausea and vomiting
- Seizures
- Syncope

## COMPLICATIONS

- Increased intracranial pressure
- Herniation
- Seizures
- Aspiration
- Contractures
- Respiratory and cardiac disturbances

## DIAGNOSTIC TESTS

- Describe each procedure, its purpose, and the normal feelings or sensations that are likely, as well as any preprocedural and postprocedural care.
  —Computed tomography or magnetic resonance imaging: to assess size of infarction, hematoma, shift of brain structures, cerebral circulation, cerebral edema
  —Electroencephalogram: to assess lesion location and brain wave activity
  —Cerebral angiography: to assess lesion size and location; to identify collateral circulation
  —Transcranial Doppler ultrasound: to assess pressure and flow in the intracranial arteries
  —Positron emission tomography: to assess cerebral metabolism and circulation
  —Phonoangiography or Doppler ultrasonography: to identify presence of bruits in the carotid arteries

—Skull x-rays: to reveal intracranial calcifications
—Lumbar puncture and cerebrospinal fluid analysis: to assess for erythrocytes, proteins, and presence of infection

## TREATMENT

*Medical*

- Therapy
  —Physical therapy
  —Occupational therapy
  —Speech therapy
  —Bowel and bladder retraining
  —Diet: may advance to fluids, pureed, soft, or chopped foods, or tube feedings depending on level of consciousness and ability to chew and swallow; low-sodium, low-fat, low-cholesterol diet may be prescribed
  —Acute care
    Intracranial pressure monitoring
    Mechanical ventilation: to maintain patent airway and adequate ventilation
    Electrocardiographic monitoring: to assess for cardiac dysrhythmias
    Hemodynamic monitoring: to assess fluid volume status
    Nasogastric tube: to aspirate gastric contents and free air
    Indwelling urethral catheter: to monitor urinary output
- Drugs
  —Anticoagulants
  —Antiplatelet agents
  —Antihypertensives
  —Diuretics
  —Corticosteroids
  —Anticonvulsants
  —Analgesics
  —Antipyretics
  —Antacids
  —H$_2$ blockers
  —Stool softeners

*Surgical*

- Cerebral artery bypass surgery: to provide collateral cerebral circulation to the area distal to the stenosis
- Craniotomy: to evacuate intracerebral hematoma, repair ruptured aneurysm, apply arterial clips

S

- Carotid endarterectomy: surgical removal of plaque in the obstructed carotid artery to increase blood supply to the brain

## HOME CARE

- Give both the patient and the caregiver *verbal* and *written* instructions. Provide them with the name and telephone number of a physician or nurse to call if questions arise.
- *General information*
  —Explain and discuss cerebrovascular accident, causes or contributing factors, care, and treatment.
- *Warning signs*
  —Review the signs and symptoms that should be reported to a physician or nurse.
    Headache, vertigo, visual disturbances
    Changes in mentation and level of consciousness
    Seizure activity
    Lack of bowel movement for more than 3 days
    Respiratory distress
    Progression of sensory-motor-perception deficits
- *Special instructions*
  —Assist the patient and caregiver in obtaining appropriate devices, such as walkers, specialty beds, and aids to safety, feeding, toileting, and grooming.
  —Discuss alternative methods to deal with chronic pain: visualization, guided imagery, meditation, relaxation, biofeedback.
  —Discuss measures to provide a safe environment.
    Orient the patient to the environment.
    Provide good lighting.
    Remove unnecessary furniture and objects, especially sharp and hazardous objects such as scissors.
    Arrange furniture to provide a clear pathway.
    Position the bed and personal objects within reach and in the unaffected visual field.
    Protect the neglected side during activities.
    Identify hazards or needed adaptations in the home, such as ramps, widening doorways to accommodate a wheelchair, rails, removal of scatter rugs, shower safety, and flat shoes.
  —Encourage the patient to use vision on the affected side.
    Gradually move objects, including meals, to the affected side.

Gradually move from the unaffected visual field to the patient's neglected side while communicating with the patient.

Encourage the patient to scan the affected visual field.

Initially place the patient with the unaffected side toward the most active part of the room. Gradually shift interactions and objects to the patient's neglected side.

—Encourage the patient to use the affected side in self-care.

Instruct the patient to include the affected extremities in performing activities of daily living.

Instruct the patient to attend to the affected site in grooming, care, and proper positioning.

Stimulate different sensations in the affected extremities with touch, scented lotions, or textured materials.

—Encourage the patient to use hearing on the affected side. Move across the patient's field to the affected side while speaking and continue to speak on that side to stimulate the patient's attention to the neglected side.

—Encourage and demonstrate use of the unaffected extremity to assist the affected side in positioning and movement.

Demonstrate positioning the affected extremities using pillows or other support aids and elevating the extremities.

Provide and demonstrate use of a sling for the affected arm to support the arm and shoulder.

Instruct the patient to support affected extremities when repositioning.

Instruct the patient to limit turning to and lying on the affected side to 1 hour.

Instruct the patient to perform range-of-motion exercises of the affected extremities, using the unaffected extremities.

Instruct the patient to watch the affected leg while walking.

Instruct the family to provide restraints or belts for support and protection if body-spatial orientation is impaired.

—Instruct the patient to protect the affected side from extreme temperatures if tactile perception is impaired.

—Instruct the patient or caregiver to supervise all activities if judgment of position, distance, or spatial orientation is impaired.

—Assist and demonstrate performing activities of daily living using the unaffected side.

—Provide and instruct the patient in use of support devices in toileting, such as raised seat, commode, handrails, and undergarments that are easy to remove and replace.

—Provide and instruct the patient in use of aids in dressing and bathing, such as Velcro closures, zippers, or elastic waists.

—Instruct the patient to plan for regular rest periods to avoid fatigue.

—Encourage physical mobility.

Encourage weight-bearing and pivoting on the stronger side.

Teach the patient to transfer toward the unaffected side. Instruct the patient to position the unaffected side next to the bed or chair to which the patient is transferring.

—Encourage effective communication.

Refer the patient to speech therapy.

Ensure that the patient is well rested when initiating communication exercises.

Stand within the patient's visual field. Maintain eye contact.

Reduce environmental distractions, such as television, music, or other conversations.

Speak to the patient in a normal voice. Do not shout or speak loudly.

Speak slowly in simple sentences and vocabulary that the patient understands. Repeat as necessary.

Use nonverbal gestures to supplement communication.

Limit each conversation to one clearly defined subject.

Use the same word each time a question or sentence is repeated.

Record the words to be used each time.

Ask yes-or-no questions.

Allow time for the patient to respond to questions.

Avoid finishing the patient's sentences.

Provide feedback. Correct errors and praise efforts. If the patient's verbal communication is unclear, ask the patient to repeat the statement or point to objects.

For a patient with right hemisphere damage, if the patient diverges from the subject of conversation, return the patient to the subject. Explain sounds that the patient hears by identifying the object producing the sounds.

For a patient with left hemisphere damage, provide objects for the patient to touch and name.

Provide flashcards with pictures and words the patient can point to for communication or a slate board if appropriate.

Avoid instructing the patient with concepts involving numbers or time.

Avoid using metaphors. Speak in clear, concrete terms.

—Assist the patient with elimination.

Offer an elimination opportunity every 2 hours and after fluid intake.

Monitor daily bowel movements.

Stress the importance of taking stool softeners as prescribed.

Provide incontinence pads or waterproof undergarments.

- *Medications*
  —Explain the purpose, dosage, schedule, and route of administration of any prescribed drugs, as well as side effects to report to the physician or nurse.

- *Activity*
  —Encourage the patient and caregiver to discuss abilities to resume occupation, recreation, and activities.
  —Advise the caregiver to encourage independent activities as much as possible.
  —Teach the caregiver and patient to perform range-of-motion exercises.
  —Assist the patient with supportive devices such as walkers and wheelchairs.
  —Assist the patient with progression of activities and ambulation. Instruct the caregiver to stand on the affected side when ambulating with the patient.

- *Diet*
  —Assist with tube feedings as ordered.
  —Assist with oral feedings as necessary.

  Position food and utensils within reach.

  Use assistive aids for self-feeding, such as large handles on utensils or a plate guard.

  —Assist the patient and family to plan a diet to include preferred foods that are thick and easy to swallow with increased bulk.

—Instruct the patient and family to avoid milk and foods that are thin and smooth.

—Instruct the patient to take small portions and chew thoroughly.

—Instruct the patient to place food on the unaffected side of the mouth.

—Position the patient on one side with the head of the bed elevated if feeding in bed.

—Encourage fluid intake up to 2 liters per day, unless contraindicated.

## FOLLOW-UP CARE

• Stress the importance of follow-up medical care with the physician, rehabilitation program, speech therapy, physical therapy, and occupational therapy. Make sure the patient and caregiver have the necessary names and telephone numbers.

## PSYCHOSOCIAL CARE

• Advise the caregiver to avoid overprotectiveness.
• Assist the caregiver to establish realistic, achievable goals.
• Praise the patient's accomplishments and progress.
• Encourage the patient and family to express concerns about adjustment to the disability: behavioral, psychosocial, and functional changes.
• Inform the patient that emotional lability and depression are common.
• Refer the patient to a social worker for further support and counseling.

## REFERRALS

• Assist the patient and family to obtain referral to support groups, government and community resources, and home health support services.
• Refer the patient to physical and occupational therapy.
• Provide referral to the National Stroke Association, 848 E. Orchard Rd., Suite 1000, Englewood, CO 80111, (303) 771-1700 or (800) 787-6537.

# Tendinitis, Epicondylitis, and Bursitis

—Tendinitis (tenosynovitis): inflammation of the tendon-covering sheath around one or a group of tendons.

—Epicondylitis: inflammation of the tendons where they insert into condyles of bones such as the humerus and femur.

—Bursitis: inflammation of a bursa, an enclosed sac between muscles and tendons and bony prominences. Tendinitis and epicondylitis generally occur together, and the symptoms are similar. The cause of these conditions is repetitive motion and overuse, which lead to tears, bleeding, edema, and pain in the affected tendons. Both conditions tend to occur in younger age groups and are often caused by sports injuries. For example, lateral epicondylitis, commonly called tennis elbow, is caused by repetitive twisting and swinging movements of the elbow that accompany swinging a tennis racket. Medial epicondylitis is called golfer's elbow because it is related to repetitive swings of the elbow made by a golfer. In older age groups epicondylitis and tendinitis are related to overuse syndromes, often from repetitive motions as in office workers, clerks, writers, and meat cutters. Tendinitis also affects people with rheumatoid arthritis and diabetes and occurs in all age groups. Bursitis is usually caused by constant friction between the skin and musculoskeletal tissues around the joint. Rarely, it results from a foreign body such as calcium or infection. Since a bursa is enclosed within other tissues, the inflammation spreads to those tissues. One or more bursae can become inflamed, but the most commonly affected are bursae of the shoulder, elbow, greater trochanter lateral to the hip, and upper tibia. Bursitis is most common in athletes who perform repetitive motions.

**T**

## SIGNS/SYMPTOMS
- Tenderness and pain around joint (increases with motion)
- Limitation of motion
- Heat, redness, swelling in joint
- Fever, malaise (if pathogen involved)

**COMPLICATIONS**

- Chronic inflammation
- Degenerative arthritis
- Avulsion tears
- Calcification in joints
- Loss of range of motion of joints
- Muscle weakness

**DIAGNOSTIC TESTS**

- Describe each procedure, its purpose, and the normal feelings or sensations that are likely, as well as any preprocedural and postprocedural care.
  - X-rays: may show enlarged bursa with or without calcified deposits (bursitis); calcified areas, tears in a specific tendon, or degenerative changes (tendinitis or epicondylitis)

**TREATMENT**

*Medical*

- Therapy
  - Ice applications to inflamed area
  - Moist heat after ice applications
  - Use of orthotics
    - Heel pads or shoe inserts for Achilles tendinitis
    - Sponge rubber knee pads (bursitis)
    - Forearm band for lateral epicondylitis (tennis elbow)
    - Application of splint to forearm (lateral or medial epicondylitis)
    - Ace or elastic bandages if bursa is accessible to reduce edema
- Drugs
  - Corticosteroids, orally or injected into the inflamed area to relieve pain and inflammation
  - Analgesic-antipyretic agents
  - Nonsteroidal antiinflammatory drugs

*Surgical*

- Excision of the bursal wall and calcified deposits
- Removal of exostosis (bone projection) around the lateral epicondyle
- Removal of the degenerated tendon sheath

## HOME CARE

- Give both the patient and the caregiver *verbal* and *written* instructions. Provide them with the name and telephone number of a physician or nurse to call if questions arise.
- *General information*
  —Describe the type of injury, explaining that it is usually managed medically with rest and medication and that surgery is seldom indicated.
- *Special instructions*
  —Instruct the patient in the use of orthotics (pads, shoe inserts), immobilizer, or splint to ease pressure on vulnerable tissues. Advise the patient where to obtain equipment.
  —Explain how to use heat and cold applications as ordered and the importance of protecting the skin from thermal injury. Teach the patient to cover the heat or cold container with a dry cotton cover.
- *Medications*
  —Explain the purpose, dosage, schedule, and route of administration of any prescribed drugs, as well as side effects to report to the physician or nurse.
  —Advise the patient not to take nonsteroidal antiinflammatory drugs on an empty stomach.
  —If the patient is given a steroid injection, explain that pain may increase after injection for the first 24 hours but is followed by significant pain relief and increasing range of motion.
- *Activity*
  —Emphasize the need to rest the affected part because this allows the inflamed tissues to begin healing. Explain that full healing takes 4-6 weeks.
  —Caution the patient to avoid activities that could prevent healing of present inflammation or cause a recurrence.
    Lower extremities: kneeling, running, aerobic exercises, especially high impact
    Upper extremities: repetitive motion: raising arms above head, swinging a golf club or tennis racket, throwing or hitting a ball
  —Instruct the patient in the importance of range-of-motion exercises to maintain function once inflammation has subsided.

## FOLLOW-UP CARE

- Stress the importance of follow-up visits. Make sure the patient and caregiver have the necessary names and telephone numbers.

# Testicular Cancer

—Testicular cancer: cancer of the testes, the most common cancer in men 15-35 years of age. Testicular cancer occurs more often in whites and in higher socioeconomic groups. The prognosis depends on cell type and stage of cancer. For stage I seminoma the cure rate is as high as 90%. Testicular cancers are most commonly seminomas or teratomas of germ cell origin. They may also be heterogeneous, nonseminomatous germ cell tumors.

## CAUSES/CONTRIBUTING FACTORS
- Cryptorchidism (undescended testes)
- Atrophic testis
- In utero exposure to diethylstilbestrol (DES) or other exogenous hormones
- Familial history of testicular cancer
- History of trauma, mumps, or orchitis

## SIGNS/SYMPTOMS
- Small, hard, painless lump in testicles (first sign)
- Sensation of scrotal heaviness
- Sudden fluid accumulation in scrotum
- Perineal pain or discomfort
- Episodic testicular pain
- Low back, groin, or abdominal ache, "dragging pain"
- Breast enlargement or tenderness (gynecomastia)
- Advanced signs
  —Cough
  —Dyspnea
  —Hemoptysis
  —Back pain

## COMPLICATIONS
- Metastases
  —Ureteral obstruction
  —Pulmonary lesion

**DIAGNOSTIC TESTS**

- Describe each procedure, its purpose, and the normal feelings or sensations that are likely, as well as any preprocedural and postprocedural care.
  - —Palpation and transillumination of testes: to detect lesion
  - —Biopsy: to detect presence of malignant cells
  - —Excretory urography: to determine placement of ureters or kidney by lesion
  - —Abdominal computed tomography, ultrasound, lymphangiography: to detect extratesticular involvement
  - —Chest x-ray, chest computed tomography, whole lung tomography: to detect presence of pulmonary metastases
  - —Serum alpha-fetoprotein (AFP), human chorionic gonadotropin (HCG): tumor markers elevated in presence of testicular cancer

**TREATMENT**

*Medical*

- Therapy
  - —Radiation therapy
       External beam; complications: fatigue, bone marrow suppression, diarrhea, decreased sperm count
  - —Chemotherapy
       For seminomas: cyclophosphamide
       For nonseminomas: PVB (cisplatin, vinblastine, bleomycin)
  - —Alternative to chemotherapy for nonseminomas: surveillance program with monthly follow-up for 12 months (physical examination, tumor markers, chest x-ray)

*Surgical*

- Inguinal exploration and orchiectomy: removal of testis, epididymis, portion of vas deferens, portion of gonadal lymphatics and their blood supply
- Bilateral retroperitoneal lymph node dissection: removal of all perivascular tissue from area bounded superiorly by renal arteries and veins, interiorly by common iliac arteries to the bifurcation, and laterally by ureters; usually unilateral

**PREPROCEDURAL TEACHING**

- Review the physician's explanation of the procedure and the reason for it; encourage the patient to ask questions and to discuss any fears or anxieties. Explain the need for informed consent.

**Review of Preprocedural Care**

- Inform the patient that the skin will be cleansed with bactericidal soap or antiseptic solution to remove bacteria.
- Explain that a complete blood count and urinalysis will be performed to check for infection and bleeding.
- Discuss the need for NPO status from midnight of the night before the procedure.

**Review of Postprocedural Care**

- Inform the patient that an orchiectomy necessitates a high inguinal incision and a retroperitoneal lymphadenectomy usually requires a transabdominal incision.
- Discuss the need for a nasogastric tube for suctioning until bowel sounds return and a Foley catheter to facilitate urinary drainage.
- Explain that vital signs will be monitored for early signs of hemorrhage and shock.
- Tell the patient that the dressing will be checked for the amount and type of drainage.
- Tell the patient that he should be prepared for a probable diminished ejaculatory ability.

**HOME CARE**

- Give both the patient and the caregiver *verbal* and *written* instructions. Provide them with the name and telephone number of a physician or nurse to call if questions arise.
- *General information*
  —Review the physician's explanation of the disease process, possible causes or contributing factors, type and stage of tumor, and prescribed treatments.
- *Special instructions*
  —For nonadvanced tumors, stress the importance of performing testicular self-examination monthly to detect new or recurrent tumors. Inform the patient that the procedure is best done after a warm shower or bath when the scrotum is relaxed. Demonstrate the procedure and permit time for practice.

  Perform the examination in a standing position.

  Place the middle and index fingers below one testis with the thumb on top.

  Gently roll the testis between thumb and fingers, palpating

for rubbery, spongy consistency. The testis should be smooth and free of lumps.

Hold one testicle in each palm and observe any difference in weight.

Report any hard painless mass (usually occur on lateral or anterior surface).

## FOLLOW-UP CARE

- Stress the importance of regular follow-up visits for medical and laboratory evaluation. Make sure the patient has the necessary names and telephone numbers.
- Explain that if the patient remains free of cancer after 1 year, follow-up examinations may be performed every 2 months for the second year, then every 6 months for life. Patients who relapse receive salvage combination chemotherapy.

## PSYCHOSOCIAL CARE

- Explain to the patient that one healthy testis can compensate for loss of function in the other testis, so male characteristics are not adversely affected.
- Discuss actual or potential sexual dysfunction associated with the prescribed treatment.
- Encourage verbalization of feelings regarding body image, self-esteem, and sexuality.
- Provide information and supportive guidance regarding sexual functioning.

# Thoracentesis

—**Thoracentesis: puncture of the chest wall with a large-gauge needle to remove air or fluid from the pleural space.**

## INDICATIONS

- Pleural effusion
- Suspected malignancy

**PREPROCEDURAL TEACHING**

- Review the physician's explanation of the procedure and the reason for it; encourage the patient to ask questions and to discuss any fears or anxieties. Discuss the need for informed consent.

## Review of Preprocedural Care

- Inform the patient that movement or coughing during the procedure is prohibited to prevent inadvertent needle damage to the lung or pleura. Tell the patient that if coughing is unavoidable, the physician should be notified so he or she can withdraw the needle slightly to prevent puncture. Explain that a cough suppressant may be given before the procedure if the patient has a troublesome cough.
- Inform the patient that a local anesthetic will be used to minimize discomfort and that only pressure will be felt when the needle is inserted.
- Explain that the patient will be positioned on the edge of the bed with the feet supported and the head and arms resting on the overbed table; if the patient is unable to sit on the edge of the bed, he or she will lie on the unaffected side with the head of the bed elevated and the arm raised over the head.

## Review of Postprocedural Care

- Explain that a bandage will be placed over the puncture site.
- Review signs and symptoms to report to the physician or nurse: bloody sputum, tachypnea, difficulty breathing, restlessness, fever.
- Inform the patient that a chest x-ray will be taken to check for pneumothorax.
- Explain that the patient will be able to resume regular activity within 1 hour if there is no sign or symptom of postthoracentesis complication.
- Teach and stress the importance of deep breathing every 2-4 hours and proper positioning to facilitate ventilatory effort.

## COMPLICATIONS

- Hemothorax
- Pneumothorax
- Air embolism
- Subcutaneous emphysema
- Pulmonary edema
- Mediastinal shift

**HOME CARE**

• Give both the patient and the caregiver *verbal* and *written* instructions. Provide them with the name and telephone number of a physician or nurse to call if questions arise.

• *General information*
—Explain the underlying cause of the procedure.

• *Warning signs*
—Review the signs and symptoms that should be reported to a physician or nurse.
    Difficulty breathing
    Chest pain
    Vertigo
    Elevated temperature
    Diaphoresis
    Uncontrollable cough
    Bloody sputum

• *Special instructions*
—Explain the importance of avoiding persons with upper respiratory tract infections.

• *Medications*
—Explain the purpose, dosage, schedule, and route of administration of any prescribed drugs, as well as side effects to report to a physician or nurse.
—Explain the need to avoid taking over-the-counter medications without checking with the physician.

• *Activity*
—Explain that after discharge the patient can resume usual activities but should avoid heavy lifting. Advise the patient to check with the physician or nurse for any specific limitations.

**FOLLOW-UP CARE**

• Stress the importance of regular follow-up visits. Make sure the patient has the necessary names and telephone numbers.

# Thrombolytic Therapy

—**Thrombolytic therapy: intravenous or intracoronary administration of a clot-dissolving drug to lyse clots, restore coro-**

nary blood flow, and limit myocardial ischemia. Thrombolytic therapy is initiated when diagnostic evidence shows that a patient is in the process of myocardial infarction.

## INDICATIONS

- Recent onset of chest pain (less than 4-6 hours)
- Acute myocardial infarction as evidenced on electrocardiogram

## PREPROCEDURAL TEACHING

- Review the physician's explanation of the procedure, the reason for it, and associated risks; encourage the patient to ask questions and to discuss any fears or anxieties. Discuss the need for informed consent for thrombolytic therapy, cardiac catheterization, percutaneous transluminal coronary angioplasty (PTCA), and coronary artery bypass grafting (CABG).
- Inform the patient and family of the possibility of emergency treatment: PTCA or CABG.

### Review of Preprocedural Care

- Explain that the procedure may last up to 3 hours.
- Review sensations to be felt during the intracoronary procedure: pressure during insertion but no discomfort with infusion.
- Explain that any uncomfortable feelings experienced as a result of thrombolytic therapy will be treated as they occur.
- Inform the patient that laboratory tests, baseline 12-lead electrocardiogram, and blood type and crossmatch will be completed before the procedure.
- Explain that at least two or three intravenous access sites will be established.
- Tell the patient that vital signs, electrocardiogram, and bleeding will be monitored during and after the procedure and that a complete neurologic assessment will be done before the procedure and repeated hourly for up to 24 hours after the infusion is completed.

### Review of Postprocedural Care

- Tell the patient that bed rest will be maintained during the procedure and for 12 hours after an intracoronary infusion; there are no restrictions after intravenous infusions.
- Explain that frequent blood sampling will be performed to monitor clotting times and that signs and symptoms of successful myo-

cardial reperfusion, coronary reocclusion, and bleeding will be monitored.
- Explain that signs of bleeding under the skin are expected and will clear with time.

## SIDE EFFECTS/COMPLICATIONS

- Bleeding
- Hemorrhage: gastrointestinal, intracranial
- Myocardial infarction

## HOME CARE

- Give both the patient and the caregiver *verbal* and *written* instructions. Provide them with the name and telephone number of a physician or nurse to call if questions arise.
- *General information*
  —Reinforce the physician's explanation regarding outcome of therapy, extent of myocardial damage, and possible need for further interventions such as PTCA and CABG.
  —Instruct the patient about the development of coronary artery disease and the potential recurrence of coronary artery occlusion.
- *Warning signs*
  —Review the signs and symptoms that should be reported to a physician or nurse.
      Chest pain: dysrhythmias, tachycardia, lightheadedness, skin cool, clammy, and diaphoretic
      Bleeding: bruising, bleeding gums, hematuria, bloody emesis, black stools, flank pain, headache
- *Medications*
  —Explain the purpose, dosage, schedule, and route of administration of any prescribed drugs, as well as side effects to report to a physician or nurse.
- *Special instructions*
  —Advise the patient to avoid vigorous toothbrushing.
  —Discuss the need to modify coronary risk factors.

## FOLLOW-UP CARE

- Stress the importance of regular follow-up visits. Make sure the patient has the necessary names and telephone numbers.
- Explain that a follow-up coronary angiography may be necessary to evaluate the patency of the coronary arteries.

# Thyroidectomy

—Thyroidectomy: surgical removal of part or all of the thyroid gland. Thyroidectomy is used in treatment of hyperthyroidism, respiratory obstruction from goiter, and thyroid cancer. Subtotal thyroidectomy, used to correct hyperthyroidism when drug therapy fails or radiation therapy is contraindicated, reduces secretion of thyroid hormone. It also effectively treats diffuse goiter. After surgery the remaining thyroid tissue usually supplies enough thyroid hormone for normal function. Total thyroidectomy may be performed for certain types of thyroid cancer, such as papillary, follicular, medullary, or anaplastic neoplasms. After this surgery the patient requires lifelong thyroid hormone replacement therapy.

## SIDE EFFECTS/COMPLICATIONS

- Hemorrhage
- Hypocalcemia: tetany
- Hypothyroidism
- Laryngeal nerve damage
- Thyroid storm

## HOME CARE

- Give both the patient and the caregiver *verbal* and *written* instructions. Provide them with the name and telephone number of a physician or nurse to call if questions arise.
- *General information*
  —Explain and discuss with the patient the thyroidectomy procedure, especially changes in thyroid function as a result of surgery.
- *Wound/incision care*
  —Teach the patient to keep the surgical site clean and dry.
  —Teach methods to conceal the surgical site without affecting healing. Suggest loosely buttoned collars, high-necked blouses, jewelry, or scarves.
  —Inform the patient that lotion may soften the healing scar and improve its appearance (if approved by the physician).

- *Warning signs*
  —Review the signs and symptoms that should be reported to a physician or nurse.

  General: respiratory distress, bleeding

  Wound infection: redness, warmth, swelling, persistent drainage from site, purulent exudate

  Total thyroidectomy: signs and symptoms of hypothyroidism and hyperthyroidism (see Hyperthyroidism, p. 380, and Hypothyroidism, p. 396).

  Parathyroid damage: signs of hypocalcemia: numbness, tingling, twitching, spasm, tetany

- *Special instructions*
  —Discuss methods of stress management.

- *Medications*
  —Explain the purpose, dosage, schedule, and route of administration of any prescribed drugs, as well as side effects to report to a physician or nurse.

  —Discuss the importance of not taking over-the-counter medications without checking with a physician or nurse.

  —If the patient has had a total thyroidectomy, explain the importance of taking thyroid replacement medication regularly.

  —If the patient has parathyroid damage, explain the need for calcium supplements.

- *Activity*
  —Encourage the patient to discuss allowances and limitations with respect to occupation, recreation, and activities.

  —Teach prescribed head and neck exercises: flexion, lateral movement, hyperextension.

  —Teach the importance of a balance between activity and rest.

- *Diet*
  —Discuss the need to maintain a well-balanced diet.

**FOLLOW-UP CARE**

- Stress the importance of regular follow-up visits. Make sure the patient has the necessary names and telephone numbers.

# Torn Knee Cartilage/Meniscectomy

—Meniscectomy: removal of menisci, C-shaped rings of cartilage covering the ends of the tibia with the knee joint. These
cartilages facilitate joint motion, while also absorbing some of
the stress placed on the joint. They are subject to wear and
tear because of trauma, or degeneration secondary to arthritis. Because cartilage has no intrinsic blood supply, it rarely
heals without developing unsatisfactory scar tissue, necessitat-
ing surgical intervention to remove the damaged or degenerated cartilage from the knee joint. Meniscectomy is performed
when torn meniscus is diagnosed; if left untreated, tears lead
to further joint degeneration and chronic arthritis of the knee
joint. The majority of meniscal tears are related to sports, particularly basketball, soccer, and football. Medial meniscal
tears, resulting from internal rotation of the knee, are the most
common; lateral meniscus tears are associated with external
rotation.

## SIGNS/SYMPTOMS
- Chronic (degenerative-osteoarthritic)
  —Joint stiffness, weakness
  —Joint pain, worsening with activity, relieved by rest
  —Joint swelling and fluid
  —Weak joint "giving way"
- Acute (occur after knee trauma)
  —Joint effusion (distention with fluid)
  —Limited range of motion
  —Locking of knee joint (inability to extend knee fully)
  —Joint pain

## COMPLICATIONS
- Chronic knee arthritis if tear is left untreated
- Weakness, atrophy of quadriceps caused by disuse of knee joint
  secondary to pain
- Joint instability, degeneration
- Postsurgical infection, hemorrhage
- Scar formation leading to future tears

- Compartment syndrome
- Hematoma or thrombus formation

## DIAGNOSTIC TESTS

- Describe each procedure, its purpose, and the normal feelings or sensations that are likely, as well as any preprocedural and postprocedural care.
  - —McMurray's test: clicks or pops accompanied by pain when the leg is extended from a flexed position
  - —Apley grinding test: grinding or crepitus elicited when the foot and lower leg are forced down on the femur from a knee flexed position
  - —Arthrogram: injection of radiopaque dye and air into the joint to outline the area of injury
  - —Arthrocentesis: extraction of synovial fluid to detect blood, indicating meniscal tear
  - —Radiologic studies
    - X-rays: to document injury
    - Magnetic resonance imaging: to show specific tissues and indicate exact injury
    - Diagnostic arthroscopy: to show meniscal and ligament injuries

## TREATMENT

*Medical*
- Drugs
  - —Analgesics for pain relief
  - —Nonsteroidal antiinflammatory drugs to reduce the inflammatory process

*Surgical*
- Meniscectomy or arthroscopy: repair of the torn areas of the meniscus is usually done arthroscopically, but more extensive surgical exposure and repair may be required, depending of the severity of the injury (a traditional meniscectomy); the repair may be done as an inpatient or outpatient procedure, usually under local anesthesia

## PREPROCEDURAL TEACHING

- Review the physician's explanation of the procedure and the reason for it; encourage the patient to ask questions and to discuss any fears or anxieties. Discuss the need for informed consent for surgery and anesthesia.

**Review of Preprocedural Care**

- Review preprocedural tests.
  - —Blood tests: to show status of electrolytes in blood; to determine presence of infection
  - —Urine tests: to document presence of infection
  - —Chest x-ray and electrocardiogram (depending on age): to provide the baseline presence of potential problems
- Explain that a shower with bactericidal soap will be necessary the night before surgery.
- Tell the patient that the incisional area will be shaved on the morning of surgery.
- Discuss the need for NPO status from midnight the night before the procedure.
- Inform the patient that weight bearing as tolerated on the affected knee is permissible before surgery; instruct the patient in crutch walking for use after surgery.

**Review of Postprocedural Care**

- Explain that knee repair is usually done on an outpatient basis but that more extensive repair may require a 1- to 2-day hospital stay.
- Discuss the need for a bandage applied to the knee and high support hose (TED hose).
- Inform the patient of the importance of elevating the operative leg and applying ice bags to the operative site to relieve swelling.
- Discuss the need for and frequency of neurovascular checks, vital signs, and peripheral pulse checks.
- Tell the patient that bed rest will be maintained for 8-24 hours as ordered, that no weight bearing on the operative leg will be permitted for 24 hours, and that ambulation with crutches will be permitted 24-48 hours postoperatively.
- Discuss the importance of beginning straight leg raising on the second or third postoperative day and active and passive range-of-motion exercises in the physical therapy department on the third to fifth postoperative day.

**HOME CARE**

- Give both the patient and the caregiver *verbal* and *written* instructions. Provide them with the name and telephone number of a physician or nurse to call if questions arise.

- *General information*
  —Review the procedure, type of injury, and contributing causes.
- *Warning signs*
  —Review the signs and symptoms of neurovascular impairment that should be reported to a physician or nurse.
    Pallor, coolness of extremity
    Numbness, tingling in toes
    Inability to use or lift leg
    Increased pain and swelling
    Decreased capillary refill of toes on affected extremity
  —Review signs of infection to report immediately.
    Fever, pain
    Swelling at incisional site
    Purulent drainage from incision
- *Special instructions*
  —Discuss methods to reduce swelling: elevation of extremity, application of ice bags to surgical site.
- *Medications*
  —Explain the purpose, dosage, schedule, and route of administration of any prescribed drugs, as well as side effects to report to a physician or nurse.
- *Activity*
  —Instruct the patient in the proper use of crutches and proper stairwalking procedures.
  —Clarify the need to refrain from sports activities that could retraumatize unhealed tissues until permitted by the physician.

**FOLLOW-UP CARE**

- Stress the importance of regular follow-up visits. Make sure the patient has the necessary names and telephone numbers.

# Tracheostomy

—**Tracheostomy: insertion of a tube into the trachea through a surgically created incision (tracheotomy).**

## INDICATIONS

- Presence of tumor
- Upper airway obstruction by foreign body, edema, or mucus
- Conjunction with laryngectomy or neck resection

## HOME CARE

- Give both the patient and the caregiver *verbal* and *written* instructions. Provide them with the name and telephone number of a physician or nurse to call if questions arise.
- *General information*
  —Explain the underlying cause and contributing factors.
  —Describe and demonstrate the type of tracheostomy tube that has been inserted, and permit time for the patient to practice removing and reinserting the outer and inner cannula.
- *Warning signs*
  —Review the signs and symptoms that should be reported to a physician or nurse.
    Stomal irritation
    Infection: elevated temperature, purulent secretions
    Persistent cough
    Inability to remove secretions
    Respiratory distress
- *Special instructions*
  —Demonstrate skin care around the stoma: use hydrogen peroxide, rinse with water, and pat dry.
  —Discuss the need to shower daily: cover tracheostomy with a stoma shield; when using a shower hose, direct spray below the neck and avoid getting soap into the stoma.
  —For male patients, discuss the need to shave with an electric razor or safety razor and to avoid getting lather into the stoma.
  —Inform the patient of the need to keep the stoma covered at all times. Suggest wearing clothing with high necklines and scarves to protect against foreign materials.
  —Teach the patient and caregiver how to use oxygen and other respiratory equipment at home. Advise them on where to obtain equipment (e.g., pharmacy, medical supply company).
  —Instruct the patient in handwashing technique, stressing the importance of washing the hands before cleaning the tracheostomy after suctioning.
  —Instruct the patient in disposal of soiled dressings and supplies.

—Demonstrate suctioning technique: take three or four deep breaths before and after suctioning if breathing spontaneously.

—Demonstrate cleaning and storage of suction catheters: rinse the catheter thoroughly with running water, soak it in hydrogen peroxide for 5 minutes, rinse thoroughly, place it in boiling water for 10-15 minutes, allow it to air dry on a clean towel, and store in a clean plastic bag. Inform the patient that catheters may be used for multiple days and discarded when secretions cannot be removed completely.

—Demonstrate care of the tracheostomy tube. Stress the importance of using clean technique when cleaning the tracheostomy. Tracheostomy dressings are not necessary unless secretions are excessive. Emphasize the importance of covering the stoma when coughing.

—Teach and demonstrate procedures for cleaning cannulas, changing tracheostomy ties, and changing dressings.

—Discuss the need to use a commercial humidifier or pan of water on the stove to add comfort and prevent encrustation. Instruct the patient to avoid extremes of temperature because they can irritate the tracheal mucosa.

—Discuss the need to avoid persons with respiratory infections and respiratory irritants (e.g., smoke, dust, fumes, aerosols, powder).

—Instruct the patient to carry some means of communication (e.g., pad and pencil, magic slate).

• *Medications*

—Explain the purpose, dosage, schedule, and route of administration of any prescribed drugs, as well as side effects to report to a physician or nurse.

—Discuss the need to avoid taking over-the-counter medications without first checking with a physician.

• *Activity*

—Advise the patient of the importance of exercising to tolerance and planning rest periods.

—Tell the patient that swimming is not permitted.

• *Diet*

—Explain that a regular diet should be followed unless contraindicated.

—Advise the patient to drink at least 3000 ml daily unless contraindicated.

### FOLLOW-UP CARE

- Stress the importance of regular follow-up visits. Make sure the patient has the necessary names and telephone numbers.
- Assist the patient to obtain a Medic-Alert band identifying the patient as a neck breather for emergency situations.
- Stress the importance of not smoking or using tobacco products and of avoiding passive smoking.

### REFERRALS

- Provide community support resources and phone numbers, for example, of Visiting Nurses Association and community home health agency.

# Tube Feeding
## (Enteral Feeding)

—Tube feeding: nutritional support provided by the enteral route for the treatment or prevention of malnutrition. Enteral products are composed of standard and modular formulas and are used for tube feeding. A gastric feeding tube or a gastrostomy tube may be used. The gastric feeding tube is placed through the naris (nasogastric) or mouth (orogastric) into the stomach. The gastrostomy tube is inserted through an opening created in the stomach. It is indicated for patients who require prolonged nutritional support. A gastrostomy button has been shown to decrease many of the disadvantages of the gastrostomy tube (e.g., leakage, mobility, catheter occlusion and expulsion).

### INDICATIONS

- Debilitated comatose patient
- Strictures of esophagus
- Malignant neoplasms

### SIDE EFFECTS/COMPLICATIONS

- Pulmonary aspiration (nasogastric tube)
- Mechanical problems: obstruction, displacement

- Metabolic problems (e.g., diarrhea, dehydration, hyperglycemia, electrolyte imbalances, vitamin and trace element deficiencies, high gastric residuals)
- Gastrostomy: skin irritation, breakdown

## HOME CARE

- Give both the patient and the caregiver *verbal* and *written* instructions. Provide them with the name and telephone number of a physician or nurse to call if questions arise.
- *General information*
  —Discuss the purpose and indication for and type of enteral feedings.
- *Warning signs*
  —Review the signs and symptoms that should be reported to a physician or nurse.
     Gastrointestinal intolerance: nausea, vomiting, abdominal distention, cramping, diarrhea
     Wound infection with gastrostomy: fever, redness, drainage, swelling, tenderness, odor
- *Special instructions*
  —Assist the caregiver to obtain formula, equipment, and supplies.
  —Teach care of the feeding tube.
     For a nasogastric tube, wash gently with soap and water and pat dry. Secure the tube to prevent tension on the patient's tissue and skin.
     For a gastrostomy, teach the patient how to change the tube. Explain that the tube can be removed after several weeks and reinserted for feedings. The skin around the tube should be inspected daily and the skin washed gently and patted dry.
  —Instruct and demonstrate how to avoid nausea and vomiting: avoid rapid infusion and adjust rate as ordered.
  —Discuss the need to flush the tube with 50-150 ml of water after each feeding or medication administration. Blocked tubes should be flushed with proteolytic enzyme papain (Adolph's Meat Tenderizer), pancreatic enzyme (Viokase), cola, or cranberry juice using a syringe.
  —Demonstrate preparation and administration of the feeding. Demonstrate use of a pump if the patient will receive continuous feedings. Permit time for practice by the caregiver.

- *Medications*
  —Explain the purpose, dosage, schedule, and route of administration of any prescribed drugs, as well as side effects to report to a physician or nurse.
  —Instruct the caregiver to substitute a liquid preparation for
  pills or to crush the pill into a fine powder and dissolve in 30
  ml of water after consulting with a physician or pharmacist.
- *Diet*
  —Discuss the prescribed type and amount of feeding. Instruct
  the patient to elevate the head of the bed more than 30 degrees during feeding and for an hour after feeding to prevent
  regurgitation or aspiration. Show the caregiver how to check
  for tube feeding residual before each feeding.
  —Tell the caregiver to administer feeding formula at room temperature. Instruct the caregiver to refrigerate all opened products and discard after 24 hours, to use clean technique when
  handling the feeding tube and enteral products, and to change
  the feeding set every 24 hours.

**FOLLOW-UP CARE**

- Stress the importance of regular follow-up medical and laboratory evaluations. Make sure the patient has the necessary names
  and telephone numbers.

# Tuberculosis, Pulmonary

—**Pulmonary tuberculosis: a chronic, acute, or subacute infectious pulmonary disease in which fibrosis and cavitation are
caused by the tubercle bacillus *(Mycobacterium tuberculosis).*
The bacilli are inhaled in airborne mucous droplets from the
sputum of persons with active disease. Less frequently they are
ingested or enter through a break in the skin. Susceptible individuals include children less than 3 years of age or adults over
65 years, the chronically ill, silicone and asbestos workers, and
malnourished and immunosuppressed persons. The incidence
is high for persons living in crowded, poorly ventilated, un-
sanitary conditions such as homeless shelters and tenements.**

## SIGNS/SYMPTOMS

- Persistent low-grade temperature
- Night sweats
- Anorexia, weight loss
- Fatigue, malaise
- Pleuritic chest pain or chest tightness
- Cough with blood-tinged or mucopurulent sputum

## COMPLICATIONS

- Atelectasis
- Hemoptysis
- Pneumothorax
- Pericarditis, peritonitis, meningitis, lymphadenitis

## DIAGNOSTIC TESTS

- Describe each procedure, its purpose, and the normal feelings or sensations that are likely, as well as any preprocedural and postprocedural care.
  - Tuberculin skin test (e.g., purified protein derivative, Mantoux test)
  - Sputum culture
  - Chest x-ray
  - Gastric washings
  - Fiberoptic bronchoscopy
  - Needle biopsy of pleura

## TREATMENT

*Medical*

- Therapy
  - Respiratory isolation as necessary
  - High-protein, high-carbohydrate diet
- Drugs
  - Isoniazid (INH)
  - Ethambutol
  - Rifampin
  - Streptomycin
  - Para-aminosalicylic acid
  - Pyrazinamide
  - Analgesics

T

*Surgical*
- Resection for persistent cavitary lesions
- Surgical intervention for massive hemoptysis, spontaneous pneumothorax, abscess drainage, intestinal obstruction, or ureteral stricture

## HOME CARE

- Give both the patient and the caregiver *verbal* and *written* instructions. Provide them with the name and telephone number of a physician or nurse to call if questions arise.
- *General information*
  —Explain the disease process, underlying causes and contributing factors, and contagiousness and transmission.
- *Warning signs*
  —Review the signs and symptoms that should be reported to a physician or nurse.
    Bloody sputum
    Chest pain
    Difficulty in breathing
    Fever
    Increased cough
    Night sweats
- *Special instructions*
  —Advise the patient on how and where to obtain supplies (e.g., drugstore, medical supply company).
  —Explain the importance of good hygiene and handwashing after handling secretions, masks, or soiled tissues to prevent transmission of disease. Instruct the patient to cough into tissue, to turn head if coughing, and to avoid direct contact with sputum. Explain how to dispose of tissues. Tell the patient to wear a mask if unable to comply with directions.
  —Review home respiratory isolation procedures as necessary: sleep in a well-ventilated room, use disposable supplies and utensils, use waterproof plastic bags for disposal.
  —Explain the need to avoid crowds and persons with upper respiratory infections.
  —Discuss the importance of avoiding close contact with others until advised by the physician.
- *Medications*
  —Explain the purpose, dosage, schedule, and route of administration of any prescribed drugs, as well as side effects (e.g., hearing loss, vertigo) to report to a physician or nurse.

—Inform the patient that antiinfective agents, most commonly isoniazid and rifampin, are given for 6-12 months. If the patient is taking rifampin, explain that body secretions (feces, saliva, tears) may appear red-orange.

—Caution a female patient that medications may interfere with the effectiveness of oral contraceptives.

—Explain the need to avoid taking over-the-counter medications without checking with a physician.

—Emphasize the importance of not stopping medication unless the physician gives approval.

• *Activity*

—Advise the patient to limit exercise and activity to tolerance, to avoid fatigue, and to plan frequent rest periods.

• *Diet*

—Discuss the need for a high-protein, high-carbohydrate diet. If the patient's appetite is poor, suggest frequent small meals.

—Instruct the patient to drink 2000-3000 ml or more daily unless contraindicated.

## FOLLOW-UP CARE

• Stress the importance of regular follow-up visits. Make sure the patient has the necessary names and telephone numbers.

• Discuss the need for the patient to inform the caregiver, friends, and all contacts to obtain skin testing at the local health department.

# Ulcer (Peptic)

U

—Peptic ulcer: circumscribed ulceration of mucous membrane that develops in the lower esophagus, stomach (gastric), or duodenum (duodenal).

## CAUSES/CONTRIBUTING FACTORS

• Gastric ulcer

—Long-term use of medications (aspirin, indomethacin, steroids)

—Chemicals (tobacco, alcohol)

—Stress
—Heredity
—Infection
* Duodenal ulcer
—Heredity
—Chemicals
—Psychosocial stressors
—Medications
—Infection

## SIGNS/SYMPTOMS

* Gastric ulcer
—Left to middle epigastric pain that may radiate to the back and occurs 60-90 minutes after eating
—Feeling of fullnesss
—Nausea and vomiting
* Duodenal ulcer
—Right epigastric pain that may radiate to the back or thorax and occurs 2-4 hours after eating or may be unrelated to food intake
—Heartburn
—Feeling of fullness after eating
—Nausea and vomiting
—Abdominal tenderness
—Belching
—Mild diarrhea with black stools

## COMPLICATIONS

* Electrolyte imbalance
* Hemorrhage
* Perforation
* Pyloric stenosis
* Shock

## DIAGNOSTIC TESTS

* Describe each procedure, its purpose, and the normal feelings or sensations that are likely, as well as any preprocedural and postprocedural care.
—Endoscopy with biopsy and cytology
—Barium studies
—Abdominal radiologic studies

—Gastric analysis
—Hematocrit; levels of hemoglobin, pepsinogen, gastrin
—Stool for melena

## TREATMENT

*Medical*
- Therapy
  —Dietary therapy
- Drugs
  —Analgesics
  —Aluminum-magnesium antacids (Delcid, Mylanta-II)
  —Cimetidine (Tagamet)
  —Ranitidine (Zantac)
  —Sucralfate (Carafate)

*Surgical*
- Pyloroplasty
- Vagotomy
- Subtotal gastrectomy
- Total gastrectomy

## HOME CARE

- Give both the patient and the caregiver *verbal* and *written* instructions. Provide them with the name and telephone number of a physician or nurse to call if questions arise.
- *General information*
  —Explain the disease process, underlying causes, and contributing factors. Assist the patient to identify factors that can exacerbate an attack and suggest measures to minimize or modify them.
- *Warning signs*
  —Review the signs and symptoms of perforation that should be reported to a physician or nurse.
    Extreme epigastric pain
    Hematemesis (frank blood or coffee-ground appearance)
    Tarry or bloody stools
    Sudden sharp epigastric or abdominal pain
    Pain radiating to shoulders
    Abdominal rigidity
    Fever

**U**

- *Special instructions*
  —Provide information for a patient undergoing surgical intervention (see Abdominal Surgery, p. 3).
    Demonstrate care of the incision line and dressing changes.
    Review signs and symptoms of wound infection to report to the physician or nurse: persistent redness, swelling, purulent drainage, local warmth, fever, foul odor.
  —Discuss the role that emotional stress plays in precipitating attacks. Assist the patient in identifying coping skills and relaxation techniques (e.g., deep breathing, meditation, guided imagery).
- *Medications*
  —Explain the purpose, dosage, schedule, and route of administration of any prescribed drugs, as well as side effects to report to a physician or nurse.
  —Explain the need to avoid taking over-the-counter medications without checking with a physician.
  —Instruct the patient to take only antacids prescribed by a physician.
  —Discuss the reason for avoiding aspirin-containing drugs, ibuprofen, and steroids, and tell the patient to read all labels.
- *Diet*
  —Review dietary allowances and restrictions. Instruct the patient to follow a bland diet, avoiding such distressing foods as black pepper; chili powder; raw, spicy, or fatty foods; fruit juices; and caffeinated beverages.
  —Emphasize the importance of avoiding alcohol.
  —Instruct the patient to eat slowly, to take small frequent meals, and to have snacks between meals.
  —Refer the patient and caregiver to a dietitian for help in modifying meals.

## FOLLOW-UP CARE

- Stress the importance of regular follow-up visits. Make sure the patient has the necessary names and telephone numbers.
- Explain the importance of not smoking and of avoiding passive smoke, since smoking stimulates gastric acid secretion. Provide information and referral to smoking and alcohol cessation programs as indicated.

# Ulcerative Colitis
## (Crohn's Disease, Inflammatory Bowel Disease)

—Ulcerative colitis: a chronic inflammatory disease of the bowel characterized by remissions and exacerbations. Ulcerative colitis produces congestion, edema, and ulcerations of the mucosa. The disease begins in the rectum and sigmoid colon but can extend the entire length of the colon. Ulcerative colitis occurs primarily between the ages of 15 and 20 years. The specific cause is unknown but may be an abnormal immune response.

### CAUSES/CONTRIBUTING FACTORS
- Bacterial infections
- Genetic factors
- Allergic reactions to certain foods
- Immunologic origin
- Emotional stress

### SIGNS/SYMPTOMS
- Cramplike right lower quadrant abdominal pain
- Diarrhea (up to 20 stools per day or more)
- Liquid stools with tenesmus: blood, mucus, pus, fat
- Anorexia, weight loss
- Fever
- Nausea, vomiting
- Malaise, weakness

### COMPLICATIONS
- Electrolyte imbalance
- Dehydration
- Malnutrition
- Anemia
- Intestinal obstruction, perforation
- Fistula
- Peritonitis
- Perianal abscess, fistula, fissure
- Hemorrhage, shock

U

## DIAGNOSTIC TESTS

- Describe each procedure, its purpose, and the normal feelings or sensations that are likely, as well as any preprocedural and postprocedural care.
  —Stool examination
  —Sigmoidoscopy
  —Colonoscopy
  —Laboratory studies
  —Biopsy
  —Barium studies
  —Liver function tests

## TREATMENT

*Medical*
- Therapy
  —Fluid replacement
  —Nutritional support
- Drugs
  —Corticosteroids
  —Antidiarrheals
  —Antimicrobials
  —Immunosuppressive agents

*Surgical*
- Total abdominal colectomy
- Mucosal proctectomy with ileoanal anastomosis
- Total proctocolectomy with permanent ileostomy

## HOME CARE

- Give both the patient and the caregiver *verbal* and *written* instructions. Provide them with the name and telephone number of a physician or nurse to call if questions arise.
- *General information*
  —Explain the disease process, underlying causes, and factors that can exacerbate an attack: stress, certain foods, fatigue, laxatives, antibiotics.
  —For ileostomy care, see p. 651.
- *Warning signs*
  —Review the signs and symptoms of perforation that should be reported to a physician or nurse.
    Unrelieved abdominal pain
    Bloating

    Distention

    Vomiting

    Abdominal rigidity

    Increase in diarrhea

    Bloody stools

- *Special instructions*
  —Discuss the need for perianal care daily and after each bowel movement.
  —Teach perianal and perineal skin care: wash gently with soap and warm water, and apply protective skin care products (e.g., ointments, gels).
  —Advise the patient on how and where to obtain supplies (e.g., drugstore, medical supply company).
  —Instruct the patient to report unrelieved irritation, bleeding, or drainage.
  —Discuss the role emotional stress plays in precipitating an attack. Assist the patient in identifying coping skills and using relaxation techniques (e.g., deep breathing, meditation, guided imagery).
  —Provide individual weight parameters. Instruct the patient to weigh daily and report any sudden or steady losses.
  —Instruct the patient to maintain a record of stools, including number, time of occurrence, color, amount, consistency, odor, and presence of mucus, blood, or pus.
- *Medications*
  —Explain the purpose, dosage, schedule, and route of administration of any prescribed drugs, as well as side effects to report to a physician or nurse.

    Analgesics

    Antiinflammatory agents

    Antiemetics

    Antidiarrheals

    Anticholinergics

  —Explain the need to avoid taking over-the-counter medications without checking with the physician.

  —Discuss the importance of not stopping steroid therapy without consulting the physician, since abrupt discontinuation may cause adrenal crisis. Review withdrawal symptoms to report to the nurse or physician: weakness, lethargy, restlessness, anorexia, nausea, muscle tenderness.

**U**

- *Activity*
  —Advise the patient to balance activity with rest, even during remission, because adequate rest is necessary to sustain remission.
- *Diet*
  —Inform the patient that a bland, high-protein, reduced-fiber, low-residue, high-calorie diet should be followed.
  —Advise the patient to avoid highly seasoned foods, raw fruits and vegetables, foods containing coarse cereals, bran, seeds, nuts, milk, fatty or fried foods, caffeine, alcohol, and carbonated beverages.
  —Encourage the patient to eat small frequent meals and to eat slowly, take small bites, and chew well.
  —Stress the importance of maintaining adequate nutrition to alleviate symptoms and prevent complications. Refer the patient and caregiver to a dietitian for assistance with modifying meals and a review of dietary allowances and restrictions.
  —Discuss the need to replace fluids. Teach the patient how to estimate fluid intake and output. Advise the patient to drink 8-10 glasses of fluid per day unless contraindicated. Instruct the patient to space the servings and to avoid fluids that are too hot or cold.

**FOLLOW-UP CARE**

- Stress the importance of keeping follow-up laboratory and medical appointments. Make sure the patient has the necessary names and telephone numbers.

**REFERRALS**

- Provide phone numbers of community support resources, such as the Crohn's and Colitis Foundation of America.

# Urinary Diversion: Urostomy/Urinary Diversion

—Urinary diversion: surgical procedure performed to provide an alternative route for urine excretion. A number of procedures may be done to divert urinary flow through a new opening on the abdomen, including urostomy, continent urinary diversion, and creation of a hemi-Kock pouch. In a *urostomy* (Bricker or ileal or colon conduit), a segment of ileum is cut away to create a receptacle or pouch to which the ureters are connected. One end is sewn closed, and the other is brought to an opening in the abdominal wall to form a stoma (opening) through which urine flows continuously into a special bag strapped to the body. An external bag must be worn at all times. In a *continent urinary diversion* (Kock puch), a segment of ileum is cut away to form a reservoir (internal pouch) for urine to which the ureters are attached. Two natural valves or "nipple valves" are created, one to prevent backflow and the other to maintain continence. Self-catheterization is required. The *hemi-Kock pouch* is a neobladder made of the intestinal pouch (see above). It is used only in men because the female urethra is too short and strong abdominal muscular pressure against the bladder is needed to urinate through the penis.

## INDICATIONS

- Cystectomy
- Severe neuropathic bladder
- Severe interstitial cystitis

## PREPROCEDURAL TEACHING

- Review the physician's explanation of the procedure and the reason for it; encourage the patient to ask questions and to discuss any fears or anxieties. Explain the need for informed consent for surgery, anesthesia, blood transfusions, and photographs if needed.

### Review of Preprocedural Care

- Explain that the patient will be admitted to the hospital 1 day before surgery.
- Explain that the enterostomal nurse will come to interview the patient, show appliances, and mark the abdomen for the ostomy site.
- Discuss bowel preparation.
    Two days before surgery the patient should ingest only clear fluids and possibly a laxative.
    The day before surgery the patient is asked to drink at least

4000 ml (1 gallon) of specially prepared solution (GoLytely) over a 6-hour period (antiemetics are given beforehand).

After bowel movements are clear, oral antibiotics are given to "sterilize the intestines."

- Tell the patient that the pubic hair may be clipped the night before and the patient may be shaved from the nipple line to midthigh, including the perineum.
- Discuss the need to shower with bactericidal soap (e.g., Hibiclens).
- Inform the patient of the need for NPO status from midnight the night before.
- Explain that intravenous hydration and intravenous antibiotics will be started.

**Review of Postprocedural Care**

- See general care under Abdominal Surgery, p. 3.
- Tell the patient that the procedure takes 3-4 hours or more and is performed with the patient under general anesthesia.
- Review the drainage tubes that may be used: urethral catheter (usually removed after 2 or more days except with a hemi-Kock procedure); two drainage tubes through the stoma from the new reservoir ("pouch"); flat Penrose drain and/or Jackson-Pratt drain near the incision; ureteral stents from kidneys.

**COMPLICATIONS**

- Urine leakage at internal connections
- Hemorrhage
- Paralytic ileus
- Wound infection
- Impotence (temporary or permanent)
- Obstruction at ureteral junction sites
- Dyspareunia
- Peristomal hernia
- Stomal necrosis
- Deep vein thrombosis
- Pulmonary embolism
- Prolonged diarrhea or bowel dysfunction
- Fistula
- Metabolic acidosis

**HOME CARE**

- Give both the patient and the caregiver *verbal* and *written* instructions. Provide them with the name and telephone number of a physician or nurse to call if questions arise.
- *Wound/incision care*
  —Provide instruction on wound care and dressing changes.
  —Discuss the care of drainage tubes. Explain that catheters remain in the stoma about 4 weeks and that a "Kock-o-gram" or "pouch-o-gram" (contrast material instilled into the pouch and x-rays taken) will be done to confirm healing of all suture lines before catheters are removed.
- *Warning signs*
  —Review the signs and symptoms of perforation that should be reported to a physician or nurse.

    Infection: redness, swelling, warm to touch, tenderness, purulent drainage

    Change in appearance of stoma: protruding, receding, bluish tint, excoriation, redness

    Acute abdominal pain or persistent pain

    Change in bowel habits: constipation, diarrhea, flatulence (gas)

    Urinary tract infection: cloudy urine, fever, malaise

    Difficulty in self-catheterization

    No urine output after 4 hours and after irrigation

    Hematuria
- *Special instructions*
  —Advise and assist the patient in obtaining supplies. Provide a list of the supplies needed, including size and type of appliance.
  —Emphasize the importance of having enough supplies and carrying supplies when traveling.
  —Stress the importance of maintaining free flow of urine (mucus will always be present in urine because the intestine normally sheds mucus; occasional flecks of blood may also be present).
  —Demonstrate catheter irrigation.

    Gather supplies: saline solution and piston syringe. Saline solution may be made by adding 1 tablespoon of salt to 1 quart of distilled water, mixing, and refrigerating, or by placing 1 quart water in a clean pan on the stove, bringing to a boil, removing and allowing to cool to room temperature, pouring the water into a clean quart-size container, adding 1 tablespoon salt and mixing, covering with a lid, and refrigerating. Any remaining solution should be discarded after 2 days.

Wash hands.

Draw up 30 ml of saline solution in the syringe and set it aside.

Clean the connection with soap and water; then rinse. Disconnect the catheter from the drainage tubing.

Insert the tip of the syringe into the catheter and inject the solution slowly (do not force).

Pull back on the syringe to remove saline solution and mucus, and discard into the toilet.

If the fluid does not return, attach the catheter to drainage tubing and let drain by gravity. (If it does not drain within 5 minutes, repeat the preceding steps using 15 ml solution.)

If the catheter is not draining well between irrigations, irrigate an extra time.

After the catheter is removed, a catheter will be inserted for daily irrigations (see catheter care under Self-Catheterization, p. 406).

The 60 ml (cc) piston syringe may be used over again. Separate the parts, wash with unscented soap and water, rinse, and let air dry. Store in a clean, dry place.

—Review the technique for self-catheterization.

Gather all supplies: paper towels, special catheter, water-soluble lubricant, piston syringe, and saline solution.

Wash hands.

Remove the dressing or bag from the stoma.

Lubricate the tip of the catheter.

Insert the catheter into the stoma until urine flows. When it stops, insert a few more inches until flow stops completely. Irrigate as described above.

Remove the catheter. Cleanse the area and reapply the dressing or ostomy bag.

Keep a catheter and supplies available even when going out.

Stress the importance of maintaining a self-catheterization schedule after the catheter is removed (other schedule may be advised).

| Week | Day | Night |
|------|-----|-------|
| 1 | Every 2 hours | Every 3 hours |
| 2 | Every 3 hours | Every 4 hours |
| 3 | Every 4 hours | Every 5 hours |
| 4 | Every 5 hours | Every 6 hours |

The goal is to reach a schedule of 4 or 5 times a day, allowing for at least 7 hours of uninterrupted sleep per night. This is influenced by the size of the pouch and amount of fluids taken in. Explain that almost all men leak urine from the penis after removal of the catheter. Kegel exercises (see Urinary Incontinence, p. 657) will decrease leakage after several weeks, but the patient may still have some leakage at night.

—Teach the patient how to change the appliance, using instructions provided by the enterostomal nurse.

Gather all supplies: paper towels, gauze, washcloth, or tampon; selected appliance with precut opening; powder (e.g., karaya or Stomahesive); skin sealant; tape; plastic bag for used items.

Wash hands.

Remove the old pouch, using adhesive solvent if necessary to loosen the seal. Since the solvent is flammable, do not smoke or be near flames when removing the pouch.

Wash the stoma with warm water and let dry. A paper towel, gauze, washcloth, or tampon may be used as a wick over the stoma until the new bag is placed.

Inspect the skin and stoma for discolored (bluish) areas, redness, irritation, excoriation, excessive swelling, or excessive hair. For mild irritation, dust the skin lightly with karaya or Stomahesive. Severe irritation may necessitate a skin barrier (wafer cut to fit around the stoma).

If no irritation is present and the skin needs shaving, shave it dry over karaya powder.

Put skin sealant on over the powder and let dry (change wick if needed).

Put the wafer in place without creases and centered around the stoma. Remove the paper.

Place the pouch or ostomy plate over the wafer or, if there is no wafer, directly on the skin. Avoid making wrinkles or creases.

Close the spout on the bag.

Place tape around all edges of the ostomy pouch to increase wearing time.

Connect the appliance to a leg bag or let it drain into an ostomy bag, but empty the bag when half full so as not to break the skin seal.

—Instruct the patient to connect the appliance to continuous closed-gravity drainage at night. Keep the drainage appliance lower than the tube.

—Stress the importance of daily inspection of the stoma, noting color and size (should be pink; size will decrease after 6 months but stoma will not be flush with the abdomen).

—Discuss sexual activity. Explain that normal activity can be resumed unless a male patient has had a cystectomy. For impotent men, discuss other methods of sexual expression and procedures available (see Erectile Dysfunction, p. 294). Advise women to use extra lubricant.

—Inform the patient that showering and bathing may be resumed as recommended by the physician.

• *Medications*
—Explain the purpose, dosage, schedule, and route of administration of any prescribed drugs, as well as side effects to report to a physician or nurse.

• *Activity*
—Encourage the patient to discuss allowances and limitations with respect to occupation, recreation, or activity (see Abdominal Surgery, p. 3).

• *Diet*
—Inform the patient that a regular diet or one prescribed by the physician for the underlying condition should be followed.

—Explain that some foods (e.g., asparagus, fish, eggs, spicy foods) cause a strong urine odor but that drops or tablets may be placed in the pouch to decrease odors.

—Encourage the patient to drink 10-12 glasses of clear fluids a day. Tell the patient that cranberry juice helps cut down on mucus. Advise decreasing fluid intake in the evening to permit uninterrupted sleep.

**FOLLOW-UP CARE**

• Stress the importance of follow-up visits. Make sure the patient has the necessary names and telephone numbers.

• Encourage or assist the patient to obtain a Medic-Alert bracelet and identification card listing diagnosis, medication, and other data.

## PSYCHOSOCIAL CARE

- Encourage the expression of feelings about the changes in body image and sexual function. Assist the patient, family, and significant other to obtain counseling if necessary.

## REFERRALS

- Assist the patient to obtain referral services (home health and support groups).
- Provide the following address as a source for further information: United Ostomy Association, 30 Executive Park, Suite 120, Irvine, CA 92714-6744, phone (800) 826-0826.

# Urinary Incontinence

—Urinary incontinence: frequent or constant involuntary loss of urine. Urinary incontinence is classified as functional (no physical impairment but associated with emotional or environmental factors such as lack of privacy, inability to read, pain, head injury, dementia, or impaired mobility); stress (when a sudden increase in abdominal pressure, such as a cough, sneeze, laugh, bending over, or lifting objects, pushes a small amount of urine out of the bladder); reflex (lack of impulse sensed by bladder fullness, usually as a result of spinal injury); urge (sensation of a full bladder and inability to reach the toilet in time); and total (constant leakage of urine).

## CAUSES/CONTRIBUTING FACTORS

- Neurologic factors
  - —Spinal cord injury and neurogenic bladder
  - —Dementia
  - —Stroke
  - —Muscular sclerosis
  - —Parkinson's disease
- Aging
- Female gender
  - —Specific anatomy

—Childbearing and weakened muscles
* Depression
* Extreme obesity
* Urologic procedure/surgery
* Pain
* Diabetic neuropathy
* Urinary tract infection
* Urinary tract obstruction
* Dehydration
* Drugs (diuretics, cardiac medications, sleeping pills)
* Radiation therapy

## SIGNS/SYMPTOMS

* Incomplete bladder emptying
* Incontinence
* Dribbling of urine
* Frequency
* Involuntary urination
* Large amounts of urine output
* Low back or flank pain
* Loss of urine with increased intraabdominal pressure
* Urgency

## COMPLICATIONS

* Urinary tract infection
* Pyelonephritis
* Septic shock
* Wound infection
* Erosion of scrotum, labia, or bladder-urethra junction (from mechanical device)
* Mechanical failure
* Dysreflexia (see Neurogenic Bladder, p. 472)

## DIAGNOSTIC TESTS

* Describe each procedure, its purpose, and the normal feelings or sensations that are likely, as well as any preprocedural and postprocedural care.
  —Urine studies
     Urinalysis: to determine kidney function and any metabolic disease (e.g., diabetes mellitus)
     Culture and sensitivity: to detect presence of bacteria

—Urodynamic studies: to determine cause and extent of incontinence

    Cystometrogram (see Glomerulonephritis, p. 335)

    Voiding cystometrogram and pressure-flow studies: to measure pressure of various areas and flow rates of urine

    Uroflowmetry: to provide information about bladder strength and ability of the urethral sphincter to open (a special pressure-sensitive commode is used and the procedure is done on an outpatient basis)

    Urethral pressure profile: use of a special catheter inserted into the urethra to measure the closing pressure of the urethra to stop the urine flow

    Sphincter electromyography: to evaluate the urinary sphincter and compare the results with those from cystometry

—Intravenous pyelogram/urogram (see Urolithiasis, p. 666)

—Postvoid residual: patient urinates normally and then is catheterized to determine how much is left in the bladder

—Cystoscopy: to determine loss of muscle elasticity

—Blood studies: to evaluate kidney function (blood urea nitrogen, creatinine)

## TREATMENT

*Medical*

- Therapy
  —Hydration to prevent infection and stone formation
  —Increased activity to help blood flow and decrease urinary stasis
  —Catheterization: continuous or intermittent (see Indwelling Catheter, p. 406)
  —Dietary therapy (see Urolithiasis)
  —Credé's method: requires arm and hand strength (see Home Care section below)
  —Pelvic muscle exercises (Kegel exercises)
  —Females: vaginal cones to improve pelvic muscle tone (see Home Care section below)
  —Males: external condom catheter or penile clamp (see Home Care section below)
- Drugs
  —Drug therapy set up for specific neurologic condition (to decrease hyperreflexivity or increase bladder tone) or for stress or urge incontinence

**U**

*Surgical*
- Procedures to restore the bladder-urethral structure
  —Urethral suspension
  —Pubovaginal sling urethroplexy
- Implantation of an artificial urinary sphincter, a hydraulically activated sphincter mechanism around the bladder neck or urethra to allow the bladder to empty; the device is activated by manually squeezing the bulbs implanted in the labia or scrotum
- Implantation of bladder pacemaker: implantation of electrodes into the sacral nerves to provide stimulation to the bladder to empty; the electrodes are connected to a device under the skin and are controlled by the patient using an external transmitter

## HOME CARE

- Give both the patient and the caregiver *verbal* and *written* instructions. Provide them with the name and telephone number of a physician or nurse to call if questions arise.
- *General information*
  —Review and discuss care of surgically implanted devices. Instruct the patient to notify the physician or nurse of wound infection, mechanical failure of device, or urinary infection.
  —Encourage the patient to notify the nurse or physician if the incontinence management program is not working.
- *Special instructions*
  —Advise the patient that protective urinary containment devices are available to protect clothing (adult diapers, pads, or undergarments; drip collector for males) and bedding. Assist the patient to choose and obtain appropriate devices from pharmacies, medical supply stores, or supermarkets.
  —Instruct the patient on the importance of skin care.
    Wash regularly with soap and water, completely dry the skin, and apply a protective skin sealant or moisture barrier.
    Change the protective undergarment as directed by the manufacturer.
    Change clothing or bedding immediately if they get wet; wash perineal area.
    If using plastic pads or sheet, avoid direct skin contact with the plastic.
    Keep the perineal area clean and change pads and undergarments to prevent odors.

—Discuss the importance of establishing a bladder training program.

  Help the patient identify usual voiding patterns. Tell the patient to keep a record of the times each day he or she urinates, measure the amount of urine at each voiding, and record the number of times and when incontinence or leakage occurs.

  Stress the importance of establishing a regular timed schedule of voiding patterns based on voiding record (i.e., every 2-3 hours, after sitting for extended periods, or self-catheterization.

  Review measures to facilitate urination at the scheduled times of day or night: finding a private location, assuming a comfortable position, listening to running water, gently pulling pubic hair, stroking the inner thigh lightly or with ice, pouring warm water over the perineum, or placing hands in warm water.

—Advise the patient to limit fluids with meals to 8 ounces; spread intake of fluids between meals, limiting amount to sips (2-3 ounces); and avoid drinking more than 2-3 ounces of fluid 2 hours before bedtime.

—Discuss the purpose of pelvic muscle (Kegel) exercises and assist the patient to initiate the exercise program.

—Instruct the patient on the correct muscle groups to exercise (those around the urethra and vagina). If a female patient has difficulty locating the muscles, place a finger or probe in the vagina and ask her to tighten the muscles around it, then do the same for the rectum. If a male patient has difficulty locating the muscles, place a finger or probe in the rectum and ask him to tighten the muscles around it. To initiate the exercise program, ask the patient to do the following.

  Schedule times and select a place for the exercises.

  Do the exercises sitting, standing, or lying down.

  Begin the sessions with 10 complete cycles, building up to 30-50 repetitions as advised by the nurse or physician. One complete cycle consists of tightening pelvic muscles for 10 seconds, followed by relaxing pelvic muscles for 10 seconds. The sessions take approximately 15 minutes.

  Do the exercises every other day (up to three times a week) as part of maintenance program.

U

—Explain that pelvic muscle exercises should not be done routinely with each voiding because of possible damage to the urethra.

—Advise the patient that biofeedback procedures are available to ensure that the patient is doing the exercises correctly. This is done by inserting a probe into the vagina (women) or rectum (men). Patches around the rectum may also be used. Lights and graphs on the recorder provide visual feedback when the patient is using the correct muscle group. Each session is 20-30 minutes long; four to six sessions are required.

—For a female patient, discuss additional procedures to strengthen pelvic muscles. A vaginal cone (wide end first) is inserted into the vagina initially. The patient is instructed to hold it in place for 15 minutes twice a day. The patient then progresses to heavier cones. Pessaries and vaginal rings may be inserted into the vagina for bladder support.

—For a male patient, discuss the use of an external condom catheter. If it is used, instruct the patient in the importance of inspecting the penis daily and maintaining good hygiene to prevent skin breakdown. Explain that care must be taken to use the correct size condom, apply tape or adhesive correctly, and change the catheter every day.

• *Medications*

—Explain the purpose, dosage, schedule, and route of administration of any drugs prescribed for stress incontinence, as well as side effects to report to a physician or nurse.

• *Diet*

—Advise the patient to drink up to 1½ quarts of fluid each day to avoid infection and formation of stones, unless fluid intake is restricted by the physician. Tell the patient to limit amounts in the evening or when planning a long trip on which bathroom stops will not be possible.

—Tell the patient to avoid carbonated beverages, caffeine drinks (e.g., colas), and alcohol.

## REFERRALS

• Refer the patient to advocacy and support groups for incontinence, such as Incontinence Restored, Inc.; Help for Incontinent People (HIP), Inc.; and the Simon Foundation for Continence.

# Urinary Incontinence Surgical Repair, Female

—Urinary incontinence surgical repair: surgical procedure to restore urinary continence. In the Marshall-Marchetti-Krantz procedure, the bladder neck and urethra are sutured to the perichondrium of the symphysis pubis or the periosteum of the superior pubic ramus using an extraperitoneal abdominal approach. In the Pereyra bladder neck suspension, a vaginal dissection and small suprapubic incision are used to access the bladder and urethra for suspension. In the Raz procedure, the bladder is elevated and suspended using tissue or inorganic material for support. The Raz procedure is performed transvaginally.

## INDICATIONS

• Urinary incontinence (see p. 657)

## PREPROCEDURAL TEACHING

• Review the physician's explanation of the procedure and the reason for it; encourage the patient to ask questions and to discuss any fears or anxieties.

### Review of Preprocedural Care

• Explain that admission is usually on the day of surgery, that the procedure lasts 2-3 hours, and that it may be done under general anesthesia or spinal anesthesia.
• Discuss the diagnostic studies for urinary incontinence (see p. 657).
• Inform the patient about the routine preoperative studies: blood and urine tests, chest x-ray, and electrocardiogram.
• Tell the patient that a clear liquid diet is usually necessary for 2 days before surgery.
• Explain that a laxative should be taken 2 nights before and an enema the night before.
• Tell the patient that a vaginal douche, usually Betadine unless the patient is sensitive to iodine, is needed the night before and the morning of surgery.

- Discuss the need for a shower and shampoo with bactericidal soap (e.g., Safeguard, Dial, Hibiclens) the night before.
- Inform the patient that the pubic hair may be shaved before the operation.
- Discuss the need for NPO status the night before surgery.

**Review of Postprocedural Care**

- Explain that the patient will remain in the hospital for 2 or more days after the procedure.
- Inform the patient that she will be required to move, turn, and deep breathe the day of surgery and will probably get out of bed the day after surgery.
- Review the drainage tubes that may be used: a urinary catheter, which is usually removed the day after surgery if a suprapubic catheter is present (may remain longer for some procedures), and a suprapubic catheter, which is usually plugged on the day after the surgery.
- Describe the purpose of the vaginal pack, which is usually removed the morning after the operation. Explain that some vaginal bleeding is possible after surgery but usually stops within a few days.
- Explain that intravenous fluids are usually stopped on the day after surgery and fluid is limited to approximately 5 glasses of clear fluid a day.
- Describe the technique of postvoid residuals (see Home Care section below).

**COMPLICATIONS**

- Urinary tract infection
- Pyelonephritis
- Septic shock
- Pulmonary problems
- Deep vein thrombosis
- Wound infection
- Difficulty in urinating

**HOME CARE**

- Give both the patient and the caregiver *verbal* and *written* instructions. Provide them with the name and telephone number of a physician or nurse to call if questions arise.

- *General information*
  —Review the type of procedure performed and the drains and catheters left in place.
- *Warning signs*
  —Review the signs and symptoms that should be reported to a physician or nurse.
    Blockage of catheter
    Fever, chills
    Continued bright red blood in urine after several days
    Leakage of urine around the catheter
    Wound infection (redness, tenderness, warm to touch, possible drainage of pus)
    Onset of or increased vaginal discharge or bleeding
- *Special instructions*
  —Review the care of catheters: indwelling (see Indwelling Catheter, p. 406) or suprapubic catheter (see Indwelling Catheter).
  —Explain the postvoid residual technique.
    Establish a time schedule (usually every 4 hours, or more often if needed).
    Sit on the toilet for at least 5 minutes and urinate normally (may take 2 or more days before normal urination).
    After urination, measure the postvoid residual by opening the suprapubic catheter and emptying into a receptacle.
    Amount of urine from the suprapubic catheter should decrease as normal urination amount increases.
    Keep a record of the amounts voided and post void.
  —Teach the patient how to unplug the suprapubic catheter.
    Wash hands.
    Wipe the connection with alcohol.
    Grasp the plug with one hand and the catheter end with the other hand.
    Gently twist the plug to loosen and remove it while squeezing the catheter with the other hand (thumb and index finger).
    Place the catheter end over the receptacle and open to drain.
    Replace the plug.
  —Discuss the importance of cleansing the perineum at least twice a day.
  —Stress the importance of cleansing the rectal area at least twice a day or after every bowel movement.

U

• *Medications*
   —Explain the purpose, dosage, schedule, and route of administration of any prescribed drugs, as well as side effects to report to a physician or nurse.

**FOLLOW-UP CARE**

• Stress the importance of regular follow-up visits. Make sure the
   patient has the necessary names and telephone numbers.

# Urolithiasis
## (Urinary Stones, Renal Calculi)

—**Urolithiasis: abnormal formation of stones in the kidney or
urinary tract. Renal calculi are classified according to composition: calcium, uric acid, phosphate, oxalate, struvite. They
vary in size and may be solitary or multiple. They occur most
commonly in men 30-50 years of age.**

**CAUSES/CONTRIBUTING FACTORS**

• Familial tendency
• Gender: females affected by some types of stone (e.g., "stag-
   horn" struvite stones) more than males
• Diet rich in calcium, oxalates, or uric acid
• Dehydration
• Geographic location: southeastern United States
• Occupation: work in industrial area; textile (cotton) worker;
   work in sedentary position
• Repeated urinary infections
• Conditions causing urinary stasis: immobility (paralysis), inabil-
   ity to empty bladder completely, inability to urinate
• Conditions causing hypercalciuria: hyperparathyroidism, kidney
   dysfunction, bone cancer, multiple myeloma, breast cancer with
   metastasis
• Renal tubular acidosis
• Long-term use (years) of indwelling catheters
• Urinary diversion or conduit

## SIGNS/SYMPTOMS

- Abrupt onset of colicky pain that usually starts in the flank and moves to the groin and lower back
- Nausea and vomiting
- Extreme restlessness
- Urine abnormality
  —Cloudy
  —Absent or scant
  —Hematuria
  —Sediment (sandlike material)

## COMPLICATIONS

- Urinary tract infection
- Pyelonephritis
- Urinary obstruction
- Hydronephrosis
- Renal failure

## DIAGNOSTIC TESTS

- Describe each procedure, its purpose, and the normal feelings or sensations that are likely, as well as any preprocedural and postprocedural care.
  —Kidney, ureter, bladder x-ray
  —X-ray with contrast dye: to show stone location or obstruction
  —Intravenous pyelogram/urogram
  —Retrograde pyelogram
  —Blood studies: to determine presence of elements (e.g., calcium, phosphorus, uric acid); infection
  —Urinalysis or 24-hour samples
  —Stone studies: chemical analysis of stones
  —Ultrasound studies
  —Radionuclide studies: to determine the presence of kidney damage

## TREATMENT

*Medical*

- Therapy
  —Hydration (oral or parenteral fluids; oral hydration with 15-20 glasses per day is used to flush out stones <4 mm)
  —Diet: changes based on stone composition

—Chemolysis to dissolve stones by oral medications or local irrigation

—Lithotripsy (stone destruction by means of external energy source; may be used with basket retrieval or flushing with irrigation fluids; method depends on size and location of stones)

—Extracorporeal shock wave lithotripsy: noninvasive procedure causing fragmentation of stones <1 inch in the kidney or upper part of the ureter by means of shock waves; stent may be placed in the ureter by cystoscope (see below) to allow passage of urine around the "sand"; same-day surgery or overnight stay

—Cystoscopic lithotripsy or basket retrieval of stones in the bladder: instrument placed through the urinary opening under local anesthetic; light sedation or none; done on an outpatient basis

—Ureteroscopic lithotripsy or basket retrieval of stones in lower ureter: an endoscopic tube is threaded up the ureter to the stone, and a smaller instrument (fiberoptic ureterscope) is threaded through; procedure is done on an outpatient basis with the patient under local anesthesia, light sedation, or no sedation

—Percutaneous nephroscopic stone lithotripsy or basket retrieval with or without irrigation of stones: a small incision is made into the flank to allow insertion of the nephroscope into the kidney; used to break up large (>1 inch) stones with an ultrasonic probe (ultrasound waves), electrohydraulic probe (electric spark gap), or laser probe (laser beam); the nephrostomy tube may remain in place temporarily and is connected to a small external drainage bag; procedure is done under local anesthetic on an outpatient basis or with an overnight stay

—"Sandwich" treatment: any combination of the above treatments, depending on size and location

*Surgical*
- Removal of stones: performed with patient under general or spinal anesthetic; patient remains in hospital 2-5 days or more (see Abdominal Surgery, p. 3)

## HOME CARE

- Give both the patient and the caregiver *verbal* and *written* instructions. Provide them with the name and telephone number of a physician or nurse to call if questions arise.

- *General information*
  —Explain urolithiasis and the reasons for it. Discuss the composition of the stone.
- *Warning signs*
  —Review the signs and symptoms that should be reported to a physican or nurse.
    Onset of colicky pain
    Decreased urine output
    Signs and symptoms of urinary tract infection: urgency, frequency, burning, low-grade fever
    Infection: redness, warm to touch, tenderness, drainage
    Leakage around nephrostomy tube
  —Assist the patient to identify early signs of an attack (restlessness, aching, flank pain) and advise the patient to notify the physician immediately. Instruct the patient to have someone drive him or her to the emergency room if pain is severe.
- *Special instructions*
  —Discuss measures to prevent recurrences, including drugs, diet, fluids (see below), regular emptying of bladder, and avoidance of or early treatment of urinary tract infections.
  —Instruct the patient in measuring and straining urine and identifying sand particles. Stress the importance of saving particles and notifying the physician or nurse. Advise the patient on how and where to obtain supplies.
  —Explain nephrostomy tube care if the tube is in place at discharge.
    The tube must be securely taped at all times.
    Change the dressing only if instructed (the dressing may be retaped).
    Monitor urine for amount, color, and smell; report decrease in or absence of urine in the bag.
    Follow clean procedure when emptying the bag: wash hands, clean connection with alcohol, disconnect cap, wash hands again after recapping.
    Use the procedure outlined when changing bags for nighttime use (see Indwelling Catheter, p. 406).
    Keep the drainage bag below the level of the kidney when up or lying down.
    If the nephrostomy tube is in place, tell the patient to confirm procedures for showering and bathing with the physician.

- *Medications*
  —Explain the purpose, dosage, schedule, and route of administration of any prescribed drugs, as well as side effects to report to a physician or nurse.
  —Discuss the need to continue a full course of antibiotics even after the patient feels well.
- *Activity*
  —Encourage the patient to discuss allowances and limitations with respect to occupation, recreation, and activities.
- *Diet*
  —Encourage the patient to increase intake of clear fluids (water, juices) to 2500 ml per day; maintenance level should be 8-10 glasses per day.
  —Explain that alcoholic beverages should be avoided.
  —Advise the patient to limit fluids sweetened with sugar or additives, which may contribute to stone formation.
  —Discuss dietary changes recommended on the basis of stone composition.
  > Calcium: decrease amounts of milk, ice cream, cheese, sardines, canned salmon, dark green leafy vegetables
  > Uric acid: decrease amounts of organ meats (kidney, liver, heart) and whole grains
  > Oxalate: decrease amount of vegetables (asparagus, beets, spinach, rhubarb), fruits (plums, cranberries, raspberries), juices (cranberry, grape, grapefruit), and nuts (almonds, cashews)

## MEDICAL FOLLOW-UP

- Stress the importance of regular follow-up visits. Make sure the patient has the necessary names and telephone numbers. Remind the patient to bring the collected stone specimens to appointments.
- Emphasize the importance of seeking medical help for stones even when traveling.

# Valve Replacement

—**Valve replacement: surgical replacement of a diseased valve, commonly the aortic or mitral valve, with either a mechanical or a tissue valve.**

## INDICATIONS
- Valve stenosis
- Valve regurgitation

## PREPROCEDURAL TEACHING
- See the discussion of preprocedural teaching in Coronary Artery Bypass Graft Surgery (p. 211).
- Review the physician's explanation of the scheduled surgery, the type of valve to be used, and associated risks and benefits. Answer any questions. Discuss the need for obtaining informed consent.

### Review of preprocedural care
- Review procedures for blood donations from the patient or family.
- Have the patient obtain dental clearance 10-14 days before surgery.
- Explain that hospital admission may be on the day of surgery.
- Instruct the patient not to eat or drink after midnight on the evening before surgery.
- Review laboratory studies, electrocardiography, and chest x-ray; check the patient's blood type and ensure crossmatch.
- Explain that the patient's skin will be cleansed and hair will be clipped.
- Teach the use of the incentive spirometer, and stress the importance of coughing and deep breathing.

### Review of postprocedural care
- Discuss postoperative care, including routines in the intensive care unit, intravenous lines, catheters, chest tubes, ventilator, fluid therapy and restrictions, and pain management.

- Stress the importance of turning, coughing, deep breathing, and early ambulation.
- Discuss the purpose of the incentive spirometer and review its use.
- Address anticipated body image changes, such as the mediastinal incision scar, activity limitations, and valve care.

## SIDE EFFECTS/COMPLICATIONS

- Perivalvular leaks
- Conduction defects or dysrhythmias
- Low cardiac output syndrome
- Endocarditis
- Hemolysis
- Malfunction or disintegration of the prosthesis

## HOME CARE

- Give both the patient and the caregiver *verbal* and *written* instructions. Provide them with the name and telephone number of a physician or nurse to call if questions arise.
- *General information*
  —Discuss the underlying valvular disease, causes or contributing factors, and care of the valve replacement.
- *Wound/incision care*
  —Demonstrate proper care of the incision site.
- *Warning signs*
  —Review the signs and symptoms that should be reported to a physician or nurse.
  
  Fever, chills, diaphoresis

  Redness, warmth, pain, swelling, purulent drainage from the incision site

  Shortness of breath, fatigue, palpitations, hemoptysis, orthopnea, exercise intolerance, syncope, dizziness, sudden weight gain

  For anticoagulation therapy: excessive bruising, bleeding from the nose, hemoptysis, hematuria, melena
- *Special instructions*
  —Discuss the type of valve inserted. For patients with a prosthetic valve, explain and stress the importance of lifelong anticoagulants to prevent systemic emboli and obstruction of the valve.
  —Explain the risk of developing endocarditis, and discuss preventive measures.

—Discuss alternative methods for dealing with pain: visualization, guided imagery, meditation, relaxation, biofeedback.
* *Medications*
  —Explain the purpose, dosage, schedule, and route of administration of any prescribed drugs, as well as side effects to report to a physician or nurse.
  —Instruct the patient on anticoagulation therapy (see Anticoagulation Therapy, p. 42).
  —Stress the importance of not taking over-the-counter medications without consulting a physician.
* *Activity*
  —Encourage the patient to discuss allowances and limitations with respect to occupation, recreation, and activities.
  —Review activity limitations.
  > Avoid heavy lifting (>10 pounds), pushing, pulling, the Valsalva maneuver, and isometric exercises for 6 weeks.
  > Avoid driving for the first 4-6 weeks.
  > Avoid sitting or driving for prolonged periods.
  > Avoid abrupt position changes from sitting and standing.
  > Increase activity gradually, as tolerated. Plan frequent rest periods to avoid fatigue.
  > Avoid sexual activity for the first 6-8 weeks, then resume as tolerated. Use positions that are comfortable and do not strain the incision.
  —Assist the patient to identify changes or adaptations that will be needed in the home, such as dealing with stairs or housekeeping activities.
  —Help the patient obtain referral to home health nursing care.
  —Discuss the importance of maintaining good oral hygiene, with daily care and regular trips to the dentist. Inform the patient of the need to wait 6 weeks after surgery before seeing a dentist.
  —Instruct patients receiving anticoagulants to use soft-bristled toothbrushes and electric razors.
  —Stress the importance of prophylactic antibiotics before procedures that predispose patients to bacteremia.
  —Provide information on contraception and pregnancy to female patients; stress the importance of planning all pregnancies and checking with the physician or nurse before conception.

- *Diet*
  —Assist the patient to plan a low-sodium, low-fat, low-cholesterol diet.
  —Advise the patient on the effects of vitamin K–rich foods if he or she is taking anticoagulants.

**FOLLOW-UP CARE**

- Stress the importance of follow-up visits for laboratory tests and medical care. Make sure the patient has the necessary names and telephone numbers.
- If the patient is taking anticoagulants, emphasize the need for adhering to the schedule for dosage and prothrombin time tests.
- Assist the patient with a prosthetic valve or taking anticoagulants to obtain a Medic-Alert bracelet and identification card.
- Instruct the patient to inform any dentists and other physicians of the valve replacement before treatment, especially childbirth or dental, genitourinary, gynecologic, or skin procedures.
- Stress the importance of not smoking. Provide referral to community resources for smoking cessation programs.

**PSYCHOSOCIAL CARE**

- Encourage the patient to express fears and concerns about the surgery, outcomes, limitations, and body image changes. Refer the patient to a social worker for further counseling, if indicated.

# Venous Thrombosis

—**Venous thrombosis: the development of a thrombus or thrombi in a vein as result of venous stasis, intimal damage, or hypercoagulability or in association with inflammation. Other terms used to describe venous thrombosis include phlebitis (inflammation of a vein), phlebothrombosis (intraluminal thrombus with minimal or no inflammatory component), thromboembolism (dislodgment and migration of a thrombus), and thrombophlebitis (acute thrombus and inflammation in a deep or superficial vein).**

## CAUSES/CONTRIBUTING FACTORS/RISK FACTORS

- Venous trauma from intravenous solutions or direct injury
- Inflammation
- Coagulopathies associated with polycythemia, anemia, steroid use, and malignancies
- Stasis of blood associated with heart failure, shock, immobility from prolonged bed rest, structural disorders of the veins, or side effects of anesthesia
- Hemoconcentration
- Recent surgery
- Use of oral contraceptives
- Obesity
- Varicose veins
- Childbirth
- Prolonged bed rest and immobility

## SIGNS/SYMPTOMS

- Leg edema
- Pain and tenderness in calf or thigh
- Erythema
- Local warmth
- Prominent superficial veins
- Increased size compared with unaffected extremity
- Heavy feeling in the affected extremity
- Cramping

## COMPLICATIONS

- Pulmonary embolism
- Chronic venous insufficiency
- Venous ulcers
- Cerebrovascular accident

## DIAGNOSTIC TESTS

- Describe each procedure, its purpose, and the normal feelings or sensations that are likely, as well as any preprocedural and postprocedural care.
  - Doppler ultrasonography: to identify area of reduced blood flow
  - Duplex imaging: to assess veins for flow and pressure

V

—Plethysmography: to assess blood flow distal to the obstruction

—I-fibrinogen scan: to detect early formation of clots and identify areas of obstruction

—Phlebography (venography): to visualize filling or absence of filling in veins

## TREATMENT

*Medical*

- Therapy
  —Bed rest during acute phase
  —Warm, moist heat
  —Antiembolic stockings
- Drugs
  —Anticoagulants
  —Fibrinolytic agents
  —Antiplatelet agents
  —Analgesics

*Surgical*

- Thrombectomy: surgical excision of a thrombus

## HOME CARE

- Give both the patient and the caregiver *verbal* and *written* instructions. Provide them with the name and telephone number of a physician or nurse to call if questions arise.
- *General information*
  —Explain the development of venous thrombosis, causes and contributing factors, care and treatment, and preventive measures.
- *Warning signs*
  —Review the signs and symptoms that should be reported to a physician or nurse.
    Venous ulceration, skin breakdown, redness
    Pain, tenderness, redness, warmth to extremities
    Pulmonary embolism: chest pain, hemoptysis, dyspnea, tachypnea
    Increased size of affected extremity
- *Special instructions*
  —Teach the patient to measure and record the size of the affected extremity daily.

—Teach the patient proper skin care.

> Use mild soap and rinse well.
>
> Dry gently and thoroughly.
>
> Avoid vigorous rubbing and massaging of the affected extremity.

—Demonstrate the use of antiembolic stockings for ambulation and periods of prolonged sitting, if prescribed. Assist the patient to obtain stockings in the proper size. Instruct the patient to remove them every 8 hours to assess the leg and skin.

—Instruct the patient on use of the bed cradle.

—Demonstrate the application of warm packs to the affected extremity.

* *Medications*
  —Explain the purpose, dosage, schedule, and route of administration of any prescribed drugs, as well as side effects to report to the physician or nurse (see Anticoagulation Therapy, p. 42).

* *Activity*
  —Teach the patient methods to prevent thrombus formation.

  > Avoid restrictive clothing, such as garters, girdles, and clothing with elastic groin bands.
  >
  > Avoid prolonged periods of standing. Alternate position by standing on the toes and then the heels.
  >
  > Elevate the legs above the level of the heart when sitting.
  >
  > Avoid dangling the legs.
  >
  > Avoid positions that restrict venous blood flow; do not use a knee gatch or cross the legs.
  >
  > Avoid nicotine and smoking.
  >
  > Avoid trauma to the extremities.

  —Encourage the patient to initiate a walking program. Provide referral to monitored exercise programs.

## FOLLOW-UP CARE

* Stress the importance of regular follow-up visits. Make sure the patient has the necessary names and telephone numbers.
* Encourage the patient to obtain a Medic-Alert bracelet and identification card listing medications, such as anticoagulants.
* Stress the importance of smoking cessation and weight loss. Provide referral to appropriate community resources.

# Desirable Weights for Men and Women

1983 Metropolitan Life Insurance Height
and Weight Table

| Height | Small frame | Medium frame | Large frame |
|--------|-------------|--------------|-------------|
| **Men\*** | | | |
| 5'2" | 128-134 | 131-141 | 138-150 |
| 5'3" | 130-136 | 133-143 | 140-153 |
| 5'4" | 132-138 | 135-145 | 142-156 |
| 5'5" | 134-140 | 137-148 | 144-160 |
| 5'6" | 136-142 | 139-151 | 146-164 |
| 5'7" | 138-145 | 142-154 | 149-168 |
| 5'8" | 140-148 | 145-157 | 152-172 |
| 5'9" | 142-151 | 148-160 | 155-176 |
| 5'10" | 144-154 | 151-163 | 158-180 |
| 5'11" | 146-157 | 154-166 | 161-184 |
| 6'0" | 149-160 | 157-170 | 164-188 |
| 6'1" | 152-164 | 160-174 | 168-192 |
| 6'2" | 155-168 | 164-178 | 172-197 |
| 6'3" | 158-172 | 167-182 | 176-202 |
| 6'4" | 162-176 | 171-187 | 181-207 |

\*Weights at ages 25 to 59, based on lowest mortality. Weight in pounds
according to frame (in indoor clothing weighing 5 lb, shoes with 1" heels).

1983 Metropolitan Life Insurance Height
and Weight Table—cont'd

| Height | Small frame | Medium frame | Large frame |
|--------|-------------|--------------|-------------|
| **Women†** | | | |
| 4'10" | 102-111 | 109-121 | 118-131 |
| 4'11" | 103-113 | 111-123 | 120-134 |
| 5'0" | 104-115 | 113-126 | 122-137 |
| 5'1" | 106-118 | 115-129 | 125-140 |
| 5'2" | 108-121 | 118-132 | 128-143 |
| 5'3" | 111-124 | 121-135 | 131-147 |
| 5'4" | 114-127 | 124-138 | 134-151 |
| 5'5" | 117-130 | 127-141 | 137-155 |
| 5'6" | 120-133 | 130-144 | 140-159 |
| 5'7" | 123-136 | 133-147 | 143-163 |
| 5'8" | 126-139 | 136-150 | 146-167 |
| 5'9" | 129-142 | 139-153 | 149-170 |
| 5'10" | 132-145 | 142-156 | 152-173 |
| 5'11" | 135-148 | 145-159 | 155-176 |
| 6'0" | 138-151 | 148-162 | 158-179 |

†Weights at ages 25 to 59, based on lowest mortality. Weight in pounds
according to frame (in indoor clothing weighing 3 lb, shoes with 1" heels).

## APPENDIX B
# Caloric Needs of Healthy Adults and Hospitalized Patients

**Healthy Adult (Resting State)**

30 kilocalories per kilogram of ideal body weight

**Hospitalized Adult**

2000-3000 calories per day

# APPENDIX C
# Therapeutic Diets

## Modification of protein intake

| Daily protein intake | Food limitations* | Practicality |
|---|---|---|
| 150 to 200 g | Meat, cheese, eggs; >10 oz/day (1 egg = 1 oz meat); starches: 5 or more servings/day; vegetables: 4 or more servings/day; fruits: 3 or more servings/day; milk, casein, shakes, eggnogs, protein supplements added | High-protein, high-fat diet |
| 100 to 140 g | Meat, cheese: 10 oz/day; starches: 5 to 6 servings/day; vegetables: 4 to 5 servings/day; fruits: 3 to 4 servings/day; milk included | Average American diet; relatively high in fat |
| 60 g (10% of total calories)† | Meat, cheese: 6 oz/day; starches: <5 servings/day; vegetables: <4 servings/day; fruits: <3 servings/day; milk in limited amounts; calories increased with sugar and fat | Generally acceptable for home use; diet fairly easily manipulated according to patient preferences |

| | | |
|---|---|---|
| 40 g (6% of calories)† | Meat, cheese: 4 oz/day; starches: 3 servings/day; vegetables: 4 servings/day; fruits: 3 servings/day; calories increased with sugar and fat | Difficult to follow at home unless patient is unusually cooperative |
| 20 g (3% of calories)† | Meat, cheese: essentially none; eggs: 2/day; starches: 2 servings/day; fruits: 2 servings/day; vegetables: 2 servings/day; calories increased with sugar and fat | Should be limited to hospital use |
| 8 to 10 g (trace) | Meat, cheese, eggs, milk: essentially none; starches, vegetables: severely limited (low-protein bread only); calories mostly as fruits, juices, sugar, and fat | For hospital use only |

*Serving sizes: most vegetables = ½ cup; most fruits = 1 piece or ½ cup; starches = 1 slice bread or approximately ⅓ to ½ cup of cooked starch.

†Percent of calories based on 2400 calories per day.

Modification of sodium intake

| Daily sodium (Na) intake* | Food limitations | Practicality |
|---|---|---|
| 5 to 6 g Na (= 12.5 to 15 g salt) | Includes table salt, heavily or visibly salted items | Average American diet |
| 4 g Na (= 10 g salt) | No additional salt on tray or at table | Practical for home use |
| 3 g Na (= 7.5 g salt) | Food only lightly salted in preparation; restrict heavily or visibly salted items (potato chips, pretzels, crackers, pickles, olives, relishes, sauces, most soups); no salt on tray | Practical for home use |
| 2 g Na (= 5 g salt) | Above limitations plus no salt in food preparation; avoid most processed foods (canned foods, dry cereals, luncheon meats, bacon, ham, cheese) unless calculated into diet; regular bread, butter, milk in limited amounts | Fairly practical for home use with cooperative patient |
| 1 g Na (= 2.5 g salt) | Above limitations plus use of only salt-free bread | Practical for home use with only unusually cooperative patient |
| 0.5 g Na (= 1.25 g salt) | Above limitations plus limitation of meat (4 oz/day), eggs, some vegetables; milk (1 pt/day) and salt-free butter allowed | Not practical for home use |

*1 g Na = 43 mEq; 1 mEq Na = 23 mg; 1 g NaCl = 2.5 g Na; 1 g Na = 0.4 g NaCl.

## HIGH-SODIUM FOODS TO OMIT ON A SODIUM-RESTRICTED DIET

### Condiments

Pickles, olives, relishes, salted nuts, meat tenderizers, commercial salad dressings, monosodium glutamate (Accent), steak sauce, ketchup, soy sauce, Worcestershire sauce, horseradish sauce, chili sauce, commercial mustard, onion salt, garlic salt, celery salt, butter salt, seasoned salt

### Breads

Salted crackers

### Meat, Fish, Poultry, Cheese, and Substitutes

Cured, smoked, and processed meats such as ham, bacon, corned beef, chipped beef, weiners, luncheon meats, bologna, salt pork, regular canned salmon and tuna; all cheese except low sodium and cottage cheese; TV dinners, pizza, frozen Italian entrees, imitation sausage and bacon

### Beverages

Commercial buttermilk, instant hot cocoa mixes

### Soups

Commercial canned and dehydrated soups (except low-sodium soups), bouillon, consommé

### Vegetables

Sauerkraut, hominy, pork and beans, canned tomato and vegetable juices

### Fats

Gravy, regular peanut butter

### Potato or Potato Substitutes

Potato chips, corn chips, salted popcorn, pretzels, frozen potato casseroles, commercially packaged rice and noodle mixes, dehydrated potatoes and potato mixes, bread stuffing

## MODIFICATION OF FOOD CONSISTENCY
### Clear Liquid Diet

This diet provides clear fluids that leave little residue and are absorbed with a minimum of digestive activity. It includes only broth, gelatin, strained fruit juices, clear beverages, and low-residue supplements. Since some of these have high osmolality, they may not be well tolerated by some patients. Clear liquids generally do not provide the RDA for any nutrients except perhaps for vitamin C. They should not be used for more than 2 or 3 days without supplementation.

### Full Liquid Diet

This diet includes foods that liquefy at room temperature; many such as whole milk, custard, pudding, strained cream soups, eggnog, and ice cream contain fat and lactose, which some patients do not tolerate well. Complete enteral supplements may be preferred in such cases or may be added to increase calories and protein. This diet can meet the RDA for all nutrients, except iron for women of childbearing age.

### Soft Diet

The soft diet contains foods that are tender but are not ground or pureed. Whole meats, cooked vegetables, and fruits of moderate fiber content are allowed. This generally excludes dried foods, most raw fruits and vegetables, and very coarse breads and cereals, and is fairly low in fiber and residue.

### Pureed or Ground Diet

This diet includes foods that are especially easy to masticate and swallow. It is useful in patients who have dysphagia or dental problems.

### Bland Diet

This is designed for patients with peptic ulcer disease. A bland diet eliminates foods suspected to be gastric irritants or to stimulate gastric secretions. It generally excludes highly spiced foods, pepper, caffeine, and alcohol.

### Low-Fiber, Low-Residue Diet

Intended to reduce fecal bulk, this diet is restricted in milk, certain vegetables, fruits, and whole-grain breads and cereals.

**High-Fiber Diet**

This diet includes unrefined starches (whole-grain bread, brown rice, potatoes, corn, beans), raw fruits, and vegetables. Bran may be added if desired.

Appendix C from Weinsier RL, Heimburger DC, Butterworth Jr MD: *Handbook of clinical nutrition,* St Louis, 1989, Mosby.

## APPENDIX D
# Food Sources of Selected Nutrients

### FOODS HIGH IN SODIUM

Processed foods: canned foods (meats, sauces, fish, vegetables), luncheon meats, dry cereals, cheese, ham, bacon, smoked or cured fish

Prepackaged foods

Salted crackers

Pickles, olives, relishes

Salty nuts, chips

Bouillon cubes

Yeast

### FOODS HIGH IN POTASSIUM

Fruits: apricots, avocado, bananas, rhubarb, melons (cantaloupe, watermelon), oranges, grapes, coconut, dried fruits, fruit juices

Vegetables: artichokes, raw carrots, tomatoes, cooked spinach, cooked potatoes, pumpkin, swiss chard, cooked sweet potato, dried beans, peas, mushrooms

Bouillon cubes

Cider, beer, wine

Nuts

Chocolate

Chili powder

Turmeric

Packaged soups

Canned spaghetti, vegetables, soups

## FOODS LOW IN POTASSIUM

Fruits: applesauce, grapefruit, canned pear, canned pineapple, plums, frozen strawberries, tangerines, cranberries, lemons

Vegetables: cooked or raw cabbage, cooked cauliflower, corn, cucumber, cooked eggplant, cooked green beans, cooked green peas, cooked onion, cooked summer squash

## FOODS HIGH IN PHOSPHORUS

Meats: brain, kidney, liver, beef (lean round, cooked), lean pork

Fish: cod, halibut

Poultry

Dairy products: milk, cheese

Whole grains: oatmeal, bran, barley

Nuts: roasted peanuts, brazil nuts, peanut butter

Vegetables: beans (kidney, white, lima), cooked green peas, dried beans and peas, cooked artichokes, white potatoes, cooked brussels sprouts

Eggs

Carbonated drinks with phosphoric acid added

## FOODS LOW IN PHOSPHORUS

Most fruits

Most vegetables

## FOODS HIGH IN CALCIUM

Dairy products: milk, cheese, ice cream

Vegetables: greens (collard, mustard, turnip), cooked spinach, cooked broccoli, cooked beans (kidney, lima, white), raw cabbage, raw carrots

Fruits: prunes, oranges, tangerines

## FOODS HIGH IN IRON

Meats: calf liver, beef liver, chicken

Boiled eggs

Vegetables: spinach, cooked beans (kidney, white, lima), asparagus, iceberg lettuce, mustard greens, cooked green peas, raw cauliflower

Fruits: watermelon, prunes, dried dates, dried apricots, raisins, blueberries, strawberries

# FOOD SOURCES OF MAJOR VITAMINS

## Vitamin A

| Food | Portion size | Amount of vitamin | |
|---|---|---|---|
| | | **RE/portion** | **RE/100 g** |
| **Meats** | | | |
| Beef liver, fried | 3½ oz | 10640 | 10640 |
| Calf liver, cooked | 3½ oz | 8116 | 8116 |
| Chicken liver, cooked | 2 livers | 7806 | 12880 |
| **Vegetables** | | | |
| Potatoes, sweet, baked | 1 medium | 2488 | 830 |
| Carrots, raw | 1 large | 2025 | 1100 |
| cooked | ½ cup | 800 | 1050 |
| Spinach, raw | 3½ oz | 810 | 810 |
| cooked | ½ cup | 737 | 657 |
| Pumpkin, cooked | ½ cup | 800 | 640 |
| Collard greens, cooked | ½ cup | 540 | 540 |
| Squash, winter | ½ squash | 420 | 420 |
| Turnip greens, cooked | ½ cup | 396 | 630 |
| Mustard greens, cooked | ½ cup | 212 | 212 |
| Lettuce, romaine | 4 leaves | 190 | 190 |
| iceberg | ¼ head | 97 | 97 |
| Broccoli, cooked | ½ cup | 110 | 250 |
| Asparagus, cooked | 5-6 medium | 90 | 90 |
| Tomatoes, raw | 1 small | 90 | 90 |
| **Fruits** | | | |
| Watermelon | 10 × 16 inch slice | 531 | 59 |
| Cantaloupe | ¼ melon | 430 | 430 |
| Apricots, raw | 3 medium | 277 | 277 |
| dried | 4 halves | 101 | 109 |
| Papaya, raw | ⅓ medium | 175 | 175 |
| Nectarines, raw | 1 medium | 165 | 165 |

One RE (retinol equivalent) = 3.33 IU from animal sources and 10 IU from plant sources.

## Thiamin (B$_1$)

| Food | Portion size | Amount of vitamin | |
|---|---|---|---|
| | | mg/portion | mg/100 g |
| **Meats** | | | |
| Pork chops, cooked | 3½ oz | 0.98 | 0.98 |
| Ham, fresh, cooked | 3½ oz | 0.96 | 0.96 |
| Beef liver, fried | 3½ oz | 0.26 | 0.26 |
| **Nuts** | | | |
| Brazil | ¼ cup | 0.82 | 1.09 |
| Pecans | ¼ cup | 0.18 | 0.73 |
| Cashew | ¼ cup | 0.11 | 0.44 |
| **Cereal Products** | | | |
| Barley cereals | ½ cup | 0.22 | 0.23 |
| Wheat germ | 1 tbsp | 0.15 | 1.68 |
| Oatmeal, cooked | ½ cup | 0.13 | 0.11 |
| **Vegetables** | | | |
| Green peas, cooked | ½ cup | 0.28 | 0.28 |
| Soybeans, cooked | ½ cup | 0.21 | 0.26 |
| Asparagus, cooked | 5-6 medium | 0.16 | 0.16 |
| Beans, cooked | | | |
| Lima | ½ cup | 0.14 | 0.18 |
| Kidney | ½ cup | 0.14 | 0.11 |
| Corn on cob, cooked | 4″ ear | 0.12 | 0.12 |
| **Miscellaneous** | | | |
| Brewer's yeast | 1 tbsp | 1.25 | 15.61 |

## Riboflavin (B$_2$)

| Food | Portion size | Amount of vitamin | |
|------|--------------|-------------------|---|
| | | mg/portion | mg/100 g |
| **Meats** | | | |
| Beef liver, fried | 3½ oz | 4.10 | 4.10 |
| Calf liver, fried | 3½ oz | 4.10 | 4.10 |
| Chicken liver, cooked | 3½ oz | 1.75 | 1.75 |
| Veal roast, cooked | 3½ oz | 0.44 | 0.44 |
| Beef, ground, cooked | 3½ oz | 0.21 | 0.21 |
| Egg, boiled | 1 large | 0.14 | 0.28 |
| **Cereal Products** | | | |
| Barley cereals | ½ cup | 0.12 | 0.13 |
| **Dairy Products** | | | |
| Milk, whole | 1 cup | 0.42 | 0.17 |
| Ice cream (1 scoop) | ½ cup | 0.17 | 0.25 |
| Cheese, cottage, low-fat, 2% | ⅓ cup | 0.14 | 0.14 |
| Blue or Roquefort | 1 oz | 0.11 | 0.39 |
| Cheddar | 1 oz | 0.11 | 0.39 |
| Brick | 1 oz | 0.10 | 0.36 |
| **Vegetables** | | | |
| Collard greens, cooked | ½ cup | 0.20 | 0.20 |
| Spinach, raw | 3½ oz | 0.20 | 0.20 |
| Broccoli, cooked | ½ cup | 0.20 | 0.20 |
| Asparagus, cooked | 5-6 medium | 0.18 | 0.18 |
| Brussels sprouts, cooked | ½ cup | 0.14 | 0.14 |
| Mustard greens, cooked | ½ cup | 0.14 | 0.14 |
| Spinach, cooked | ½ cup | 0.13 | 0.14 |
| **Miscellaneous** | | | |
| Brewer's yeast | 1 tbsp | 0.43 | 4.30 |

## Niacin (B₃)

| Food | Portion size | Amount of vitamin mg/portion | Amount of vitamin mg/100 g |
|------|-------------|------------------------------|----------------------------|
| **Meats** | | | |
| Calf liver, fried | 3½ oz | 16.5 | 16.5 |
| Beef liver, fried | 3½ oz | 14.4 | 14.4 |
| Chicken, cooked | 3½ oz | 6.6 | 6.6 |
| Beef, ground, cooked | 3½ oz | 5.7 | 5.7 |
| Chicken liver, cooked | 3½ oz | 4.5 | 4.5 |
| Haddock, cooked | 3½ oz | 2.1 | 2.1 |
| **Nuts** | | | |
| Peanuts, roasted | 1 oz | 5.6 | 2.0 |
| Peanut butter | 2 tbsp | 4.8 | 15.8 |
| **Vegetables** | | | |
| Green peas, cooked | ½ cup | 1.7 | 2.3 |
| Potatoes, white, baked | 1 medium | 1.7 | 1.7 |
| Asparagus, cooked | 5-6 medium | 1.4 | 1.4 |
| Corn on cob, cooked | 4″ ear | 1.4 | 1.4 |
| Peas, black-eyed | ½ cup | 1.1 | 1.4 |
| Collard greens, cooked | ½ cup | 1.2 | 1.2 |
| Lima beans, cooked | ½ cup | 1.0 | 1.3 |
| **Miscellaneous** | | | |
| Brewer's yeast | 1 tbsp | 3.8 | 38.0 |

## Pyridoxine (B$_6$)

| Food | Portion size | Amount of vitamin | |
|---|---|---|---|
| | | mg/portion | mg/100 g |
| **Meats** | | | |
| Salmon, broiled | 3½ oz | 0.70 | 0.70 |
| Chicken, baked | 3½ oz | 0.52 | 0.52 |
| Beef, ground | 3½ oz | 0.39 | 0.39 |
| Pork chop, broiled | 3½ oz | 0.35 | 0.35 |
| Beef liver, fried | 3½ oz | 0.35 | 0.35 |
| Tuna, canned | 3 oz | 0.34 | 0.40 |
| Turkey, baked | 3½ oz | 0.27 | 0.27 |
| **Vegetables** | | | |
| Potato, baked | 1 medium | 0.70 | 0.70 |
| Spinach, cooked | ½ cup | 0.22 | 0.14 |
| Broccoli, cooked | ½ cup | 0.15 | 0.14 |
| Turnip greens | ½ cup | 0.13 | 0.13 |
| Asparagus | ½ cup | 0.13 | 0.13 |
| **Fruits** | | | |
| Banana | 1 medium | 0.66 | 0.58 |
| Figs, dried | 10 | 0.42 | 0.23 |
| Watermelon | 1 cup | 0.23 | 0.14 |
| Cantaloupe | 1 cup | 0.18 | 0.11 |
| Orange | 1 medium | 0.08 | 0.07 |
| **Miscellaneous** | | | |
| Brewer's yeast | 1 tbsp | 0.40 | 4.00 |

Folic acid

| Food | Portion size | Amount of vitamin | |
| --- | --- | --- | --- |
| | | μg/portion | μg/100 g |
| **Meats** | | | |
| Chicken liver | 3½ oz | 770 | 770 |
| Beef liver, fried | 3½ oz | 175 | 175 |
| **Vegetables** | | | |
| Spinach, cooked | ½ cup | 131 | 131 |
| Asparagus, cooked | 5-6 medium | 89-140 | 89-140 |
| Turnip greens, cooked | ½ cup | 86 | 106 |
| Kale, cooked | ½ cup | 34 | 51 |
| Endive, raw | 20 long leaves | 27-63 | 27-63 |
| Broccoli, cooked | ½ cup | 26 | 34 |
| Escarole, raw | 4 large leaves | 26 | 26 |
| Okra, cooked | 8-9 pods | 24 | 24 |
| Brussels sprouts, cooked | ½ cup | 20 | 27 |
| Mustard greens, cooked | ½ cup | 17-38 | 17-38 |
| Acorn squash, cooked | ½ medium | 17 | 17 |
| Cauliflower, cooked | ½ cup | 16 | 29 |
| **Nuts** | | | |
| Walnuts | 8-10 halves | 12 | 77 |
| Filberts | 10-12 nuts | 10 | 67 |
| Peanuts | 1 tbsp | 9 | 57 |
| Almonds | 12-15 nuts | 7 | 46 |
| Pecans | 12 halves | 4 | 27 |

## Vitamin B$_{12}$

| Food | Portion size | Amount of vitamin | |
| --- | --- | --- | --- |
| | | μg/portion | μg/100 g |
| **Meats** | | | |
| Beef liver, fried | 3½ oz | 31-120 | 31-120 |
| Beef round | 3½ oz | 3.4-4.5 | 3.4-4.5 |
| Ham | 3½ oz | 0.9-1.6 | 0.9-1.6 |
| Haddock | 3½ oz | 0.6 | 0.6 |
| Egg, whole | 1 large | 0.6 | 1.3 |
| **Dairy Products** | | | |
| Milk, whole | 1 cup | 1.3 | 0.6 |
| Cheese, Swiss | 1 oz | 0.5 | 1.7 |
| American | 1 oz | 0.2 | 0.7 |

Tables from Weinsier RL, Heimburger DC, Butterworth Jr MD: *Handbook of clinical nutrition,* St Louis, 1989, Mosby.

## APPENDIX E
# Pain Management Techniques

### RELAXATION

Relaxation relieves pain by easing muscle tension. This can also help you feel less tired and nervous and help other pain-relieving methods work better.

#### How to Relax

Sit or lie down in a quiet place. Be sure you are comfortable. Do not cross your legs or arms. Take a deep breath, and tense your muscles (you may tense up your whole body or concentrate on one set of muscles at a time, such as your facial muscles or those in your arms and hands).

Hold your breath and keep your muscles tense. Release your breath and your muscles at the same time. Let your body go limp (repeat for other muscle areas if you are concentrating on one set at a time).

You can add imagery or music to help you relax. Relaxation tapes are available from your health care agency or local music store.

Do not be discouraged if relaxation does not help immediately. Practice the relaxation technique for at least 2 weeks before you give it up. If you find that it aggravates your pain, try another method.

## IMAGERY

Imagery involves using your imagination to create mental scenes that use all your senses: sight, sound, touch, smell, and taste. You can imagine exotic locations or revisit one of your favorite places. You can create stories and characters to add to your scenes. Imagery can take your mind off your fear, boredom, and pain.

### How to Use Imagery

Close your eyes. A few moments of the relaxation technique (see above) will help your body and mind prepare for imagery. Let your mind begin forming its image. The following is an example of imagery: Imagine that you are at the seashore. You are sitting in the wet sand; the afternoon sun is warm on your shoulders. The ocean rolls into the shore in gentle waves, and the water laps teasingly at your toes. A hungry pair of seagulls cry overhead and take swift, darting dives at a dog that is scavenging along the shore. Your tension lessens with each wave that touches your toes and retreats. You close your eyes and take a deep, slow breath of air. You are completely relaxed. Stay on the beach as long as you like. To end the image, count to three and open your eyes. Resume your regular activities slowly.

## DISTRACTION

A distraction is any activity that takes your mind off your pain and focuses your attention elsewhere. Doing crafts, reading a book, watching television, or listening to music through headphones can distract your mind. Distraction works well when you are waiting for drugs to take effect or if you have brief bouts of pain. Sometimes people can take their minds off their pain for long periods, especially if the pain is mild.

## SKIN STIMULATION

Skin stimulation is used to block pain sensation in the nerves. Pressure, massage, hot and cold applications, rubbing, and mild electrical current are all ways to stimulate the skin. If you are having radiation therapy, consult your physician before applying any skin stimulation. You can do the stimulation at the site of the pain, near it, or on the side opposite the pain. For example, stimulating the left wrist when the right wrist is in pain can actually ease the pain in the right wrist.

### Pressure

Using your entire hand, the heel of your hand, your thumb, your knuckles, or both hands, apply pressure for at least 15 seconds at the point where you feel pain. Keep trying spots around the painful area if you find no relief the first time. You may extend the time you apply pressure to 1 minute.

### Massage

You or someone else can perform the slow, circular motions of massage. The feet, back, neck, and scalp can be massaged to relieve tension and pain anywhere in the body. Some people prefer to use oils or lotions during the massage. If deep massage is too uncomfortable, try light stroking. Do not massage red, raw, or broken skin.

### Heat and Cold

Some people prefer cold; others prefer heat. Use whichever works better for you. A convenient way to use cold is to freeze gel-filled packs and wrap them in towels. Ice cubes can also be used. Heat can be applied with a heating pad; hot, moist towels; or a hot water bottle or by taking a hot bath. Be careful not to burn your skin with water that is too hot or to go to sleep with a heating pad on. Do not expose your skin to intense cold for long.

## TRANSCUTANEOUS ELECTRICAL NERVE STIMULATION

TENS can be used to eliminate or ease pain. A TENS unit is a pocket-sized, battery-operated device that provides a mild, continuous electrical current through the skin by the use of two to four electrodes taped to the skin. Lead wires connect the electrodes to the device. It is this mild electrical current that blocks or modifies the pain messages and replaces them with a buzzing, tingling sensation. TENS is also thought to stimulate the body's production of endorphin, a natural pain reliever.

**APPENDIX F**
# Care of a Urinary Diversion

The most common type of urinary diversion is the ileal conduit, in which a piece of small bowel is used as a passage (conduit) for urine to the surface of the skin. This piece of bowel is closed at one end. The other end is brought to the surface of the abdomen to form a stoma (opening). The ureters are attached inside the abdomen so that urine drains through the ileal conduit and out through the stoma. Other urinary diversions include colon conduit (the sigmoid colon is used as the passage), ureterostomy (the ureters are brought through the abdominal wall to form stomas), and vesicotomy (an opening into the bladder).

## APPLYING AN OSTOMY POUCH

- Peel back the paper from the adhesive faceplate. Center the pouch opening over the stoma, and press all around the faceplate to ensure that it is firmly attached to the skin. Attach the belt for additional security if you wish.
- Press the air out of the pouch. Clamp the bottom.

## REMOVING AN OSTOMY POUCH

Explain the need to change the ostomy pouch every 5 to 7 days. Instruct the patient to gather the following equipment before beginning: adhesive solvent, gauze pads, powder (if desired), towel, and scissors. Describe the procedure:

- While standing, hold the skin around the stoma taut and begin peeling off the adhesive square that holds the pouch to the skin. Peeling from top to bottom works best. If the pouch does not peel off, use adhesive solvent to loosen the edges.
- Wipe away excess drainage from around the stoma with gauze pads.
- Wash the area around the stoma with soap and water. Dry thoroughly. Apply powder if the skin is irritated. You may also want to apply a skin barrier.

## COLLECTING URINE FOR CULTURE AND SENSITIVITY

The nurse or physician will remove the external pouch and insert a sterile catheter into the stoma to collect a sterile specimen.

## SPECIAL ASPECTS OF CARE

Use a skin barrier or liquid film to protect the skin from irritation. Drink at least eight glasses of water a day. Test urine pH regularly, using a freshly voided specimen before a meal. The pH should be 4.5 to 8. Test sticks are available at drugstores. Vitamin C works well for keeping an acid urine. Odor may indicate an alkaline urine, which can cause stones to form or a urinary tract infection to develop.

## APPENDIX G
# Pulse-taking Diary

My heart rate should be: _____.

| DATE | TIME | HEART RATE | NOTES |
|------|------|------------|-------|
|      |      |            |       |
|      |      |            |       |
|      |      |            |       |
|      |      |            |       |
|      |      |            |       |
|      |      |            |       |
|      |      |            |       |
|      |      |            |       |
|      |      |            |       |
|      |      |            |       |
|      |      |            |       |
|      |      |            |       |
|      |      |            |       |

## APPENDIX H
# Patient Resources

Phone numbers for local offices and divisions are listed in the white pages of the telephone book.

Acoustic Neuroma Association
P.O. Box 12402
Atlanta, GA 30355
(404) 237-8023

AIDS Clinical Trials Information Service
1-800-874-2572 (English/Spanish)
1-800-243-7012 (hearing impaired)

AIDS Treatment Information Service
1-800-448-0440 (English/Spanish)
1-800-243-7012 (hearing impaired)

Alcoholic Center for Information and Drug Dependency
c/o National Council on Alcoholic and Drug Dependency
12 W. 21st St.
New York, NY 10010
(212) 206-6770

Alcoholics Anonymous World Services
P.O. Box 459
Grand Central Station
New York, NY 10163
(212) 870-3400

Alzheimer's Association
919 N. Michigan Ave, Suite 1000
Chicago, IL 60602
(312) 335-8700

American Brain Tumor
3725 N. Talman
Chicago, IL 60618
(312) 286-5571
1-800-886-2282

American Cancer Society
National Center
1599 Clifton Rd. NE
Atlanta, GA 30329
(404) 329-7651
1-800-227-2345

American Diabetes Association
National Center
1660 Duke St.
Alexandria, VA 22314
1-800-232-3472 (general information)
1-800-DIABETES (patient literature)

American Heart Association
7272 Greenville Ave.
Dallas, TX 75231
(214) 373-6300
1-800-AHA-USA1

American Lung Association
National Headquarters
1740 Broadway
New York, NY 10019
(212) 315-8700

American Parkinson's Disease Association
1250 Hylan Blvd.
Staten Island, NY 10305-1943
1-800-223-2732

American Red Cross
National Headquarters
2025 E St.
Washington, DC 20006
(202) 728-6500

Arthritis Foundation
1314 Spring St., NW
Atlanta, GA 30309
(404) 872-7100
1-800-283-7800 (patient information)

Cancer Information Service
1-800-4-CANCER (Spanish available)
1-800-638-6070 (Alaska)
1-800-524-1234 (Hawaii)

CDC National AIDS Hotline
P.O. Box 13827
Research Triangle Park, NC 27709
1-800-342-AIDS
1-800-344-7432 (Spanish)
1-800-243-7889 (TTY/TDD)

Crohn's and Colitis Foundation of America
444 Park Ave. South
New York, NY 10016-7374
(212) 685-3440
1-800-343-3637

Cystic Fibrosis Foundation
6931 Arlington Rd.
Bethesda, MD 20814
(301) 951-4422
1-800-FIGHT CF

Epilepsy Foundation of America
4351 Garden City Dr., Suite 500
Landover, MD 20785
(301) 459-3700

Guillain-Barré Syndrome Foundation International
P.O. Box 262
Wynnewood, PA 19096
(610) 667-0131

Head Injury Foundation
1140 Connecticut Ave. SW, Suite 812
Washington, DC 20054
(202) 296-6443

Help for Incontinent People
P.O. Box 544
Union, SC 29379
(803) 579-7900

National Association for Continence
P.O. Box 8310
Spartanburg, SC 29305-8310
(803) 579-7900

Information Center for Individuals with Disabilities
29 Stanhope Street
P.O. Box 256
Boston, MA 02117
(617) 450-9888

International Association of Laryngectomees
c/o American Cancer Society
1599 Clifton Rd. NE
Atlanta, GA 30329-4251
(404) 329-7651

Leukemia Society of America, Inc.
National Headquarters
600 Third Ave.
New York, NY 10016
(212) 573-8484
1-800-955-4572

Lupus Foundation of America
4 Research Place, Suite 180
Rockville, MD 20850-3226
(301) 670-9292

Meals on Wheels
Local Offices

Medic-Alert
P.O. Box 1009
Turlock, CA 95381-1009
(209) 668-3333
1-800-344-3226

The Mended Hearts, Inc.
7320 Greenville Ave.
Dallas, TX 75231
(214) 373-6300

Multiple Sclerosis Society
National Headquarters
733 3rd Ave.
New York, NY 10017-3288
(212) 986-3240
1-800-FIGHT MS

Muscular Dystrophy Association
National Headquarters
3300 E. Sunrise Dr.
Tucson, AZ 85718-3208
1-800-572-1717

Myasthenia Gravis Foundation
222 So. Riverside Plaza, Suite 1540
Chicago, IL 60606
(312) 258-0522
1-800-541-5454

National Association for Home Care
228 7th St. SE
Washington, DC 20003
(202) 547-7424 (ask for Public Information Line)

National Association of People with AIDS
1413 K Street NW
7th Floor
Washington, DC 20005
(202) 898-0414
(202) 898-0435 (FAX)

National Heart, Lung, and Blood Institute
Information Center
P.O. Box 30105
Bethesda, MD 20824
(301) 251-1222
(301) 496-4236 (for general public)

National Hemophilia Foundation
110 Greene Street, Suite 303
New York, NY 10012
(212) 219-8180
800-42-HANDI (Spanish available)

National Information Center on Deafness
Gallaudet University
800 Florida Ave. NE
Washington, DC 20002-3695
(202) 651-5051

National Institute of Allergies and Infectious Diseases
31 Central Drive
Building 31, Room 7A50
Bethesda, MD 20892-2520
(301) 496-5717

National Institute of Neurological Disorders and Stroke
Office of Scientific and Health Reports
(pamphlets on stroke)
Building 31/RM 8A16
31 Center Drive, MSC 2540
Bethesda, MD 20892-2540
(301) 496-5751

National Jewish Center for Immunology & Respiratory Medicine
Denver, Colorado
(303) 398-1477
Lung Disease Hotline
1-800-222-LUNG

National Kidney Foundation
30 E. 33rd St., 11th Floor
New York, NY 10016
(212) 889-2210
1-800-622-9010

National Marrow Donor Program
3433 Broadway Street, NE, Suite 400
Minneapolis, MN 55413
(414) 257-8325
1-800-MARROW2

National Multiple Sclerosis Society
733 3rd Ave., Third Floor
New York, NY 10017
(212) 986-3240

National Rehabilitation Information Center
8455 Colesville Rd., Suite 935
Silver Spring, MD 20910
(301) 588-9284

National Stroke Association
848 E. Orchard Rd., Suite 1000
Englewood, CO 80111
(303) 771-1700
1-800-787-6537

Parkinson Disease Foundation
710 W. 168th St.
New York, NY 10032
1-800-344-7872

Project Information
(For AIDS patients and clinicians)
1965 Market St., Suite 220
San Francisco, CA 94103
1-800-822-7422

Public Health Service's Agency for Health Care Policy and Research
Publications Clearinghouse
P.O. Box 8547
Silver Spring, MD 20907
1-800-358-9295
(patient guidelines for urinary incontinence in adults, angina pectoris, heart failure; available in English or Spanish)

Self Help for Hard of Hearing People
National Office
7910 Woodmont Ave., Suite 1200
Bethesda, MD 20814
(301) 657-2248

Simon Foundation for Continence
P.O. Box 835
Wilmette, IL 60091
(708) 864-3913
1-800-23-SIMON

Stroke Clubs International
805 12th St.
Galveston, TX 77550
(409) 762-1022

United Ostomy Association
36 Executive Park, Suite 120
Irvine, CA 92714-6744
(714) 660-8624
1-800-826-0826

## APPENDIX I
# Patient Instructions for Use of an Oral Inhaler

1. Remove the mouthpiece and cap from the inhaler. Insert the metal stem of the inhaler into the small hole on the side of the mouthpiece, and then shake the device five times.
2. Purse your lips and exhale fully. Hold the inhaler upside down, and close your lips and teeth around the mouthpiece. Tilt your head back slightly; take a slow, deep breath. As you do, firmly press the inhaler against the mouthpiece *once only,* to release one dose of medication. Breathe in until your lungs feel full of air.
3. Remove the mouthpiece from your mouth, and hold your breath for a count of 3 to 5. Purse your lips and exhale slowly. Your heart may beat faster or you may feel slightly dizzy for a few minutes the first couple of times you use the inhaler, but this should pass. If it persists, notify your physician or a nurse.
4. Clean your inhaler once a day. Take it apart and rinse the mouthpiece and cap under warm, running water for 1 minute. Allow the parts to dry completely, and then reassemble them.

# Bibliography

Aegerter E, Kirkpatrick JA: *Orthopedic diseases,* Philadelphia, 1975, WB Saunders.

Beare PG, Myers JL: *Principles and practice of adult health nursing,* ed 2, St Louis, 1994, Mosby.

Belcher AE: *Mosby's clinical series: cancer nursing,* St Louis, 1992, Mosby.

Brundage D: *Mosby's clinical series: renal disorders,* St Louis, 1993, Mosby.

Buckwald E: *Physical rehabilitation for daily living,* New York, 1952, McGraw-Hill.

Canobbio MM: *Mosby's clinical series: cardiovascular disorders,* St Louis, 1990, Mosby.

Carey LC: *The surgical clinics of North America,* Philadelphia, 1983, WB Saunders.

Cheitlin MD, Sokolow M, McIlroy MB: *Clinical cardiology,* ed 6, Norwalk, Conn, 1993, Appleton & Lange.

Chipps E, Clannin N, Campbell V: *Mosby's clinical series: neurologic disorders,* St Louis, 1992, Mosby.

Ferri FF: *Practical guide to the care of the medical patient,* ed 3, St Louis, 1994, Mosby.

Garrick JG, Webb DR: *Sports injuries,* Philadelphia, 1990, WB Saunders.

Giloth BE: *Managing hospital-based patient education,* Washington, DC, 1993, American Hospital Publishing Inc.

Gray M: *Mosby's clinical series: genitourinary disorders,* St Louis, 1992, Mosby.

Griffith H, Dambro M: *The five minute clinical consultant,* Philadelphia, 1993, Lea & Febiger.

Grimes DE: *Mosby's clinical series: infectious diseases,* St Louis, 1991, Mosby.

Groenwald SL, Frogge MH, Goodman M, et al: *Cancer nursing: principles and practice,* ed 3, Boston, 1993, Jones & Bartlett.

Hamilton HK, Rose MB: *Diseases,* Nurse's Reference Library, Springhouse, Penn., 1984, Springhouse.

*Handbook of medical surgical nursing,* Springhouse, Penn, 1994, Springhouse.

Holloway N: *Medical surgical care planning,* ed 2, Springhouse, Penn, 1993, Springhouse.

Ignatavicius DD, Batterden RA, Hausman KA: *Pocket companion for medical-surgical nursing,* Philadelphia, 1992, WB Saunders.

Isselbacher K, Braunwald E, Wilson J, et al: *Harrison's principles of internal medicine,* ed 13, New York, 1994, McGraw-Hill.

Jaffe MS, Skidmore-Roth L: *Home health: nursing care plans,* ed 2, St Louis, 1993, Mosby.

Kniesl CR, Ames SW: *Adult health nursing: a biopsychosocial approach,* Reading, Mass, 1986, Addison-Wesley.

*Mosby's patient teaching guides,* St Louis, 1995, Mosby.

Mourad LA: *Mosby's clinical series: orthopedic disorders,* St Louis, 1991, Mosby.

Mudge-Grout CL: *Immunologic disorders,* St Louis, 1992, Mosby.

*Nurses desk reference: diagnostics: a comprehensive manual of laboratory tests and diagnostic procedures,* Springhouse, Penn, 1994, Springhouse.

*Nurses desk reference: diseases,* ed 2, Springhouse, Penn, 1988, Springhouse.

Onion D: *The little black book of primary care: pearls and references,* New York, 1993, WW Norton.

Otto SE: *Oncology nursing,* ed 2, St Louis, 1994, Mosby.

Pagana K, Pagana T: *Mosby's diagnostic and laboratory test reference,* St Louis, 1992, Mosby.

Palandri MK, Sorrentin CR: *Pocket companion: Luckmann and Sorensen's medical surgical nursing,* ed 4, Philadelphia, 1993, WB Saunders.

*Professional guide to diseases,* ed 4, Springhouse, Penn, 1992, Springhouse.

Redman BK: *The process of patient education,* ed 7, St Louis, 1993, Mosby.

Rothman RH, Simeone FA: *The spine,* Philadelphia, 1975, WB Saunders.

Rutherford, RB: *Vascular surgery,* ed 3, Philadelphia, 1989, WB Saunders.

Stillwell S: *Mosby's critical care nursing reference,* St Louis, 1992, Mosby.

Swearingen PL: *Manual of medical-surgical nursing care,* St Louis, 1994, Mosby.

*Taber's cyclopedic medical dictionary,* Philadelphia, 1993, FA Davis.

Thompson J, McFarland G, Hirsch J, Tucker S: *Clinical nursing,* ed 3, St Louis, 1993, Mosby.

Tucker SM, Canobbio MM, Paquette EV, Wells MF: *Patient care standards,* ed 6, St Louis, 1996, Mosby.

Wagner MM: Pathophysiology related to peripheral vascular disease, *Nurs Clin North Am* 21(2):195-206, 1986.

Weinsier RL, Heimburger DC, Butterworth CE: *Handbook of clinical nutrition: clinician's manual for prevention, diagnosis, and management of nutritional problems,* ed 2, St Louis, 1989, Mosby.

Whitman NI et al: *Teaching in nursing practice: a professional model,* ed 2, Norwalk, Conn, 1992, Appleton & Lange.

Wilson SF, Thompson JM: *Respiratory disorders,* St Louis, 1993, Mosby.

# Index

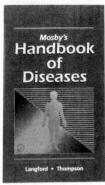